DATE DUE

Unless Recalled Earlier			
NOV - 7 1997			
9-4-01			
MAR - 7 2002			

DEMCO 38-297

ESSENTIALS OF OXYGENATION

The Jones and Bartlett Series in Nursing

ESSENTIALS OF OXYGENATION
IMPLICATION FOR CLINICAL PRACTICE

Thomas Ahrens, DNS, RN, CCRN

Critical Care Clinical Nurse Specialist
Barnes Hospital at Washington University Medical Center
St. Louis, Missouri

Kim Rutherford, MSN, RN, CCRN

Critical Care Clinical Nurse Specialist
Louisville, Kentucky

Jones and Bartlett Publishers
Boston   London

Editorial, Sales, and Customer Service Offices
Jones and Bartlett Publishers
One Exeter Plaza
Boston, MA 02116

Jones and Bartlett Publishers International
PO Box 1498
London W6 7RS
England

Library of Congress Cataloging-in-Publication Data
Ahrens, Thomas.
    Essentials of Oxygenation
    Critical concepts in oxygenation: Implication for clinical practice /
    Thomas Ahrens, Kim Rutherford.
      p.   cm.
    Includes bibliographical references and index.
    ISBN 0-86720-332-3
    1. Respiration. 2. Tissue respiration. 3. Oximetry.
  4. Respiratory intensive care. 5. Impaired oxygen delivery.
  6. Respiratory organs—Diseases—Nursing. I. Rutherford, Kim.
  II. Title.
    [DNLM: 1. Biological Transport. 2. Oxygen—pharmacokinetics.
  3. Oxygen—physiology. 4. Oxygen Consumption—physiology.
  5. Respiratory Insufficiency—therapy.   QV 312 A287e]
  QP121.A52 1993
  612.2′2—dc20
  DNLM/DLC
  for Library of Congress   92-17567
                    CIP

Printed in the United States of America
96 95 94 93 92   10 9 8 7 6 5 4 3 2 1

To the children in each of our families: Tom, Matt, Dave and Maggie from my family and Erin and Greg from Kim's. For all the times we were tied up writing the book, thanks for waiting. Now all those times we said "wait till the book was done" are over and our time is now your time.

Contents

PART IV. Treatment of Oxygenation Disturbances

Preface

Oxygenation is one of the most exciting clinical concepts to be involved with due to the many developments and improvements in the area. Perhaps the most commonly assessed area in critical care (including ICUs and subacute areas) is the concept of oxygenation. Despite the critical role of oxygenation in assessment of the acutely ill, oxygenation is frequently not well understood by many practicing clinicians.

The lack of understanding of the concept of oxygenation is easy to grasp. Educational programs in most health care professions generally do not teach the concept of oxygenation, but instead teach separate systems such as cardiac and pulmonary. One of the most important aspects of oxygenation, which is often overlooked in both education and clinical practice, is the multiple systems involved in oxygenation. Oxygenation is not simply an assessment of the pulmonary system. Oxygenation is the key to any assessment of all cellular (and organ) function. It is frequently overlooked that oxygenation is the primary reason for assessing hemodynamics, pulmonary, and neurologic function as well as aspects of hematology and metabolism. Only through assessing all aspects of oxygenation can the clinician really make an intelligent assessment of cellular oxygenation status.

In addition, only through assessment of oxygenation can the effect of many common clinical therapies be evaluated. For example, adding dobutamine to raise the cardiac index in the patient with congestive heart failure can only be evaluated for its effectiveness by evaluating the impact on oxygenation. Another example would be with the addition of positive end-expiratory pressure (PEEP) or inverse ratio ventilation (IRV). While these therapies primarily elevate the Pa_{O_2} and Sa_{O_2} level, their effect can only be assessed through analyzing all aspects of oxygenation, not just the assessment of the Pa_{O_2} or Sa_{O_2} level.

Because of the crucial role oxygenation plays in critical care, this text is designed to help fill the gap in knowledge regarding oxygenation. Considering the importance of oxygenation in clinical practice, one would think concepts involving oxygenation are covered in undergraduate and graduate education. If this were the case, the clinician could recall answers to basic oxygenation questions such as:

1. What is the normal oxygen transport and consumption levels?
2. What is the most important component of oxygen transport?
3. If you could have one measurement to assess oxygen transport, what parameter would you choose?
4. How does venous oxygen content and saturation reflect cellular oxygenation?
5. Is the assessment of oxygen transport and consumption adequate to understand the cellular oxygenation state?
6. Can any one parameter assess oxygenation?
7. What is the most effective way of improving oxygenation, administering oxygen therapy or reducing oxygen consumption?
8. Does pulse oximetry reveal more information regarding oxygen transport or intrapulmonary shunting?

9. Is treating the cardiac output in the patient with left ventricular failure a more effective method for improving oxygenation or is the administration of nasal cannula more important?

These questions can serve as a basis for readers to assess their understanding of oxygenation (all nine questions are addressed in the text). These questions are not advanced questions but may be difficult to answer due to the lack of consistent teaching of principles of oxygenation. If you found any of these questions difficult, consider yourself normal. One of the exciting aspects of this text is the attempt to aid the clinician in more sophisticated assessment of oxygenation and to correct some of the educational gaps most of us have experienced.

Outside the area of formal education, the concept of oxygenation has received increasing attention in the literature, although much of this information is not designed for practical, clinical application. Despite increasing attention to the area of oxygenation, common errors in clinical practice are present regarding the assessment and evaluation of oxygenation as well as the correct use of new technology. For example, how often is an oxygenation assessment made by obtaining blood gases (to obtain a Pa_{O_2} value) or using pulse oximetry (Sp_{O_2})? In an assessment of oxygenation, both Pa_{O_2} and Sa_{O_2} levels play relatively small roles. Only through understanding the overall role of oxygen in energy generation can individual parameters be placed in perspective regarding their role in oxygenation.

Due to the application of oxygenation principles in all acute care settings, this text is intended for use in intensive care units, telemetry areas, emergency rooms, operating and postanesthesia recovery areas. The text is designed for all clinicians, including nurses, physicians, and respiratory therapists. Due to our background in nursing, some of the orientation to the book is toward nursing. However, all aspects of the text can readily be applied to any clinician involved with the assessment and treatment of oxygenation.

The format of the text is to present the reader with the molecular basis for assessing oxygenation. The molecular foundation for oxygenation is important in order to understand the role of oxygen in energy generation and how to best assess potential abnormalities. Following molecular oxygen are sections addressing the assessment of oxygen transport (D_{O_2}). Oxygen transport components address the most commonly assessed areas in oxygenation, such as the Pa_{O_2} and pulse oximetry. In this section, the emphasis is on identifying and prioritizing individual components of oxygen transport. Some common myths and misconceptions are addressed in this area. The third section addresses oxygen consumption and integration of oxygen transport and consumption. The integration of oxygen transport and consumption also addresses the issue of cellular oxygenation, or factors which alter cellular utilization of oxygen independent of oxygen supply and demand. Included in this section is a brief presentation of exciting developments in the future assessment of oxygenation. The fourth section of the text addresses treatments for disturbances in oxygenation.

Through the organization of the text, material will be presented that is relevant and clinically applicable. The format of the book is designed for the busy, practicing clinician. Each chapter is designed to accomplish four specific goals:

1. contain clinically relevant material
2. provide a brief theoretical background to the clinical content
3. present examples of clinical situations utilizing the material in the chapter
4. present the material in short, manageable segments.

We would like to say the material is presented in an easy-to-read format. While we have tried to present the material whenever possible in such a manner, some of the material regarding oxygenation is not easy to simplify. For this reason, the chapters are short and have examples illustrating how to utilize the material in clinical settings.

Another feature of the text is the attempt to address economic issues that have an impact in areas of oxygenation. For example, should pulse oximetry replace blood gases or should Sv_{O_2} catheters replace cardiac output measurements? While not all chapters address economic issues, the goal of adding economic considerations to some chapters is to increase the awareness of the clinician to issues they may have to address in practice.

The last goal of the text is to increase the understanding of oxygenation in a text that is enjoyable to read. Attempts at humor are occasionally employed to ease the technical nature of the text. If you can enjoy reading this book as well as learning principles of oxygenation, we will feel as if a key goal has been accomplished.

This text is not centered on the concept of nursing diagnosis, partially due to the multidisciplinary audience the text is intended to address. However, we recognize the importance of the nursing diagnosis concept. In an effort to meet the nursing audience's use of nursing diagnosis, we have included in the Appendix common nursing diagnoses associated with disturbances in oxygenation. We hope this will prove beneficial in the nursing application of oxygenation disturbances.

No text can address all aspects of oxygenation in the depth required for complete understanding. This text is no exception. We hope the material in the text is useful, however, and can improve your assessments of patients with disturbances in oxygenation.

We thank the Barnes Hospital Nursing Service for their support during the writing of this book.

Thomas Ahrens
Kim Rutherford

Contributors

Thomas Ahrens, DNS, RN, CCRN
Critical Care Clinical Nurse Specialist
Barnes Hospital at the Washington University Medical Center
St. Louis, Missouri

Cathy McGrath, BSN, RN
Nurse Clinician—Respiratory ICU
Barnes Hospital at the Washington University Medical Center
St. Louis, Missouri

Ann Padwojski, MSN, MBA, RN
Critical Care Clinical Nurse Specialist
St. Johns Medical Center
St. Louis, Missouri

Kim Rutherford, MSN, RN, CCRN
Critical Care Clinical Nurse Specialist
Deaconess Hospital
St. Louis, Missouri

Pamela Weilitz, MSN, (R), RN
Pulmonary Clinical Specialist
Barnes Hospital at the Washington University Medical Center
St. Louis, Missouri

Part I
Cellular Oxygenation

1
The Cellular Basis for Oxygenation

Oxygenation is a major component of the process of energy generation. Subsequently, when an assessment of oxygenation is made, what is really being assessed is the ability for energy generation to take place. The aim of this chapter is to accomplish three objectives: (1) to illustrate oxygen's role in energy generation, (2) to demonstrate how oxygen functions in a biochemical relationship with other elements in order to give the basis for oxygen's role in cellular metabolism, and (3) to present this biochemical material in such a way as to be understandable and practical to the practicing clinician. As this chapter is presented, it is important to keep in mind that the concepts of biochemistry are not usually one of the strong features of clinical education. That does not mean this concept should be unclear to clinicians, particularly in regard to key aspects of metabolism such as oxygenation. But as this chapter is presented, aspects of biochemistry will be presented in ways that are simple and relatively easy to understand. The chapter will not go to the depth that is required to understand the actual relationships between chemical components as is necessary for a true in-depth understanding of oxygenation. The information that is presented will be understandable and useful, and should give a better insight into the actual assessment of oxygenation. This first chapter may be a little difficult, stick with it though, because it is important for the clinical application of oxygenation concepts.

Oxygen has been involved in the process of energy generation for about one-half the history of the world (a few billion years). A common thread through all animal life forms, from dinosaurs to humans, is the use of oxygen as the key method for the formation of energy.

The process by which oxygen works in this energy-generation system can be seen in the molecular characteristics of oxygen. Over the next few paragraphs, key concepts in the molecular behavior of oxygen will be presented. During this presentation, descriptions and definitions involving oxygen are given which form the basis for understanding oxygen's role in energy generation. By understanding oxygen's role in energy generation, the subsequent clinical applications of oxygen will become more clear.

MOLECULAR OXYGEN

The key to understanding oxygen's role in clinical practice is the knowledge of oxygen's role in electron movement. The oxygen molecule has six electrons in orbit although a more stable orbit is achieved with eight electrons (Figure 1.1). Oxygen has a tendency to acquire electrons from other molecules due to this increased stability with eight electrons. The process of acquiring electrons

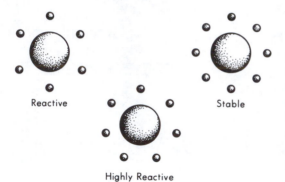

Reactive

Stable

Highly Reactive

FIGURE 1.1. Oxygen's reactivity varies with different electron configurations. Six-electron orbits are reactive while eight-electron orbits are stable. Seven-electron orbits are the most reactive, oxidizing most molecules they come into contact with.

from other molecules is termed *oxidation* of the molecule losing electrons. The substance gaining electrons, in this case oxygen, is *reduced*. The oxidation-reduction reactions that occur with oxygen are referred to as *redox* reactions.[1]

Oxygen frequently completes the stable eight-electron orbit by sharing two electrons with a second oxygen molecule. The pairing of the two oxygen molecules, or diatomic oxygen, is represented by the familiar symbol, O_2. As long as the eight-electron orbit is achieved, oxygen does not react actively with other substances. For example, hydrogen peroxide (H_2O_2) is a relatively stable element. If, however, hydrogen peroxide dissociates to OH (hydroxyl radical), an extremely reactive oxygen reaction is created.

Oxygen Radicals

If only one electron is acquired by oxygen (a seven-electron configuration), a very strong attraction to other electrons is created. For example, if hydrogen (which has one electron) is combined with oxygen, a hydroxyl radical (OH) is formed. The hydroxyl radical rapidly oxidizes the nearest molecule, creating an electron imbalance in the oxidized molecule.[2] The process of oxidizing molecules from hydroxyl radicals is an example of the potential clinical danger from oxygen. If hydroxyl radicals are released near healthy tissue, destruction of the tissue will result (Figure 1.2). The oxidation capability of oxygen radicals may contribute to many clinical conditions, including aging, sepsis, and ARDS.[3–7]

The action of oxygen radicals is not all bad. Immune mechanisms, for example, neutrophil action, are based partially on exposing antigens (foreign substances) to toxic oxygen radicals. Neutrophils and other elements can generally control the damage done to healthy tissues by oxygen radicals through the production of neutralizing substances such as superoxide dismutases, catalase, and peroxidases.[8]

OXYGEN'S ROLE IN ENERGY GENERATION

The affinity oxygen possesses for electrons is the basis for its role in energy generation. Oxygen acts as the terminal electron acceptor in a process that passes electrons

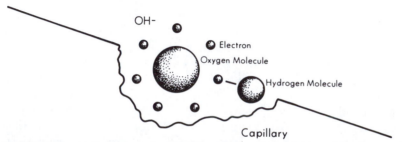

OH-

Electron

Oxygen Molecule

Hydrogen Molecule

Capillary

FIGURE 1.2. Hydroxyl radicals are highly reactive, taking electrons from any nearby molecule. If the nearest molecule is part of normal tissue, the normal tissue will be damaged. In this case, a capillary wall is injured by a nearby hydroxyl radical.

obtained from substrates (food). During this process, energy is created through electron transfer. A review of the electron-transfer mechanism will clarify oxygen's role in energy generation.

Given an understanding of the process of energy generation, one can identify oxygenation as a mechanism from which energy is generated. With this understanding, the role that oxygen plays in the formation of energy stores in the body is readily apparent. To illustrate this point, analyze the basic processes by which energy is formed.

Substrate Utilization

All substrates such as fats, carbohydrates, and proteins that are available for energy generation are metabolized for their energy potential through the removal of hydrogen (Figure 1.3). Most of these reactions occur inside the mitochondria. Hydrogen is removed from each substrate, usually through a dehydrogenase enzyme (e.g., lactate dehydrogenase or LDH) which initiates the hydrogen release from the substrate.[9] The hydrogen then enters into a series of metabolic pathways. As hydrogen is removed from the substrate, it becomes a source of energy due to the electrons which are available in the hydrogen molecule. The electrons from hydrogen are taken by the coenzyme of dehydrogenase, nicotinamide adenine dinucleotide (NAD).[10] NAD is reduced (accepts electrons) to NADH after receiving an electron from hydrogen. Another substance besides NAD can act to accept the hydrogen electron. This substance is flavin adenine dinucleotide (FAD). FAD is reduced to $FADH_2$ as it accepts two electrons from hydrogen molecules removed from substrates. Electrons from NADH and $FADH_2$ are entered into a process of electron transfer.

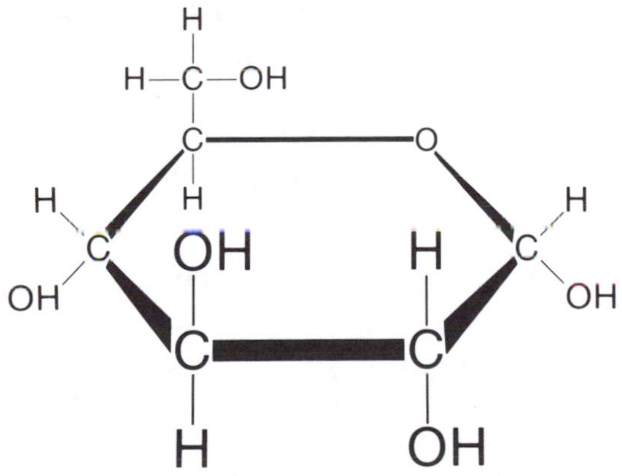

The electron-transfer process occurs through coupling with a series of iron compounds called cytochromes (Figure 1.4). Electrons from NADH and $FADH_2$ are passed down a series of cytochrome reactions in a sequential manner. As the electrons are passed down this cytochrome pathway, energy is released at intervals and adenine triphosphate (ATP) is synthesized from adenine diphosphate (ADP). As the electrons are passed down this pathway, the last cytochrome available for electron transfer is cytochrome a_3. Cytochrome a_3 is the only cytochrome that has the ability to transfer electrons to oxygen. Approximately 80% of all oxygen is utilized through cytochrome a_3.[11] Oxygen acts as the final electron acceptor in this cytochrome pathway. After oxygen accepts the electrons from hydrogen, it combines with hydrogen to form water. Oxygen's affinity for electron acceptance is valuable as it allows the energy-generation process an outlet for the transference of electrons.

Energy Generation Through Phosphorylation

Conversion of ADP to ATP is termed *phosphorylation*. If the phosphorylation takes place during the cytochrome transfer process, it is referred to as *oxidative phosphorylation*. The oxygen pathway utilized during cytochrome transfer is crucial since most of the energy stores in the body (up to 90%) are the result of oxidative phosphorylation. In other words, the synthesis of ATP from ADP is done, for the vast major-

FIGURE 1.3. Hydrogen molecules in food substrates. Hydrogen is the key component for energy generation. The removal of hydrogen from substrates initiates the energy process. Adapted from McArdle D, Katch FI, Katch V. *Exercise Physiology*, 3rd ed. Philadelphia: Lea & Febiger, 1991.

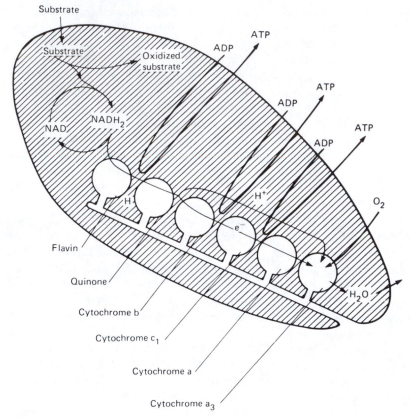

FIGURE 1.4. The cytochrome pathway is the primary mechanism for ATP generation during oxidative phosphorylation. Adapted from Nunn JF. *Applied Respiratory Physiology,* 3rd ed. Stoneham, Mass.: Butterworth, 1987.

ity of cases, through the use of the oxidative phosphorylation pathway (Figure 1.5). Energy generated through use of oxidative phosphorylation (with oxygen) is termed *aerobic energy.* Anaerobic energy generation occurs without the use of oxygen.

ADP levels are the primary stimulus for oxygen utilization. The greater the ADP level, the greater the demand for oxygen. If ADP levels are low (assuming normal phosphate and adenosine levels), adequate generation of ATP has occurred. If adequate levels of ATP exist, the need for oxygen is reduced. ADP is not the only source of energy in the body, but, in critical care settings, it is by far the most utilized. Other energy sources, such as creatine phosphate (PCr), can also serve as temporary energy stores (Figure 1.6).

The role of creatine phosphate is primar-

ily in the area of sudden energy requirements; ATP is much more likely to be used for long-term requirements. Creatine phosphate stores are limited in comparison to ATP. Creatine phosphate can be utilized, however, when ATP production cannot proceed aerobically. The PCr reaction is illustrated below:

$$PCr + ADP + H \leftrightarrow ATP + Cr$$

Two potentially important aspects of the phosphorylation using creatine phosphate have been proposed. One, in the presence of an acidosis, creatine phosphate can create ATP and simultaneously remove a hydrogen ion from the environment. Two, research has indicated that as the creatine phosphate levels decrease, energy stores fall to dangerously low levels.[12-13] The use of

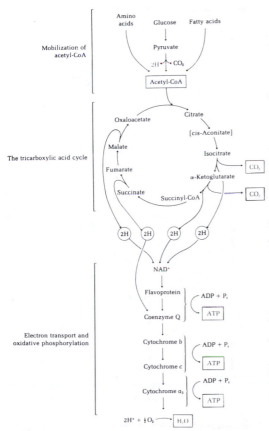

FIGURE 1.5. ATP generated primarily through oxidative phosphorylation.

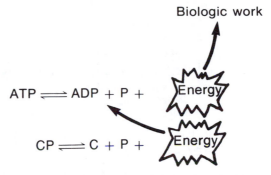

FIGURE 1.6. Creatine phosphate is a key short-term energy source. Creatine phosphate can act as a temporary source of energy, particularly in the absence (or reduction) of ATP stores. Adapted from McArdle D, Katch FI, Katch V. *Exercise Physiology*, 3rd ed. Philadelphia: Lea & Febiger, 1991.

PCr may be a mechanism for measuring cellular oxygenation. This will be addressed again in the discussion of magnetic resonance imaging of PCr (Chapter 9).

The purpose of forming ATP is to create energy stores within cells. Energy storage within cells is necessary in order to perform all biochemical reactions that occur in the human body. For example, energy is necessary to change cellular ion concentrations, such as with the sodium/potassium pump. All of these cellular processes require energy. Without the energy stores usually provided by ATP, the cellular processes would break down and not function. ATP releases energy for these functions through in a process called hydrolysis.[14] Hydrolysis is when the phosphate bond of ATP is broken and

reduced to a new bond—ADP. ADP is capable of regenerating to ATP during phosphorylation and thereby acts as a potential energy source. ATP also can be broken down into adenosine monophosphate (AMP). The most common hydrolysis, however, is into ADP. Complete hydrolysis can occur after AMP with the release of adenosine and inorganic phosphate (Pi). Adequate levels of both adenosine and Pi are necessary for cellular energy generation in the form of AMP/ADP → ATP to occur.

All foods or substrates ingested undergo hydrogen removal at the molecular level. Electrons removed from the foods may be utilized in the reductions of NAD to NADH and FAD to $FADH_2$. Once NADH and $FADH_2$ are formed, the electron-transfer process is able to continue and energy can be generated. The Krebs cycle initiates the reactions of NADH and $FADH_2$ from fats and proteins (Figure 1.7). As NADH and $FADH_2$ are generated from fats and proteins, they can enter the oxidative phosphorylation pathway and the cytochrome electron-transfer pathway. As presented, this pathway terminates with oxygen's acceptance of the electrons and then results in the formation of water. During the Krebs cycle, another important byproduct, carbon dioxide, is produced. Carbon dioxide production will be important during the discus-

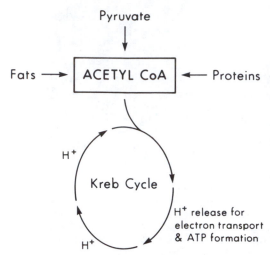

FIGURE 1.7. Acetyl-CoA is the entry point in the Krebs cycle for fats and carbohydrates.

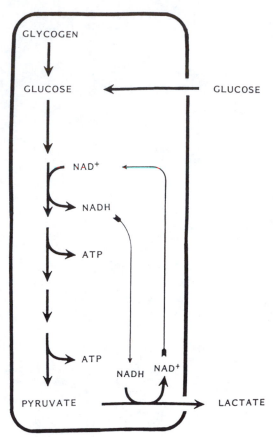

FIGURE 1.8. Carbohydrates are the only substrates that can release energy in the absence of oxygen. Anaerobic metabolism can occur only in the presence of carbohydrates. Both fats and proteins require oxygen for energy generation. Adapted from Kruse JA, Carlson RW. "Lactate metabolism." *Crit Care Clin* 1987;5:727.

sion of the use of oxygen consumption and carbon dioxide production as an indicator of the type of substrate utilization occurring (Chapter 8).

Carbohydrate is the only substrate that can generate ATP without oxygen (anaerobic metabolism). Anaerobic metabolism can take place through the catabolism of glucose (Figure 1.8). During the catabolism of glucose, four ATP molecules are created while two ATP molecules are consumed (Figure 1.9). The anaerobic pathway during the catabolism of a mole of glucose is much less efficient than aerobic energy generation. The aerobic energy pathway results in 36 molecules of ATP being created using the oxidative phosphorylation pathway; the anaerobic metabolism pathway produces only 2 ATP molecules.

LACTATE AND PYRUVATE

The end result of glucose breakdown is the formation of lactate and pyruvate, generally favoring the production of pyruvate. Pyruvate production is necessary for the formation of acetic acid, that is, acetyl-CoA.[15] Acetyl-CoA allows the glucose metabolism to use pyruvate and begin the Krebs cycle (Krebs cycle is also called the *citric acid,* or *tricarboxylic acid cycle*) (Figure 1.10).

If insufficient stores of oxygen are avail-

able, energy transfer or energy production through the oxidative phosphorylation pathway eventually will cease. At that point, formation of pyruvate is stopped and the formation of lactate increases. Lactate formation by itself is not to be viewed as an abnormal or adverse event. Lactate can be converted back to pyruvate once oxygen stores have been reestablished and can also be converted to glucose in tissues that lack the ability to perform oxidative phosphorylation, that is, mitochondria and erythrocytes.[16] Most cellular tissues can perform the conversion of lactate to pyruvate.

Lactate is formed in preference to pyruvate in conditions of hypoxia (lack of oxy-

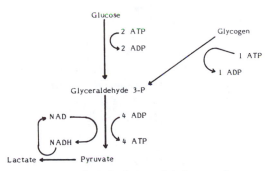

FIGURE 1.9. Carbohydrate metabolism produces four ATP molecules while consuming two. Adapted from Dantzker D. "Oxygen delivery and utilization in sepsis." *Crit Care Clin* 1989;83.

gen). Pyruvate is metabolized by the enzyme lactate dehydrogenase (LDH) to lactate. The normal level of lactate (1–2 mMol per liter) increases in these conditions. Increased lactate allows for the accumulation of hydrogen which is taking place during the catabolism of substrates, particularly glucose. As lactate is formed, two events occur: (1) a molecule of ATP is formed

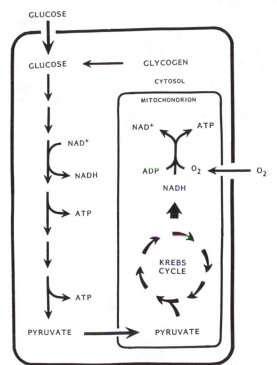

FIGURE 1.10. Acetyl-CoA ends glucose metabolism and enters the Krebs cycle. Adapted from Kruse JA, Carlson RW. "Lactate metabolism." *Crit Care Clin* 1987;5:726.

through anaerobic metabolism, and (2) a hydrogen ion is released. The frequent use of anaerobic metabolism will eventually result in excessive hydrogen ion release, generating an acidosis. Excessive reliance on the lactate system for energy can eventually result in the development of an acidosis as well as being an inefficient mechanism for producing ATP. This acidosis is usually referred to as a lactic acidosis.

Some organs rely heavily on lactate for normal oxygenation. Examples of these organs include the heart and kidneys.[17] As mentioned, lactate can be reconverted into glucose, primarily in the liver, through a process called gluconeogenesis. However, with increasing amounts of lactate generation, the potential exists for cell hypoxia. Without further formation of pyruvate, acetyl-CoA is not formed and other substrates, particularly fat, are not able to enter the Krebs cycle.

More than one type of lactic acidosis can exist and these are classified according to the Cohen–Woods classification system (Table 1.1).[18] For the purpose of this text, the only type of lactic acidosis which will be addressed is type A.

Defects in Energy Production Not Due to Oxygen

Its use in the development of ATP is clearly the primary value of oxygen. Understanding the cellular need for oxygen allows

TABLE 1.1. Cohen–Woods Classification of Hyperlactatemia

1) Type A
   Result of lack of oxygen at cellular level, i.e., tissue hypoxia.

2) Type B1
   Result of a predisposing disease not due to lactic acidosis (Type A) but may be associated with Type A. Includes liver disease, sepsis, diabetes, pancreatitis.

3) Type B2
   Result of pharmacologic agents or toxins.

4) Type B3
   Due to inborn errors of metabolism, such as pyruvate deficiency or problems in oxidative phosphorylation.

for clinical application of oxygen assessment and interventions. There are, however, other substances and conditions that affect the generation of energy. The term "dysoxia" will probably increase in its application in critical care.[18] Dysoxia refers to either an inability to use oxygen or an abnormality in other aspects of energy generation in the cell. For example, conditions that would affect the use of oxygen at the molecular level include an abnormal functioning of cytochrome a[3], which would inhibit the final transfer of electrons to oxygen. Cyanide poisoning is a clinical example of the blocking of cytochrome a[3]; it prevents the transfer of final electrons and inhibits any further oxidative phosphorylation.[19] Abnormal oxygenation could also result from diminished cellular concentrations of needed elements, such as phosphate, or changes in the environmental pH owing to excessive hydrogen ion concentration. The acidosis may prevent the normal coupling which would occur during oxidative phosphorylation.[20]

REGULATION OF OXYGEN SUPPLY TO THE TISSUE

In order for oxygen to be utilized at the cellular level, adequate supplies of oxygen are required. The main determinants of oxygen supply are presented in the next several chapters. One key determinant of oxygen supply will be presented here, that is, local blood flow and factors that influence its regulation.

Local blood flow is the key determinant of adequate oxygen supply. Several factors help determine the adequacy of local blood flow, including vessel-wall strength, intra- and extravascular hydrostatic and osmotic pressures, ion concentration (e.g., hydrogen and potassium), blood gases (e.g., P_{O_2} and P_{CO_2}), neurohumoral factors, and local vasoactive substances. While it is beyond this text to explain each of these factors in-depth, a brief review of how these factors can influence local blood flow will be useful.

In addition, keep in mind that different organ systems may respond in a different manner to similar substances. As a rule, however, the factors affecting local blood flow will cause generally similar organ responses. For the purpose of this text, individual organ responses will not be addressed.

Vascular Effects

Blood flow into a local capillary area is controlled by a variety of mechanisms. The blood-vessel wall is partially held open by the inherent strength of the vessel as well as by the hydrostatic and osmotic pressures inside and outside the vessel (Figure 1.11).[21] If intravascular hydrostatic pressure decreases or extravascular hydrostatic pressure increases, blood flow may be reduced. Intravascular osmotic-pressure increases can actually help blood flow be maintained if they are able to pull adequate vascular volume into the vessel. On the other hand, increased extravascular osmotic pressure tends to pull fluid out of the vessel and can reduce blood flow. An example of this may occur in capillary leak syndromes, that is, ARDS. If fluid is pulled out of the blood vessel (increased extravascular osmotic pressure) or allowed to seep out of the vessel (decreased intravascular osmotic pressure), the net effect may be to compress the vessel and reduce blood flow.

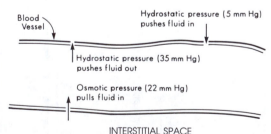

INTERSTITIAL SPACE

FIGURE 1.11. Hydrostatic and osmotic pressures influencing fluid movement out of the blood vessel. A slight net movement of fluid out of the blood vessel occurs due to hydrostatic pressure in vessel overcoming pressures keeping fluid in the vessel. Higher pressure in the vessel aids in maintaining vessel patency.

Another factor which reduces blood flow due to the loss of perfusion pressure is the presence of microemboli.[22] Microemboli may develop for a variety of reasons and obstruct local blood flow. When this occurs, no blood will be supplied to the area (Figure 1.12). Microembolization will be further discussed in the section on prostaglandins.

Neurohumoral Effects

Neurohumoral control of vascular tone is regulated partially by both the sympathetic and parasympathetic nervous systems.[23] Sympathetic stimulation or parasympathetic inhibition can cause vasoconstriction. On the other hand, sympathetic inhibition or parasympathetic stimulation can cause vasodilation. For example, in a patient with a low systemic vascular resistance, that is, vasodilation, a sympathetic stimulant such as norepinephrine (Levophed) can act to increase the vessel tone and increase vasoconstriction properties.

Ions and Gases

Local ions, such as hydrogen (H+) and potassium (K+) act to change vessel tone. Increases in H+ or K+ will cause a reduction in vessel tone and result in vasodilation. Decreases in either of the ions may lead to vasoconstriction.[24] Changes in local gas concentration can also alter vascular tones. Severely low oxygen levels at the local level (perhaps less than 10 mm Hg) can cause vasodilation.[25] Increased P_{CO_2} levels, probably through an increase in hydrogen-ion concentration via the Henderson–Hasselbach reaction, also act to cause vasodilation.

Osmolality

Another factor that alters vessel tone is the concentration of solutes in the area (osmolality). A concentration of solutes or a local osmolality can serve to cause vasodilation. A decreased concentration of solutes can cause vasoconstriction. The decreased concentration of solutes may be secondary to a lack of active metabolic activity in the area which would by nature decrease requirements for blood flow. A decreased requirement for blood flow is an indicator that cellular activity is not prominent and that the cellular production of solutes is not increasing.

Prostaglandins

The subject of prostaglandins is both a complex and actively changing area in regard to current knowledge of their role. While prostaglandins were identified approximately 60 years ago, the mechanisms of action and their role in various disease states are still being studied. However, it is important to understand the key role of the prostaglandins in the regulation of local muscle and vessel tone in order to understand potential problems in oxygenation. Over the next several paragraphs, a brief review of prostaglandins and their role in local blood flow will be reviewed.

Prostaglandins were originally thought to be generated in the human prostate.[26] While this has subsequently been shown not to be true, since prostaglandins are synthesized in most all body tissues except for red blood cells, the name reflects this original idea. Prostaglandins and elements similar to prostaglandins, such as thromboxane and leukotrienes, are frequently referred to

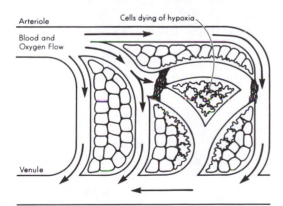

FIGURE 1.12. Pericapillary shunting. Several conditions can restrict capillary blood flow, including precapillary sphincter closure, microemboli, and vasoconstriction. This illustration indicates the impact of blood flow with microembolic formation.

by the term "eicosanoid." The origin of all the eicosanoids can be seen in Figure 1.13.

All the eicosanoids are generated from phospholipids in the cell membrane. The key element produced in the development of the phospholipid conversion is arachidonic acid. Arachidonic acid can take one of two pathways in the further conversion to other substances. Arachidonic acid can be converted in a lipooxygenase cycle into leukotrienes. The most common leukotrienes are leukotriene C_4 (LTC$_4$) and leukotriene D_4 (LTD$_4$). The leukotrienes generate vasoconstriction, increase cell membrane permeability, and can act to stimulate leukocyte aggregation. Arachidonic acid can also be converted through cyclooxygenase into one of two substances: thromboxane A_2 or prostacyclin. Thromboxane A_2 (A_2 coming from arachidonic acid) works in mechanisms very similar to the leukotrienes. However, one key aspect of thromboxane A_2 (TxA$_2$) is the marked tendency to promote platelet aggregation as well as vasoconstriction.

If arachidonic acid is converted through cyclooxygenase cycles into prostacyclin, then the result is markedly different from TxA$_2$. Prostacyclin can be converted into several prostaglandin substances. Prostacyclin (also referred to as PGI$_2$) acts to prevent platelet aggregation and produces vasodilation. These effects are basically opposite to those of thromboxane A_2. Other prostaglandins synthesized through prostacyclin include (although many more exist) prostaglandin E_2 (PGE$_2$) and prostaglandin E_1 (PGE$_1$). The prostaglandins E_2 and E_1 also cause vasodilation, inhibit to some extent platelet aggregation, and may have a role in the inhibition of the release or formation of free oxygen radicals. The role of the eicosanoids and their effect on oxygenation can be seen in the properties of each of these substances. For example, the release of thromboxane A_2 has been hypothesized to be a major component in microembolization and the reduction of local blood flow. Agents that act to reduce cyclooxygenase activity and thereby prevent the conversion of arachidonic acid into thromboxane A_2 have been proposed to help treat conditions where microembolism may be taking place, e.g., sepsis. Agents such as indomethacin and ibuprofen have been suggested as possibly improving outcome in sepsis because of the inhibition of thromboxane A_2. The use of agents that inhibit leukotrienes has also been proposed as a mechanism to reduce capillary permeability that may be seen in conditions such as sepsis and ARDS.

Agents that may actually help offset thromboxane A_2, such as prostaglandins E_1, E_2, and prostacyclin, have been utilized with some success in altering the effects of sepsis and ARDS.[27-30] The key point to remember is that prostaglandins, thromboxane A_2, and leukotrienes can act either to reduce local blood flow (thromboxane A_2 and leukotrienes) or to improve local blood flow (prostacyclin, prostaglandins E_1 and E_2).

All of the above agents can have an interactive effect on regulating local blood flow. It is unlikely that any single agent will cause a dominant effect to offset all other actions. For example, it is unlikely that neurohumoral stimulation alone would offset the vasoactive substances and hydrostatic and colloidal osmotic pressures (both intra- and extravascularly). It is the complex interaction between these mechanisms which makes the understanding and control of lo-

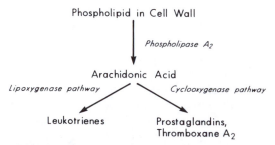

FIGURE 1.13. Origin of eicosanoids. Eicosanoids originate from the cell membranes. From eicosanoids, arachidonic acid is generated. Arachidonic acid has the potential to produce leukotrienes, thromboxane A_2, and prostaglandins, depending on the pathway selected (either lipooxygenase or cyclooxygenase).

cal blood flow regulation relatively difficult. However, understanding the mechanisms influencing local blood flow is crucial to understanding and developing new treatments to enhance cellular oxygen delivery through maintaining local blood flow.

SUMMARY

Maintenance of Cellular Oxygenation

Aspects of oxygenation which are important in regard to energy generation generally center on maintaining normal quantities of oxygen (i.e., oxygen transport), and maintaining normal cellular utilization of oxygen (i.e., O_2 consumption). In order to transport oxygen adequately to the cells, the normal components of oxygen transport must be maintained. These components will be the focus of the next several chapters. However, in addition to getting oxygen to the cells, a couple of points should be kept in mind. As the components of oxygenation are presented, specifically oxygen transport and O_2 consumption and to a lesser extent the cellular use of oxygen, it is important to keep in mind that oxygenation is the concept of using oxygen for energy generation. Measurements of values that reflect only part of the oxygenation process, such as oxygen transport or O_2 consumption, are clearly insufficient to assess overall energy needs of the cells. This first chapter's value is to help illustrate how oxygen plays a role in the generation of energy.

The role oxygen plays in total energy generation is limited to one small aspect of overall energy generation. Many other features, independent of oxygen, can affect energy generation. In the assessment of oxygenation, the clinician has the responsibility not to be too narrow in the overall view of oxygenation. It is important to remember no single test currently is available to assess clinical oxygenation status. Ideally, tests for oxygenation may be measurement of ATP stores at the cellular level or of concentrations of NADH and $FADH_2$. Until these types of measurements are available, the cli-

nician must rely on much more global concepts of oxygenation, such as assessment of factors of oxygen transport and the relationship with oxygen consumption. As you read the rest of this text, keep in mind as each component of oxygenation is presented, the clinician is trying to make sure oxygen is available in quantities adequate for oxidative phosphorylation. Remember concepts such as the level of ADP is the primary stimulus generating the need for oxygen. As ADP levels increase, more oxygen is required by the cells. As we make our assessment of oxygenation, keep in mind that we are not measuring specific oxygenation factors, such as ADP levels. This should keep us more knowledgeable in our clinical interpretation of oxygenation.

If you stuck with this first chapter, congratulations. The rest of the text is more clinically focused.

REFERENCES

1. Masterton WL, Slowinshi EJ. *Chemical Principles.* Philadelphia: WB Saunders, 1969, 377.
2. Bersten A, Sibbald WJ. "Acute lung injury in septic shock." *Crit Care Clin* 1989;5:69.
3. Cone JB. "Cellular oxygen utilization." *In Oxygen Transport in the Critically Ill.* Chicago: Yearbook Medical Pub, 1987, 157.
4. Cochrane C, Spragg R, Revak S, et al. "The presence of neutrophil elastase and evidence of oxidation activity in bronchoalveolar lavage fluid of patients with adult respiratory distress syndrome." *Am Rev Respir Dis* 1983;127:S25.
5. Hammond B, Doutos HA, Hess ML. "Oxygen radicals in the adult respiratory distress syndrome, in myocardial ischemia and reperfusion injury, and in cerebral vascular damage." *Can J Physiol Pharmacol* 1985;63:173.
6. Machlin LJ, Bendich A. "Free radical tissue damage: Protective role of antioxidant nutrients." *FASEB J* 1987;1:441.
7. McCord JM, Fridovich I. "The biology and pathology of oxygen radicals." *Ann Intern Med* 1978; 89:122.8.
8. Mecca RS. "Complications of therapy." *In* Kirby RT, Taylor RW (eds). *Respiratory Failure.* Chicago: Yearbook Medical Pub, 1986, 584.
9. McArdle WD, Katch FI, Katch VL. *Exercise Physiology: Energy, Nutrition and Human Performance.* Philadelphia: Lea & Febiger, 1981, 65.
10. Kaminski MV. *Hyperalimentation: A Guide for Clinicians.* New York: Marcel Dekker, 1985, 6.

11. Kariman K, Hempel FG, Jobsis FF. "In vivo comparison of cytochrome aa$_3$ redox state and tissue PO$_2$ in transient anoxia." *J Appl Physiol* 1983; 55:1057.

12. Hilberman M, Subramanian H, Haselgrove J, et al. "In vivo time resolved brain phosphorus nuclear magnetic resonance." *J Cerebr Blood Flow Metab* 1984;4:334.

13. Masterton WL, Slowinshi EJ. *Chemical Principles.* Philadelphia: WB Saunders, 1969.

14. Lorenz A. "Lactic acidosis: A nursing challenge." *Crit Care Nurse* 1989;9:64.

15. Frommer JP. "Lactic acidosis." *Med Clin North Am* 1983;67:815.

16. Kruse JA, Carlson RW. "Lactate metabolism." *Crit Care Clin* 1987;5:725.

17. Cohen RD, Woods HF. *Clinical and Biochemical Aspects of Lactic Acidosis.* Oxford: Blackwell Scientific Pub, 1976.

18. Robin ED. "Of men and mitochondria: Coping with hypoxic dysoxia." *Am Rev Resp Dis* 1980; 122:517.

19. Singh BM, Coles N, Lewis P, et al. "The metabolic effects of fatal cyanide poisoning." *Postgraduate Medical Journal* 1989;65:923.

20. Jeffers L. "The effects of acidosis on cardiovascular function." *J Am Assn Nurse Anes* 1986;54:148.

21. Groer ME, Shekleton ME. *Basic Pathophysiology: A Conceptual Approach.* St. Louis: CV Mosby, 1979, 260.

22. Landau SE, Alexander RS, Powers SR Jr, et al. "Tissue oxygen exchange and reactive hyperemia following microembolization." *J Surg Res* 1982; 32:38.

23. Boyd JL, Stanford GG, Chernow B. "The pharmacotherapy of septic shock." *Crit Care Clin* 1989;5:65.

24. Bruns FJ, Fraley DS, Haigh J, et al. "Control of organ blood flow." *In Oxygen Transport in the Critically Ill.* Chicago: Yearbook Medical Pub, 1987, 92.

25. Shepherd, JT. "Circulation to skeletal muscle." *In* Shepherd JT, Abbound FM, Geiger SR (eds). *Handbook of Physiology, Vol. 3: The Cardiovascular System.* Bethesda: American Physiological Society, 1983, 3xx.

26. Reines HD, Halushka RV. "Arachidonic acid metabolites—The eicosanoids." *In* Shoemaker WC, Ayres S, Grenvik A, et al. (eds). *Textbook of Critical Care.* 2nd Ed. Philadelphia: WB Saunders, 1989, 1028.

27. DeMaria A, Heffernan JJ, Grindlinger GA, et al. "Naloxone versus placebo in treatment of septic shock." *Lancet* 1985;1:363.

28. Appel P, Shoemaker W. "Hemodynamic and oxygen transport effects of prostaglandin E1 in patients with adult respiratory distress syndrome." *Crit Care Med* 1984;12:528.

29. Jacobs ER, Bone RC. "Therapeutic implications of acute lung injury." *Crit Care Clin* 1986;2:615.

30. Bihari D, Smith M, Gimson A, Tinker J. "The effects of vasodilation with prostacyclin on oxygen delivery and uptake in critically ill patients." *N Engl J Med* 1987;317:397.

2
Clinical Application of Arterial Oxygen Tensions (Pa$_{O_2}$)

When examining the tests used in the assessment of oxygenation, the arterial blood gas P_{O_2} continues to rank as one of the most frequently employed tests. While this will certainly change as oximetry devices are more commonly employed, one must ask why the Pa_{O_2} is such a common test in the assessment of oxygenation. This is an important question since the Pa_{O_2} contributes only a minor role in the delivery of oxygen to the cells. In many cases, an assessment of oxygen delivery can take place without a Pa_{O_2} measurement. In this chapter, we will explore the clinical application of Pa_{O_2} values in patient care situations. Through clinical situations presented in this chapter, the answer to the question of why the Pa_{O_2} is such a common test can be answered.

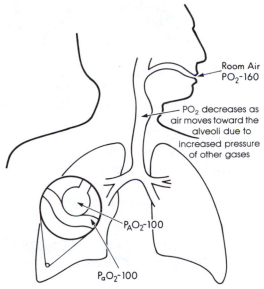

FIGURE 2.1. Changes in the Pa_{O_2} from room air to the alveoli.

DEFINITION OF Pa$_{O_2}$

The Pa_{O_2} refers to the amount of oxygen physically dissolved in arterial blood. The normal Pa_{O_2} is 80–100 mm Hg at sea level, although clinically acceptable values range from 60–100 mm Hg.[1] The actual Pa_{O_2} is determined by the alveolar oxygen concentrations (Figure 2.1). Pa_{O_2} levels are a function of several factors: $F_{I_{O_2}}$, barometric pressure (Pb), and other alveolar gases. While more on the determination of Pa_{O_2} levels will be presented under intrapulmonary shunting, one factor determining the Pa_{O_2}, Pb, can be used to illustrate the role played by the Pa_{O_2} in the delivery of oxygen (D_{O_2}). Residents of Denver, due to the higher altitude and lower barometric pressure, have lower than normal Pa_{O_2} levels.[2] The normal Pa_{O_2} in Denver is 65–80 mm Hg rather than 80–100 mm Hg. This example helps illustrate why clinical normals are accepted as low as 60 mm Hg.

OXYGEN DELIVERY AND Pa$_{O_2}$

The amount of oxygen dissolved in the blood contributes minimally to the amount of oxygen delivered to the tissues. In humans, oxygen is transported by hemoglobin rather than dissolved in the blood. A small amount of oxygen does reach the cells from the oxygen dissolved in the blood, but not much. Many years ago physiologists determined that the amount of oxygen reaching the cells in the free floating form accounts for less than 3% of the total amount of oxygen arriving at the cells.[3]

To illustrate the amount of oxygen carried to the cells by the Pa_{O_2} in comparison to hemoglobin, consider the following analogy. Assume you need a system to measure how many people pass through an intersection. Most people pass through the intersection in cars or buses. Few are pedestrians. Yet if one were to use a system of measurement that relied on actually seeing people, the only ones visible would be the pedestrians. While this is an accurate representation of people visible on the street, it is not an accurate representation of the people passing through the intersection. In many ways, this is the same situation as measuring the Pa_{O_2}. The Pa_{O_2} refers to the oxygen floating in the blood, unattached to hemoglobin. Minimal amounts of oxygen reach the cells unattached to hemoglobin.

DETERMINING AMOUNT OF OXYGEN DELIVERED BY THE Pa_{O_2}

The actual amount of oxygen supplied by the Pa_{O_2} can be computed by applying the oxygen-solubility coefficient. The oxygen-solubility coefficient refers to the amount of oxygen that will dissolve in a given solution at a given pressure. In blood, oxygen dissolves at a rate of .003 cc/dl per mm Hg. Rather than describe how to calculate how much oxygen is carried by the Pa_{O_2}, Table 2.1 contains sample calculations over several clinically relevant Pa_{O_2} levels. Table 2.2 illustrates the practical application of Pa_{O_2} and the dependence of the amount of oxygen transported on the cardiac output. Table 2.2 contains the more relevant values since it reflects the variation common in clinical situations.

TABLE 2.1. Determination of Oxygen Carried by the Pa_{O_2}

If the P_{O_2} is,		Then the Amount Carried is
40 mm Hg	$\dfrac{5000^*}{40 \times .003 \times 100}$	6 cc
60 mm Hg	$\dfrac{5000}{60 \times .003 \times 100}$	9 cc
100 mm Hg	$\dfrac{5000}{100 \times .003 \times 100}$	15 cc
300 mm Hg	$\dfrac{5000}{300 \times .003 \times 100}$	45 cc

*Assume a cardiac output of 5000 cc/min (5 LPM). The cardiac output is divided by 100 (dl), the amount of blood utilized in the oxygen-solubility coefficient calculation.

The computations in Table 2.2 are particularly interesting considering that the normal oxygen transport ranges from 600 to 1000 cc/min. For significant amounts of oxygen to be carried by the Pa_{O_2} method, the cardiac output must be high. If the cardiac output is low, the Pa_{O_2} must be very high (> 300 mm Hg) to have any clinical value. Under most clinically encountered values (Pa_{O_2} < 100 mm Hg), very little oxygen is carried in the blood by the Pa_{O_2}. Clinically, this concept has several implications. Consider the following clinical examples.

TABLE 2.2. Influence of the Cardiac Output of Oxygen Carried by the Pa_{O_2}

P_{O_2} Level	Cardiac Output	Amount of O_2 Carried by Pa_{O_2}
40 mm Hg	3 LPM	3.6 cc/min
	4 LPM	4.8 cc/min
	6 LPM	7.2 cc/min
60 mm Hg	3 LPM	5.4 cc/min
	4 LPM	7.2 cc/min
	6 LPM	10.8 cc/min
100 mm Hg	3 LPM	9.0 cc/min
	4 LPM	12.0 cc/min
	6 LPM	18.0 cc/min
300 mm Hg	3 LPM	27.0 cc/min
	4 LPM	36.0 cc/min
	6 LPM	54.0 cc/min

A patient admitted with congestive heart failure has a room-air blood gas with a Pa$_{O_2}$ of 63 mm Hg (normal pH and Pa$_{CO_2}$). The physician requests oxygen therapy. What is the value of such a treatment? If the Pa$_{O_2}$ increases from 63 to near 100, what benefit has been obtained? From Table 2.2, one can see that the improvement in oxygen transport (if the CO stays the same) is only a few cc. This represents only about a 1% improvement in oxygen transport. The value of such a therapy appears very limited. As can be seen in Table 2.2, the amount of oxygen carried by the Pa$_{O_2}$ is probably clinically insignificant. However, the amount of oxygen delivered to the cells actually is higher than the values in Table 2.2 imply. More oxygen is delivered as the Pa$_{O_2}$ increases due to the relationship Pa$_{O_2}$ values have with oxyhemoglobin (S$_{O_2}$) levels. The Pa$_{O_2}$ is the primary factor in determining the amount of oxyhemoglobin (the hemoglobin species which carries oxygen). While changes in the Pa$_{O_2}$ will not markedly change oxygen delivery, changes in oxyhemoglobin values can have a larger impact on oxygen delivery. Oxyhemoglobin's role in oxygen delivery will be presented in more depth in Chapter 4.

The cost of initiating oxygen therapy in the above example is twofold. First, (unless an arterial line is present) there is pain associated with testing the blood gases. Most critical care nurses are very aware of the discomfort associated with blood gas sampling. Second, blood gas sampling is costly. Costs will be discussed later, but blood gas charges range from $50 to $100. From a nursing and patient perspective, it would be wise to question oxygen therapy as a routine application.

The above example can be applied to any situation where the Pa$_{O_2}$ is to be used. Some of these situations are common and may indicate inappropriate use of blood gases or oxygen therapy. For example, consider the patient with chest pain (from angina or myocardial infarction). If the Pa$_{O_2}$ is normal, the administration of small amounts of oxygen therapy is of little value. Only when the Pa$_{O_2}$ falls under 60 mm Hg would oxygen therapy be of value and then for reasons less associated with oxygen transport than with hypoxemic stimulation to breathe and the development of pulmonary hypertension.

Why is oxygen therapy such an integral part of treating a patient with chest pain? There has been no clear research determining that oxygen therapy reduces myocardial injury patterns.[4-6] Perhaps oxygen therapy is commonly used because we have not developed better methods to improve myocardial oxygenation, so an increased reliance is placed on any method that may provide some benefit. Oxygen therapy probably does little to improve myocardial oxygenation, but it may provide a minor improvement in D$_{O_2}$. Perhaps the psychological value it provides to both the patient and clinicians gives some concrete value to the use of oxygen in uncomplicated chest pain.[7] However, the key point is that as long as the Pa$_{O_2}$ is over 60 mm Hg, little value will be obtained from oxygen therapy since oxygen therapy only elevates the Pa$_{O_2}$ (and Sa$_{O_2}$), and the Pa$_{O_2}$ does not transport oxygen in significant quantities.

EMPIRICAL EVIDENCE SUPPORTING THE MINIMAL CONTRIBUTION OF THE Pa$_{O_2}$ IN D$_{O_2}$

Given the minimal role in oxygen transport played by the Pa$_{O_2}$, it is surprising that so much emphasis is given to its use. Many nurses have encountered physicians and other health care providers anxious to treat clinically acceptable Pa$_{O_2}$ levels, e.g. between 60 and 80 mm Hg. Is this appropriate? One obvious example why it is usually not appropriate is the previously mentioned Pa$_{O_2}$ level in Denver. If it is appropriate to treat Pa$_{O_2}$ levels in the 60 to 80 range, then most everyone in Denver should be on oxygen.

An interesting illustration of the limited value of the Pa$_{O_2}$ can be seen in exercise studies. In people with normal lung function, increasing the Pa_{O_2} through breathing oxygen has not been demonstrated to significantly change exercise performance.[8-11] For example, athletes, such as football players completing long runs, frequently come back to the bench and breathe oxygen. Does this help? Based on the oxygen solubility coefficient and increase in cardiac output, perhaps a 1–2% increase in D_{O_2} occurs, yet few studies support the contention that this therapy helps the athlete. Why is it done? Perhaps because if an athlete who is paid $1,000,000 a year to perform *thinks* breathing oxygen improves performance, then the best course may be to supply the oxygen, considering no demonstrable harm comes from short-term oxygen therapy.

A third example of the restricted value of treating Pa_{O_2} levels is more common clinically, particularly in trauma/surgical settings. A patient with hypovolemia secondary to blood loss of a nonpulmonary nature will have normal or elevated Pa_{O_2} levels, provided lung function has not been altered. This type of patient will have cellular deficits of oxygen and can die of the reduced blood volume. At the same time however, the Pa_{O_2} will be normal.[12] This scenario further illustrates the limitation of using Pa_{O_2} levels to assess D_{O_2}. Use of the blood gas to assess oxygen transport in this situation will result in inaccurate assessments and could potentially delay needed treatments. The clinician who relies on the Pa_{O_2} to assess oxygen transport will be in error more times than is acceptable.

This last example has nothing to do with clinical situations but is interesting and illustrative of the value of not relying on Pa_{O_2} for D_{O_2}. What would an animal look like if it existed completely on the Pa_{O_2} for D_{O_2}? The answer can be found in comparative physiology, specifically that of insects. Insects do not rely on a cardiac output or Hgb to transport oxygen. Instead, they have openings throughout their body which have tubes similar to tracheas (Figure 2.2). These tubes must virtually come into contact with

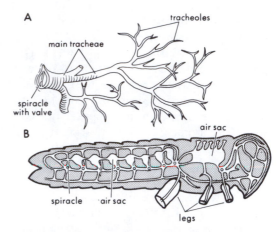

FIGURE 2.2.   Insect respiration. Insects do not rely on lungs as humans do. The insect body is permeated with respiratory tubes (tracheoles) since all cells are required to be in contact with air due to the absence of an adequate internal lung system.

all cells in their body or oxygen will not diffuse to them. Such a system limits the size to which the insect can grow. The oxygen-transport system of insects also limits the size to which they can grow (Figure 2.3). The oxygen supply system of the insect is insufficient to support a body much larger than a few inches (despite what might be seen in motion pictures). Oxygen cannot be transported efficiently without a heart (circulatory system) or hemoglobin.

POTENTIAL VALUE IN THE Pa_{O_2}

There are potential values for the P_{O_2} which have not been discussed. One of these will be presented in more depth in Chapter 5 on hemoglobin saturation (S_{O_2}). P_{O_2} values have three potential contributions to the interpretation of S_{O_2} levels. First, the P_{O_2} can be used to estimate S_{O_2} levels through the oxyhemoglobin dissociation curve. Clinically this can have some value (Table 2.3). Second, while the Pa_{O_2} does not transport oxygen in substantial quantities, Sa_{O_2} levels do start to have an impact on D_{O_2}. Interpretation of the Pa_{O_2} should always consider the Sa_{O_2} role in D_{O_2}. A third value relative to Sa_{O_2} is in regard to assessing the carrying capacity of hemoglo-

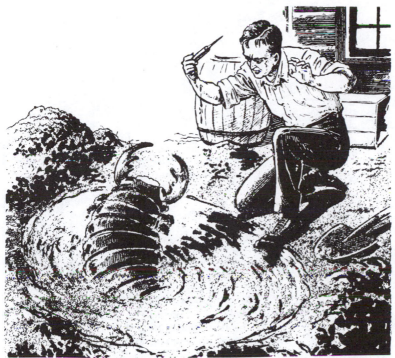

FIGURE 2.3. Can giant insects exist? Have you ever been working in your yard only to find giant insects coming out of the ground? While this gentleman is obviously taken aback by such an occurrence, no such insects can exist in real life. An insect's oxygen-transport system cannot support the presence of any body system larger than a few inches. Adapted from Haining P. "Terror: A history of horror illustrations from the pulp magazines." Peter Haining & Pictorial Presentations.

based on clinical factors such as changing pH, Pa_{O_2}, and temperature, P_{O_2} levels can be used to aid in identifying clinically significant changes.

In addition, two other potential uses of the Pa_{O_2} exist independent of Sa_{O_2} values. The first is in regard to patients with limited

TABLE 2.3.   Relationship Between Pa_{O_2} and Sa_{O_2}

If the Pa_{O_2} is,	Then the Approximate Sa_{O_2} is
20 mm Hg	33%
27 mm Hg	50%
40 mm Hg	75%
60 mm Hg	90%
80 mm Hg	94%
100 mm Hg	98%

CO and hemoglobin levels. It is possible, if the Pa_{O_2} is increased to very high levels, that a small improvement in oxygen transport can occur. While under most circumstances this is not important, in patients with a diminished CO and/or Hgb level, this increase may be of slight benefit. Such a treatment should only be temporary however, while a problem such as a low CO or Hgb is addressed. In order to achieve Pa_{O_2} levels high enough to help, F_{IO_2} levels must be elevated to near toxic ranges. More on oxygen toxicity will be presented in Chapter 12.

Another possible value is one that is difficult to measure but has theoretical value. This value is relative to the driving pressure exerted by arterial oxygen tensions. If the Pa_{O_2} is high, a larger pressure difference exists between cellular and arterial oxygen, potentially facilitating oxygen transfer to the cells (Figure 2.4). Research has not substan-

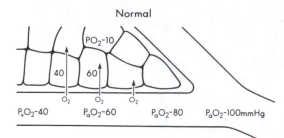

Normal

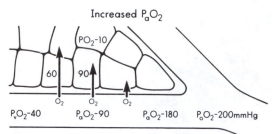

Increased Pa_{O_2}

FIGURE 2.4. Increased Pa_{O_2} can potentially increase oxygen movement into the cell.

tiated the theory that values higher than normal contribute significantly to improving gas transfer, yet such a potential does exist.

Clinical Application of Pa_{O_2} Values

1. A patient is admitted with an acute MI. He is in no distress, chest pain is absent, and breathing is unlabored. Your unit has a policy of starting oxygen at 4 LPM on all patients admitted. Your patient is uncomfortable with the oxygen in place and is worried that it will make his wife and children more anxious when they visit. In your opinion, is it clinically necessary to keep the oxygen in place?

ANSWER

While the oxygen therapy is probably not hurting him and may provide minimal benefit, the improvement in oxygen transport is so small as to be clinically negligible. If your unit allows the nurse discretion in applying oxygen, he would probably be safe if it were discontinued. Otherwise, contacting the physician to waive the routine order is appropriate.

2. A patient with left ventricular failure has a Pa_{O_2} of 52, Sa_{O_2} .83, pH 7.38, hemoglobin 13 Gm/dl, and a cardiac output of 3.2 LPM. The physician orders the $F_{I_{O_2}}$ to be increased from .30 to .40. The Pa_{O_2} returns at 76 and the Sa_{O_2} is .93 with other parameters unchanged. How much improvement in oxygen transport occurred with therapy? If oxygen therapy is to be used to increase oxygen transport, was the increase in $F_{I_{O_2}}$ adequate?

ANSWER

The increase in the Pa_{O_2} from 52 to 76 would have improved transport by only 5–10 cc/min from the Pa_{O_2} method. The increased hemoglobin saturation increased transport by 56 cc (D_{O_2} of 462 to 518 cc/min). The increase in oxygen transport was helpful, but not as useful as increasing the cardiac output. If oxygen therapy is to be used, the $F_{I_{O_2}}$ should be temporarily increased to high levels (> 50%) while attempting to increase the cardiac output. For any substantial increase in oxygen transport to occur, the Pa_{O_2} must be elevated to very high levels. Of course, oxygen toxicity dangers must also then be considered.

3. A patient on 40% oxygen has a Pa_{O_2} of 93 (Sa_{O_2} .96). Current BP is 126/82, P 87, RR 17. The hemoglobin value is 12 GM/dl. The physician orders the $F_{I_{O_2}}$ to be lowered to .30. The Pa_{O_2} on .30 is 66 (Sa_{O_2} .91). Vital signs are BP 128/80, P 84, RR 16. Upon receiving this information, the physician requests that the $F_{I_{O_2}}$ be increased back to .40, stating that the Pa_{O_2} is too low on the new $F_{I_{O_2}}$. Is this request appropriate?

ANSWER

Without information on the cardiac output, we can assume that no substantial change has occurred since the vital signs are similar. A fall of the Pa_{O_2} from 93 to 66, at virtually all normal cardiac outputs, will result in minor changes in oxygen transport (between 5 and 10 cc/min) from the Pa_{O_2} change. The loss of hemoglobin saturation may produce a larger decrease (up to 20–40 cc), depending on the cardiac output. However, the change generally is not clinically significant. Subsequently, the request to increase the $F_{I_{O_2}}$ is not justified in this instance.

ECONOMIC ASPECTS ASSOCIATED WITH Pa_{O_2} USE

The application of oxygen transport concepts when interpreting Pa_{O_2} levels will usually result in a reduction in the number of blood gases requested. Blood gas tests ordinarily do not cost the institution much to perform, yet charges are frequently high. It is difficult to determine how much a blood gas actually costs, but it is probably only about $^1/_{10}$ of the charge. If a gas is charged at $50, the cost is probably $5. It is important to remember, however, the patient or third party will be paying the charge. The hospital would benefit if the reimbursement is of a fixed nature (prospective payment) since any reduction in costs improves the income/expense ratio. Table 2.4 shows the projected economic impact of reducing blood gases in both an individual and in a unit. The figures listed are easy to attain if concepts in oxygen transport are applied to clinical settings.

SUMMARY

While the Pa_{O_2} is one of the most commonly tested factors in the assessment of oxygenation, it is of little value in actually improving oxygen transport. The Pa_{O_2} should be analyzed and maintained at levels in excess of 60 to prevent problems such as increased work of breathing and development of pulmonary hypertension, and to maintain hemoglobin saturation and im-

prove oxygenation. Pa_{O_2} levels generally are less valuable in assessing oxygen transport than are other components of oxygenation. When assessing oxygenation status, keep in mind that Pa_{O_2} values are limited in usefulness and can be misleading if used as a primary assessment tool.

REFERENCES

1. Shoemaker WC. "Physiologic monitoring of the critically ill patient." *In* Shoemaker WC, Ayres S, Grenvik A, et al. (eds). *Textbook of Critical Care.* 2nd Ed. Philadelphia: WB Saunders, 1989, 151.
2. Albert RK. "Physiology and management of failure of arterial oxygenation." *In* Fallat RJ, Luce JM. *Cardiopulmonary Critical Care Management.* New York: Churchill Livingstone, 1988, 37.
3. Von Rueden KT. "Cardiopulmonary assessment of the critically ill trauma patient." *Crit Care Nurs Clin N Am* 1989;1:33.
4. Rawles JM, Kenmure ACF. "Controlled trial of oxygen in uncomplicated myocardial infarction." *Br Med J* 1976;1:10121.
5. Snider GL, Fairley HB, Fulmer JD, Weg JG. "Scientific basis of oxygen therapy." *Chest* 1984; 86:236.
6. Ganz W, Donoso R, Marius H, et al. "Coronary hemodynamics and myocardial oxygen metabolism by oxygen therapy in patients with and without coronary artery disease." *Circ* 1972;45:763.
7. American Heart Assn. *Textbook of Advanced Cardiac Life Support.* 1987, 12.
8. Shapiro BA, Cane RD "Interpretation of blood gases." *In* Shoemaker WC, Ayres S, Grenvik A, et al. (eds). *Textbook of Critical Care.* 2nd Ed. Philadelphia: WB Saunders, 1989, 305.
9. Winter FD, Snell PG, Stray-Gundersen J. "Effects of 100% oxygen on performance of professional soccer players." *JAMA*, 1989;262:227.
10. Titlow LW. "The effects of oxygen administration during simulated athletic competition." *J Sports Med* 1982;22:323.
11. Bjorgum RK, Sharkey BJ. "Inhalation of oxygen as an aid to recovery after exertion." *Res Q* 1965; 37:462.
12. Harper R. *Guide to Respiratory Care.* Philadelphia: JB Lippincott, 1981, 129.

TABLE 2.4. Economic Value of Avoiding Blood Gases

Number of Blood Gases Reduced	Cost	Charges
Individual Patient		
1 per day	$5	$50
5 per ICU stay	$25	$250
Unit Admissions (150)		
1 per day	$750	$7,500
5 per ICU stay	$3,750	$37,500
Unit Admissions (450)		
1 per day	$2,250	$22,500
5 per ICU stay	$11,250	$112,500

3
Intrapulmonary Shunting (Qs/Qt)

One of the most interesting clinical aspects of obtaining arterial blood gases is the potential misuse of the arterial oxygen pressure (Pa_{O_2}) for use in assessing oxygen transport. A key value of the Pa_{O_2} lies in its ability to estimate intrapulmonary shunting, not in the assessment of oxygen transport. Intrapulmonary shunting (Qs/Qt) refers to the pulmonary blood flow that does not come into contact with functioning alveoli (Qs) in comparison to total pulmonary blood flow (Qt). Intrapulmonary shunting is the primary mechanism by which the arterial P_{O_2} level will change in clinical settings. As such, Qs/Qt can be used in several ways: (1) to detect the degree of pulmonary dysfunction from a given clinical condition, (2) to identify changes in clinical status based either on interventions or changing clinical conditions, or (3) to understand the amount of oxygenation support required by the lungs. In this chapter, the use of the intrapulmonary shunt in clinical practice will be reviewed.

The intrapulmonary shunt has one primary clinical effect, that is, to alter the Pa_{O_2} level. The reduction in Pa_{O_2} with an increasing Qs/Qt can have the additional effect on oxygen transport of lowering the hemoglobin saturation level. Subsequently, this chapter will focus on the effects of the intrapulmonary shunt on Pa_{O_2} and Sa_{O_2} levels.

Another major focus of this chapter is to demonstrate mechanisms by which intra-pulmonary shunts can be approximated. Under many clinical circumstances, Qs/Qt measurements are unavailable. However, estimates of Qs/Qt, through Pa_{O_2} analysis, are possible. These estimates must be used carefully, though, due to potential inaccuracies. The use and limitation of these Qs/Qt estimates will be presented.

NORMAL OXYGENATION OF THE BLOOD

In the human lung, oxygen enters the blood from the alveoli. The amount of oxygen that enters the blood is dependent on the partial pressure of oxygen in the alveoli (Figure 3.1).

Room air contains 20.9% (.21) oxygen, about 78.9% nitrogen, with less than 1% of other gases making up the total barometric pressure (P_B). Carbon dioxide makes up about .003 of the P_B. Barometric pressure is normally near 760 mm Hg. A room-air gas sample can be analyzed for the pressure exerted by each of the gases based on this information. Room-air P_{O_2} is about 160 mm Hg (.21 × 760) and the P_{CO_2} is near 2 mm Hg (.003 × 760). If an air bubble contaminates a blood-gas sample, the P_{O_2} rises toward 160 and the P_{CO_2} falls toward 2 mm Hg.

As a person inspires, the oxygen concentration of the inhaled air will reach the alveoli. The blood perfusing the alveoli will

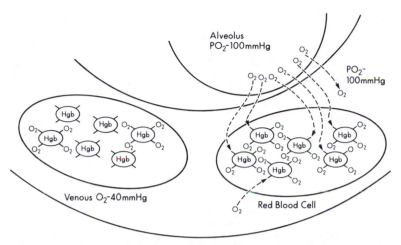

FIGURE 3.1. Alveolar oxygen pressures determine arterial pressures and hemoglobin saturation.

immediately exchange the venous oxygen tension with the oxygen in the alveoli (Figure 3.2).

The oxygen concentration in the alveoli will determine how much hemoglobin is loaded with oxygen. The hemoglobin loading is primarily based on the behavior of the oxyhemoglobin-dissociation curve. Deoxyhemoglobin in the venous blood will pick up oxygen from the lungs to become oxyhemoglobin in the pulmonary capillary (and eventually the artery).

If for any reason the alveolar gas concentrations are less than normal, the arterial blood level will be less than expected. Determining the level of alveolar concentration of oxygen (PA_{O_2}) can be computed from the alveolar air equation (Tables 3.1 and 3.2). Alveolar oxygen tensions are lower than room air due to increased carbon-dioxide and water-vapor pressures in the alveoli. Based on the alveolar oxygen tension of room air (which is approximately 100 mm Hg) (Table 3.3), if the lung functioned perfectly, all the oxygen in the alveoli would equilibrate with the blood in the pulmonary capillaries. This equilibration of gases between the alveoli and pulmonary capillaries would result in an oxygen level in the artery equal to that in the alveoli. Unfortunately, several factors exist that limit how close the Pa_{O_2} can ap-

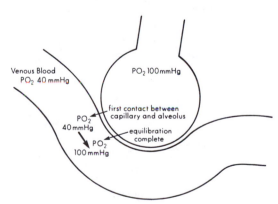

FIGURE 3.2. Gas transfers between the alveolus and capillary almost instantaneously. Equilibration is almost complete before the blood is more than one third across the alveolar/capillary surface area.

TABLE 3.1. Measuring Alveolar Oxygen Tensions (PA_{O_2})

The alveolar air equation is determined by the following:

$$PA_{O_2} = F_{I_{O_2}} (Pb - P_{H_2O}) - \frac{Pa_{CO_2}}{r}$$

where

$F_{I_{O_2}}$ = fraction of inspired oxygen
Pb = barometric pressure
P_{H_2O} = water vapor pressure
Pa_{CO_2} = pressure of arterial carbon dioxide
r = respiratory quotient (V_{CO_2}/V_{O_2})

TABLE 3.2.   Assumptions of the Alveolar Air Equation

The alveolar air equation (below) uses the following assumptions:

$$PA_{O_2} = F_{I_{O_2}} (Pb - P_{H_2O}) - \frac{Pa_{CO_2}}{r}$$

Values are assumed to be:

$F_{I_{O_2}}$ varies with each situation
Pb = 760 mm Hg (except at non–sea-level areas)
P_{H_2O} = 47 mm Hg
Pa_{CO_2} varies with each patient
r = .8 (clinically, could vary between .7–1)

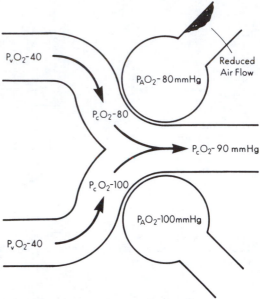

FIGURE 3.3.   Arterial P_{O_2} will almost equal ideal alveolar P_{O_2} under most circumstances. PA_{O_2} = 100 mm Hg is the ideal alveolar oxygen level in this example.

proximate the alveolar oxygen concentration.

Theoretically, arterial oxygen levels should equal alveolar oxygen levels (Figure 3.3). However, several anatomic variations exist that prevent arterial oxygen tension from actually equaling alveolar tension. For example, thebesian and bronchial veins empty directly into the left-heart circulation, which then causes a decrease in arterial oxygen tension (Figure 3.4). Owing to these anatomic limitations, arterial oxygen levels do not actually equal alveolar gas concentrations. However, alveolar gas concentrations are usually within very close ap-

proximation of arterial oxygen since these anatomic shunts comprise only a small part of total blood flow.

In addition to anatomic structure limiting the Pa_{O_2} level, the lung does not always

TABLE 3.3.   Examples of Calculating Alveolar Oxygen Tensions

Given the following information, the alveolar oxygen tension is computed as follows:

Example 1
$F_{I_{O_2}}$ is .21 (room air) Pa_{CO_2} is 40

The alveolar air equation is:

$$PA_{O_2} = .21 (760 - 47) - \frac{40}{.8}$$
$$PA_{O_2} = .21 (713) - 50$$
$$PA_{O_2} = 150 - 50$$
$$PA_{O_2} = 100$$

Example 2
$F_{I_{O_2}}$ is .50 Pa_{CO_2} is 40

The alveolar air equation is:

$$PA_{O_2} = .50 (760 - 47) - \frac{40}{.8}$$
$$PA_{O_2} = .50 (713) - 50$$
$$PA_{O_2} = 357 - 50$$
$$PA_{O_2} = 307$$

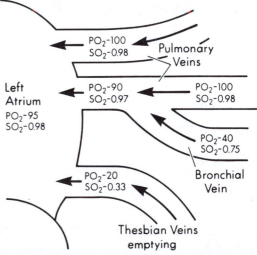

FIGURE 3.4.   Anatomic shunts produce arterial oxygen levels lower than pulmonary capillary oxygen levels.

have maximal alveolar function. Under normal circumstances, not all alveolar units are in full function. The failure of alveolar units to be open while they are perfused with venous blood causes a small amount of venous blood to enter the arterial circulation (Figure 3.5). Again, under normal circumstances, only a small part of the total alveoli are not functioning. The effect on the oxygenation of the blood due to these nonfunctioning alveoli is relatively small. Recruitment of these nonfunctioning alveoli can occur during deep breathing (exercise, yawning); therefore, the effect of nonfunctioning alveoli is even less during episodes of deep breathing.

Venous blood mixing with arterial blood is referred to by several names, one being a "venous admixture." Another common description is that of an intrapulmonary shunt. No actual intrapulmonary shunt exists, that is, no blood is being shunted away from the lung. However, venous blood has not come into contact with functional alveoli and is, in essence, being "shunted" past the lungs. Since blood is bypassing the lung, the term intrapulmonary shunt is utilized to describe the phenomenon. The intrapulmonary shunt is normally quite low; it accounts for less than 5% of the total blood flow to the lung (see Table 3.4).

Intrapulmonary shunts are a form of a low V/Q ratio. Whenever perfusion (Q) exceeds ventilation (V), inadequate oxygenation of the venous blood will occur. High V/Q ratios also exist (ventilation in excess of perfusion) in conditions such as pulmonary emboli and chronic lung disease. In clinical practice, it is common to have both high and low V/Q ratios in different parts of the lung. However, high V/Q ratios have less of an effect on Pa_{O_2} levels and more of an effect on Pa_{CO_2} values. For the purpose of this chapter, only low V/Q ratios (or intrapulmonary shunts) will be presented.

REASONS FOR CHANGE IN ARTERIAL P_{O_2} LEVELS

Based on both the intrapulmonary and anatomic shunts, alveolar oxygen levels are always higher than arterial oxygen levels. This actually is useful when the clinician starts to analyze the severity of the intrapulmonary shunt.

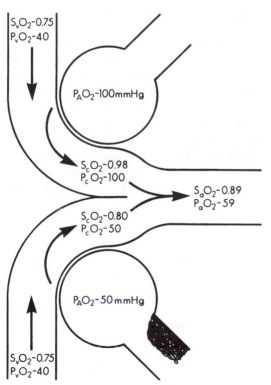

FIGURE 3.5. Ventilation of alveoli at levels below perfusion will result in abnormal Pa_{O_2} levels. Note that the equilibration of pulmonary-capillary hemoglobin saturations produce a mixed arterial hemoglobin saturation and oxygen tension.

TABLE 3.4. Values for Qs/Qt

		Characteristics
Normal	2–5%	No clinical symptoms.
Mild	5–15%	Shortness of breath, particularly on exertion.
Major	15–30%	Resistant hypoxemia, requires substantial oxygenation support.
Severe	>30%	Difficulty with spontaneous breathing, may require mechanical ventilation.

The Pa_{O_2} level can decrease to levels less than normal for several reasons: (1) a decrease in barometric pressure; (2) the development of a true anatomic shunt; (3) a diffusion defect; (4) hypoventilation; and (5) an intrapulmonary shunt.[1] With the exception of an intrapulmonary shunt, which is by far the most common, a change in the P_{O_2} level caused by any of these mechanisms is not common in clinical practice. A brief review of all of these mechanisms will help illustrate their potential impacts on the Pa_{O_2} (and subsequently Sa_{O_2}) levels.

Decreases in barometric pressure (P_B) will cause a decrease in the alveolar oxygen concentrations (Table 3.5). A decrease in alveolar oxygen concentrations, such as seen at high altitudes, will directly cause a reduction in Pa_{O_2} levels. For example, people who live in high altitudes, such as Denver, routinely will have lower Pa_{O_2} levels — the normal Pa_{O_2} in Denver is 65–80 mm Hg.[2] The lower Pa_{O_2} level by itself does not cause any known long-term harmful effects on residents of high altitudes. However, the lower (P_B) will cause a reduction in Pa_{O_2}.

A second factor that might cause the Pa_{O_2} to fall is a true anatomic shunt. Anatomic shunts are clinical conditions such as an intraventricular septal defect. The septal defect may allow venous blood from the right ventricle to mix with arterial blood from the left ventricle. This mixture of blood causes the arterial oxygen level to fall, reflecting the influence of the venous oxygen blood contamination. The anatomic shunt, like decreased barometric pressure, is not a common problem in adult critical care settings.

The third mechanism that can cause the Pa_{O_2} to decrease is a diffusion barrier. Diffusion barriers are actual obstructions between the pulmonary capillaries and the alveoli. These barriers, such as pulmonary fibrosis, are generally not sufficient to obstruct gas transfer completely. The usual effect is to slightly obstruct gas transfer. The obstruction becomes evident primarily during exercise or high cardiac-output states. As the flow of blood increases past the alveoli, the oxygen exchange rate between the alveoli and capillaries may become insufficient. In clinical practice, however, the high cardiac-output state, which makes the diffusion barrier evident, is usually not a major clinical problem.

Hypoventilation is a more common problem than are the first three causes of hypoxemia (Table 3.6). Hypoventilation may occur when a reduction in alveolar ventilation (V_a) occurs. If alveolar ventilation is reduced, the person will be unable to clear the carbon dioxide produced during substrate catabolism. As the level of carbon dioxide increases, it displaces oxygen. The displacement of oxygen occurs since of the gases that are present in the alveolus, only carbon dioxide and oxygen are biologically active. Nitrogen and water-vapor pressures, which are also in the alveoli, are relatively constant and are not affected by changing Pa_{CO_2}

TABLE 3.5. Hypoxemia Induced by Barometric Pressure

	Altitude		
	0 ft	5,000 ft	10,000 ft
Pa_{O_2}	95	70	40
PA_{O_2}	100	75	45
Pa_{CO_2}	40	40	40
Pb	760	640	500

TABLE 3.6. Hypoxemia Induced by Hypoventilation

	Time		
	1000	1400	1600
Pa_{O_2}	70	50	80
Pa_{CO_2}	35	55	65
pH	7.38	7.22	7.14
$F_{I_{O_2}}$	.30	.30	.40

Note as the Pa_{CO_2} increases, the Pa_{O_2} level falls proportionately. An increase in the $F_{I_{O_2}}$ will prevent a further decrease in the Pa_{O_2} but will not stop the increase in Pa_{CO_2} levels.

levels. As the Pa_{CO_2} level rises, the Pa_{O_2} level falls proportionately. For example, if a person has an initial P_{CO_2} of 40 mm Hg and a P_{O_2} of 70 mm Hg, an increase in the Pa_{CO_2} of 20 mm Hg would make the P_{O_2} fall by 20 mm Hg. In other words, if the Pa_{CO_2} changed from 40 to 60 mm Hg, the Pa_{O_2} would be expected to fall from 70 to 50 mm Hg. Sudden changes in Pa_{CO_2} have the potential to cause a decrease in Pa_{O_2} levels. Clinically, this effect of the Pa_{CO_2} decreasing the Pa_{O_2} is easily altered or offset by increasing the F_{IO_2} through oxygen therapy. The oxygen that is added will displace a portion of the nitrogen in the alveoli. As nitrogen is displaced, the Pa_{O_2} levels increase through the increasing alveolar oxygen concentration. The elevation in the alveolar oxygen concentration will correct the Pa_{O_2} level but will not correct the Pa_{CO_2} level. The failure to improve the cause of the Pa_{O_2} fall, that is, the Pa_{CO_2} increase, can be a major clinical error. A person can have serious problems with the development of respiratory acidosis owing to the Pa_{CO_2} rise, and it is the change in Pa_{CO_2} that should be treated in hypoventilation, not the change in Pa_{O_2}. Failure to correct the acidosis produced by the rising Pa_{CO_2} level can cause marked cellular dysfunction, eventually leading to a respiratory arrest.

INTRAPULMONARY SHUNT

The intrapulmonary shunt is by far the most common reason for change in the Pa_{O_2} levels (and Sa_{O_2} values as well). The reasons for change in the Pa_{O_2} level from an intrapulmonary shunt are important for the clinician to understand in order to assess clinical conditions correctly.

As blood returns to the lung from the veins, it is exposed to alveolar concentrations of oxygen that are higher than the venous oxygen tension. The oxygen tension rapidly transfers from the alveoli to the veins and pulmonary capillaries, elevating the venous oxygen to the same level as the alveolar oxygen. As mentioned earlier, if the lung is functioning perfectly, the arterial gas concentration flowing from the lungs will equal the alveolar gas concentrations. In an intrapulmonary shunt, the venous blood is not exposed to a functional alveolar unit. The lack of exposure of venous blood to a functioning alveolar unit will result in the venous blood being mixed with other alveolar samples that have adequate blood flow (Figure 3.6). As the venous blood empties

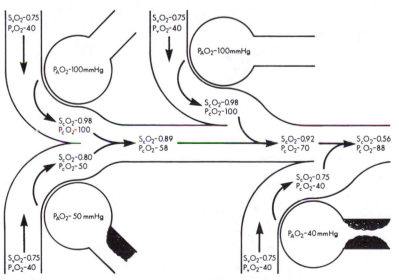

FIGURE 3.6. The greater the ventilation reduction relative to the perfusion, the lower the Pa_{O_2} level.

into the pulmonary capillary system which does have adequate perfusion, the arterial gas mixture will become decreased. The degree of the venous admixture will determine the net effect on the arterial blood. For example, the larger the amount of intrapulmonary shunt that exists, the larger the effect will be on lowering the Pa_{O_2} level (Figure 3.7). As alveolar function is reduced and more venous blood is exposed to fewer functioning alveoli, the Pa_{O_2} level will progressively decrease. This increase in intrapulmonary shunt causes a progressively larger difference between alveolar and arterial oxygen concentrations.

Measuring the Intrapulmonary Shunt

The intrapulmonary shunt can actually be measured through many mechanisms, including equations and inhalation of marked gases. The most common clinical mechanism is the use of the classic shunt equation (Table 3.7). The classic shunt equation requires measurement of the capillary, arterial, and venous oxygen contents. From these levels, the oxygen level in the pulmonary capillary (Cc_{O_2}), the oxygen content leaving the lung (Ca_{O_2}), as well as the oxygen content entering the lungs from the venous system ($C\bar{v}_{O_2}$) will be known. Mea-

TABLE 3.7.   Classic Shunt Equation

$$\frac{Cc_{O_2} - Ca_{O_2}}{Cc_{O_2} - C\bar{v}_{O_2}}$$

Where
Cc_{O_2} = pulmonary-capillary oxygen content
Ca_{O_2} = arterial oxygen content
$C\bar{v}_{O_2}$ = mixed-venous oxygen content
Sc_{O_2} = pulmonary-capillary oxygen saturation
Sa_{O_2} = arterial oxygen saturation
$S\bar{v}_{O_2}$ = mixed-venous oxygen saturation

Calculations:
Cc_{O_2} = 1.34 × Hgb × Sc_{O_2} + (PA_{O_2} × .003)
Ca_{O_2} = 1.34 × Hgb × Sa_{O_2} + (Pa_{O_2} × .003)
$C\bar{v}_{O_2}$ = 1.34 × Hgb × $S\bar{v}_{O_2}$ + ($P\bar{v}_{O_2}$ × .003)

surement of the shunt fraction through the shunt equation is the preferred method of determining Qs/Qt. Examples of calculating Qs/Qt are provided in Tables 3.8 and 3.9. Measurement of the intrapulmonary shunt by the classic shunt equation has limitations due to the need to measure mixed venous blood gas levels.

In the absence of mixed venous blood gas concentrations, the clinician can rely on estimates of intrapulmonary shunts through such measures as oxygen-derived variables and clinical shunt equations. The next several paragraphs will discuss how to ap-

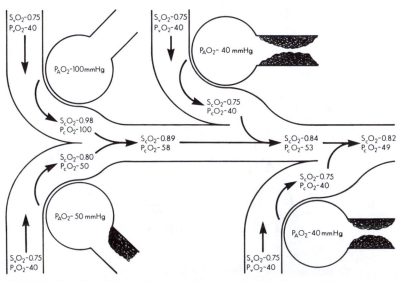

FIGURE 3.7.   The effect on the Pa_{O_2} of a major disruption in ventilation.

TABLE 3.8. Calculation of the Intrapulmonary Shunt (Qs/Qt)

Given the following information, the intrapulmonary shunt can be calculated:

Pa_{O_2} = 78
Sa_{O_2} = .94
$P\bar{v}_{O_2}$ = 35
$S\bar{v}_{O_2}$ = .62
Hgb = 12
$F_{I_{O_2}}$ = .40

Cc_{O_2} = 1.34 × 12 × 1.00 + (241 × .003) = 16.8
Ca_{O_2} = 1.34 × 12 × .94 + (78 × .003) = 15.3
$C\bar{v}_{O_2}$ = 1.34 × 12 × .62 + (35 × .003) = 10

$$Cc_{O_2} = 16.8$$
$$Ca_{O_2} = 15.3$$
$$C\bar{v}_{O_2} = 10$$

$$Qs/Qt = \frac{16.8 - 15.3}{16.8 - 10} = .22$$

ply these estimates of the intrapulmonary shunt.

Estimating Intrapulmonary Shunt from Oxygen-Derived Variables

The intrapulmonary shunt can be estimated by noting the degree of difference between the Pa_{O_2} levels and the alveolar oxygen (PA_{O_2}). As presented, in theory, a normal functioning lung will have equal arterial and alveolar oxygen levels. Despite the pres-

TABLE 3.9. Clinical Application of the Intrapulmonary Shunt (Qs/Qt)

A 60-year-old man complains of shortness of breath at 0900 following admission (at 0700) to the ICU with the diagnosis of pneumonia. Based on the following information, calculate the change in intrapulmonary shunting that has occurred with the shortness of breath.

	0700	0900
Pa_{O_2}	95	74
$P\bar{v}_{O_2}$	30	35
Sa_{O_2}	.97	.93
$S\bar{v}_{O_2}$	.54	.60
Hgb	11	12
$F_{I_{O_2}}$	.50	.40
Qs/Qt	$\frac{15.7 - 14.6}{15.7 - 8.1}$ = .15	$\frac{16.8 - 15.2}{16.8 - 9.8}$ = .23

ence of small anatomic and intrapulmonary shunts, the Pa_{O_2} level should approximate the PA_{O_2}. As a guideline, the normal Pa_{O_2} (80–100 mm Hg) differs from a normal PA_{O_2} by 0–20 mm Hg.[3] The maximal discrepancy of the Pa_{O_2} from PA_{O_2} is about 40 mm Hg (assuming a normal acceptable clinical Pa_{O_2} is 60–100 mm Hg). Knowing that the maximal difference of Pa_{O_2} from PA_{O_2} is 40 mm Hg forms the basis for some estimates of intrapulmonary shunting.

Estimates of Qs/Qt

There are four measures commonly used to estimate intrapulmonary shunting. These include the alveolar-to-arterial gradient (A-a gradient), the arterial-to-alveolar ratio (a/A ratio), the $Pa_{O_2}/F_{I_{O_2}}$ ratio, and the respiratory index (RI).[4–7] Of these methods to estimate alveolar oxygen concentrations, the most accurate is either the $Pa_{O_2}/F_{I_{O_2}}$ or the a/A ratio.[8–10] The least accurate is the A-a gradient.[11,12] In order to use these estimates of Qs/Qt, the PA_{O_2} may need to be determined (Table 3.1).

The A-a gradient is one of the most common clinical methods employed to estimate intrapulmonary shunting. However, it is inaccurate for one primary reason: the A-a gradient does not take into account the normal increasing alveolar-to-arterial oxygen concentration difference as a function of changing the fraction of inspired oxygen ($F_{I_{O_2}}$). The higher the $F_{I_{O_2}}$, the larger the increase in the A-a gradient without changing the intrapulmonary shunts (Table 3.10). The A-a gradient is a measure that should be restricted in its clinical use and should not be the primary mechanism by which intrapulmonary shunts are estimated.

The two most common and accurate measures of intrapulmonary shunt include the $Pa_{O_2}/F_{I_{O_2}}$ ratio and the a/A ratio. Of these, the $Pa_{O_2}/F_{I_{O_2}}$ ratio is the easiest to compute, thus making it an attractive option for the clinician.[13] Examples of the $Pa_{O_2}/F_{I_{O_2}}$ ratio computations are provided in Table 3.11. The normal $Pa_{O_2}/F_{I_{O_2}}$ is

TABLE 3.10.   Example of the Alveolar-arterial (A-a) Gradient Inaccuracy with Changing F_{IO_2}

	Time	
	1130	1400
Pa_{O_2}	58	106
Pa_{CO_2}	37	37
F_{IO_2}	.30	.50
A-a	$168 - 58 = 110$	$307 - 106 = 201$
a/A	.345	.345

Note how the A-a gradient is increasing although no change in the a/A ratio (a measure which includes F_{IO_2}) has taken place. The increasing A-a gradient is a function of the increasing alveolar oxygen tension.

greater than 350, although levels as low as 286 may be clinically acceptable.

$$\frac{Pa_{O_2}}{\text{Room Air } F_{IO_2}} \quad \frac{60}{.21} = 286$$

When using the Pa_{O_2}/F_{IO_2} ratio, remember, the lower the Pa_{O_2}/F_{IO_2} ratio, the larger the Qs/Qt.

The a/A ratio is a commonly used estimate of Qs/Qt.[14,15] The a/A ratio is useful since it takes into account changes in the F_{IO_2} and Pa_{CO_2}. Normal a/A ratio values are listed in Table 3.12.

The arterial-to-alveolar ratio (a/A) has one advantage over the Pa_{O_2}/F_{IO_2} ratio, which makes it preferable in some circumstances. The a/A ratio accounts for changes in the Pa_{CO_2} levels, unlike the Pa_{O_2}/F_{IO_2} ratio. In a patient who does not have

TABLE 3.11.   Calculation of the Pa_{O_2}/F_{IO_2} Ratio

Pa_{O_2}	70	91
F_{IO_2}	.21	.60
$\dfrac{Pa_{O_2}}{F_{IO_2}}$	$\dfrac{70}{.21} = 333$	$\dfrac{91}{.60} = 152$

The normal Pa_{O_2}/F_{IO_2} ratio is greater than 350. In this example, the first person has a near normal Qs/Qt, whereas the second has an increased Qs/Qt. The lower the Pa_{O_2}/F_{IO_2} number, the more severe the Qs/Qt disturbance.

TABLE 3.12.   Guidelines for Use of arterial-Alveolar Ratio

a/A ratio is obtained by the equation

$$\frac{Pa_{O_2}}{PA_{O_2}}$$

where
Pa_{O_2} = arterial oxygen pressure
PA_{O_2} = alveolar oxygen pressure

Normal, > .60, usually indicates no oxygen therapy is necessary.

Levels less than .60 indicate worsening shunt.

The lower the a/A ratio, the worse the Qs/Qt.

Takes into account changes in F_{IO_2} and Pa_{CO_2}.

changes in the Pa_{CO_2} level, the Pa_{O_2}/F_{IO_2} ratio is probably the preferred method for estimating intrapulmonary shunt. The a/A ratio should be used if the Pa_{CO_2} is not stable. Tables 3.13 and 3.14 contain examples of how to use the a/A ratio and illustrate the effect of changing Pa_{CO_2} levels.

The respiratory index is a less commonly used measure and will not be presented although the mechanism for its calculation is provided in Table 3.15.

Some authors have questioned the accuracy of oxygen-derived variables and have indicated that their use in clinical settings is not always accurate.[16,17] The estimates of Qs/Qt, or oxygen-derived variables, will not always be accurate owing to the inability to assess venous oxygen content. The follow-

TABLE 3.13.   Calculation of the arterial-Alveolar (a/A) Ratio

Given
F_{IO_2} = .60
Pa_{O_2} = 91
Pa_{CO_2} = 41

Then the a/A ratio is determined by the following steps:

(1) Calculate the PA_{O_2}:

$$PA_{O_2} = .60 \,(713) - \frac{41}{.8} = 377$$

(2) Determine the a/A ratio from the PA_{O_2} and Pa_{O_2}:

$$\frac{Pa_{O_2}}{PA_{O_2}} = \frac{91}{377} \qquad a/A = .24$$

TABLE 3.14.   Limitation of the $Pa_{O_2}/F_{I_{O_2}}$ Ratio with Changing Pa_{CO_2} Levels

	Time	
	0800	1600
Pa_{O_2}	88	62
Pa_{CO_2}	36	52
$F_{I_{O_2}}$	.28	.21
$\dfrac{Pa_{O_2}}{F_{I_{O_2}}}$	314	295
a/A	$\dfrac{88}{155} = .57$	$\dfrac{62}{85} = .73$

Qs/Qt has improved as noted by the a/A but not by the $Pa_{O_2}/F_{I_{O_2}}$.

Example 1 Limitations of the Oxygen Tension Estimates of Intrapulmonary Shunting

In the following sets of blood gases, no overt clinical change has taken place. Computing the estimates of intrapulmonary shunt, however, fails to detect the improvement in lung function that is revealed when the Qs/Qt calculation is performed.

PaC_{O_2}	40	45
Pa_{O_2}	91	89
Sa_{O_2}	.96	.97
$F_{I_{O_2}}$	.50	.50
Hgb	12	10
$S\bar{v}_{O_2}$	.62	.50
$P\bar{v}_{O_2}$	35	27
Ca_{O_2}	15.7	13.3
$C\bar{v}_{O_2}$	10.1	8.1

Estimates of Qs/Qt

a/A	.30	.30	(remained same)
$Pa_{O_2}/F_{I_{O_2}}$	182	178	(remained about the same)

Qs/Qt Calculation

Cc_{O_2}	17	14.3
Ca_{O_2}	15.7	13.3
$C\bar{v}_{O_2}$	10.1	7.44
Qs/Qt	.19	.13

$$.19 = \frac{17-15.7}{17-10.1} \qquad .13 = \frac{14.3-13.3}{14.3-7.44}$$

---

ing example illustrates a situation where the estimates of intrapulmonary shunting, the $Pa_{O_2}/F_{I_{O_2}}$ and a/A ratios, do not change although the intrapulmonary shunt is actually improving (Example 1).

This inaccuracy of oxygen variables has led to the proposal of other methods for estimating intrapulmonary shunt, such as the clinical shunt equation.[18] The clinical shunt equation (see Table 3.16) provides a closer proximation to the actual classic shunt equation. This approximation by the clinical shunt equation to Qs/Qt is provided by estimating the normal arterial to venous oxygen content difference. Examples of the clinical shunt equation are provided in Table 3.17.

Whichever method is used to estimate the intrapulmonary shunt, it should be noted that the value of estimating the shunt is in its ability to help identify changes in

lung dysfunction. A change in intrapulmonary shunt can indicate an improvement in the patient if the shunt is decreasing. If the shunt is increasing, the clinical condition may be deteriorating. The use of intrapulmonary-shunt estimates allows the clinician to more routinely analyze changes in the patient's pulmonary status. Without estimating the intrapulmonary shunt, the clinician is limited in understanding how much of a discrepancy exists between how

TABLE 3.15.   Calculation of the Respiratory Index (RI)

$$\frac{PA_{O_2} - Pa_{O_2}}{PA_{O_2}}$$

where

PA_{O_2} = alveolar oxygen tension
Pa_{O_2} = arterial oxygen tension

Normal, $< .4$

The greater the value over .4, the worse the intrapulmonary shunt.

TABLE 3.16.   Calculation of the Clinical Shunt Equation

$$\frac{Cc_{O_2} - Ca_{O_2}}{(Cc_{O_2} - Ca_{O_2}) + 3.5\ mg/dl}$$

where

Cc_{O_2} = pulmonary-capillary oxygen content
Ca_{O_2} = arterial oxygen content
3.5 is an assumed A − V content difference

TABLE 3.17. Application of the Clinical Shunt Equation

Given the following information, use the clinical shunt equation to determine if the intrapulmonary shunt has changed.

	Time	
	1530	1730
Pa_{O_2}	83	69
Sa_{O_2}	.94	.92
Pa_{CO_2}	38	40
F_{IO_2}	.40	.30
Hgb	12	12

Clinical shunt equation (Qs/Qt) $\dfrac{Cc_{O_2} - Ca_{O_2}}{(Cc_{O_2} - Ca_{O_2}) + 3.5 \text{ mg/dl}}$

Time: 1530

$PA_{O_2} = .40(713) - \dfrac{38}{.8} = 237$

$Cc_{O_2} = 1.34 \times 12 \times 1.00 + (.003 \times 237) = 16.8$
$Ca_{O_2} = 1.34 \times 12 \times .94 + (.003 \times 83) = 15.4$

$Qs/Qt = \dfrac{16.8 - 15.4}{[16.8 - 15.4] + 3.5} = .29$

Time: 1730

$PA_{O_2} = .30(713) - \dfrac{40}{.8} = 164$

$Cc_{O_2} = 1.34 \times 12 \times 1.00 + (.003 \times 164) = 16.6$
$Ca_{O_2} = 1.34 \times 12 \times .92 + (.003 \times 69) = 15.0$

$Qs/Qt = \dfrac{16.6 - 15.0}{[16.6 - 15.0] + 3.5} = .31$

Based on the clinical shunt equation, the Qs/Qt worsened between 1530 and 1730.

TABLE 3.18. Conditions That Will Increase the Intrapulmonary Shunt

Pulmonary Origins
Adult respiratory distress syndrome
Asthma (severe)
Atelectasis
Chronic Bronchitis
Mucous plugging of airways
Pneumonias
Pulmonary emboli (large)

Cardiovascular Origins
Pulmonary edema from
    Left-ventricular failure
    Mitral stenosis
    Hypervolemia
    Low colloidal osmotic pressure

well the lungs are presently oxygenating the blood versus how well they should be oxygenating the blood. This understanding is important based on the levels of clinical support being given, that is, increased F_{IO_2}, PEEP, and mechanical ventilation. In addition, use of shunt estimates helps the clinician avoid simply looking at a Pa_{O_2} level. The shunt estimates encourage at least simultaneous analysis of F_{IO_2} and Pa_{O_2}.

Many conditions or diseases can cause increases in the intrapulmonary shunt. Any condition that reduces ventilation relative to perfusion will increase the Qs/Qt. Examples of these conditions are listed in Table 3.18. It is important to remember that measurement of intrapulmonary shunt does not identify what condition exists. Measurements of intrapulmonary shunt only reveal the extent of the pulmonary dysfunction induced by a clinical condition. As such, the intrapulmonary shunt is not a diagnostic tool but is used in the assessment of changes in lung function.

$S\bar{v}_{O_2}$ Influences on Pa_{O_2} and Qs/Qt

One other factor that can affect the Pa_{O_2} and Sa_{O_2} levels without changing the intrapulmonary shunt is the venous oxygen content, primarily the $S\bar{v}_{O_2}$.[19,20] As the venous oxygen content returns to the lung, some of the venous blood will enter the arterial system without being exposed to functional alveoli, thereby reducing the Pa_{O_2} slightly from normal. As long as the intrapulmonary shunt is low, changes in venous oxygen levels will not affect the arterial P_{O_2} level (Figure 3.8). However, as the intrapulmonary shunt increases, changes in the venous oxygen content can start to affect the Pa_{O_2} level. For example, if a large intrapulmonary shunt exists and the venous oxygen content changes, the arterial oxygen content will be affected (Figure 3.9). The decrease in the venous oxygen content will cause the arterial oxygen content to change independently of any change in the intrapulmonary shunt. The clinician must be aware that changes in the $S\bar{v}_{O_2}$ (in the presence of an increased intrapulmonary shunt) may make

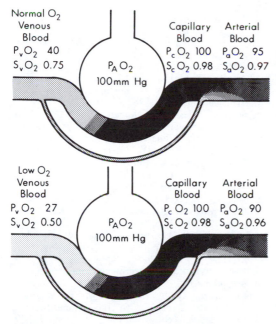

FIGURE 3.8.   Changes in $S\bar{v}_{O_2}$ have little effect on Pa_{O_2} and Sa_{O_2} values when Qs/Qt is normal. Adapted from Ahrens TS, Rutherford KA. "The new pulmonary math. Use of the a/A ratio." *Am J Nurs* 1987;87:337A.

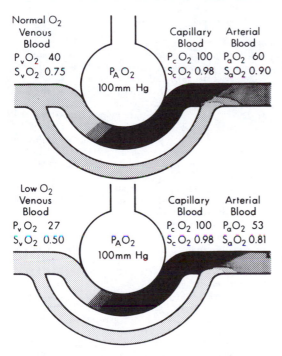

FIGURE 3.9.   Changes in $S\bar{v}_{O_2}$ have a major effect on Pa_{O_2} and Sa_{O_2} values when Qs/Qt is elevated. Adapted from Ahrens TS, Rutherford KA. "The new pulmonary math. Use of the a/A ratio." *Am J Nurs* 1987;87:337A.

the Pa_{O_2} level fall, even though the Qs/Qt has not changed. The change in the Pa_{O_2} level caused by a decrease in $S\bar{v}_{O_2}$ does not indicate a worsening lung function, although it may indicate worsening cellular oxygenation. Unfortunately, the only way to determine why the Pa_{O_2} changes is to continually measure the $S\bar{v}_{O_2}$. If the $S\bar{v}_{O_2}$ is measured continuously, it can be used to continuously estimate the intrapulmonary shunt. (See Chapter 10.)

If the patient has an unstable oxygenation status, such as a reduction in cardiac output or hemoglobin, or increased oxygen consumption, the clinician should be careful in the use of estimates of the intrapulmonary shunt. In these situations, the actual measurement of the intrapulmonary shunt is preferred. This practice of actually measuring Qs/Qt presents a dilemma to the clinician, since many situations exist in which estimating the intrapulmonary shunt measurement will not be feasible. The best way to address this problem is to estimate the intrapulmonary shunt as often as possible, but be aware that changes in intrapulmonary shunt may be caused by worsening cellular oxygenation status.

Pulse oximetry can also be used to assess, to some extent, the change in intrapulmonary shunt owing to the relationship between the Pa_{O_2} and Sa_{O_2} levels. The use of pulse oximetry is explained more in Chapter 5.

SUMMARY

The Qs/Qt is the most common reason for the Pa_{O_2} to decrease. Since blood gases, and particularly the Pa_{O_2}, are commonly measured clinical parameters, understanding the intrapulmonary shunt is useful. Through understanding the Qs/Qt, the clinician can avoid errors associated with using only the Pa_{O_2} level in regard to assessing lung function. For example, based on the first set of blood gases given below, the physician orders that the F_{IO_2} be reduced to .40. The second set of blood gases is obtained following the F_{IO_2} change. Upon seeing these blood gases, the physician requests an increase in the F_{IO_2} because the lung function has worsened. Is the increase in F_{IO_2} necessary based on the Qs/Qt changes?

Pa_{O_2}	98	61
Pa_{CO_2}	36	38
F_{IO_2}	.60	.40
a/A	98/383 = .26	61/237 = .26

No, the Pa_{O_2} fall was a result of the decrease in F_{IO_2}. A second example also illustrates the use of shunt estimates. Assume you are to start weaning trials on a patient today but the physician states that the chest x-ray has worsened. Has the worsening chest x-ray had any effect on the Qs/Qt? Should the weaning trial be delayed?

	Data before x-ray	Data after x-ray
F_{IO_2}	.40	.30
Pa_{CO_2}	39	37
Pa_{O_2}	86	61
a/A	86/236 = .36	61/166 = .37

No, since the Qs/Qt has probably not changed.

Estimates of Qs/Qt are available when actual measurement of Qs/Qt is not possible. The most accurate of these estimates are the clinical shunt equation and the Pa_{O_2}/F_{IO_2} and a/A ratios. All of these are useful although their abilities to accurately predict Qs/Qt changes suffer when the $S\bar{v}_{O_2}$ changes. Use of the estimates of Qs/Qt, however, make the Qs/Qt concept of practical value of the clinician.

REFERENCES

1. Burrows B. *Respiratory Insufficiency*. Chicago: Year Book Medical Pubs, 1984.
2. Albert RK "Physiology and management of failure of arterial oxygenation." *In* Fallat RJ, Luce JM. *Cardiopulmonary Critical Care Management*. New York: Churchill Livingstone, 1988, 37.
3. Kanber GJ, King FW, Eshchar YR, et al. "The alveolar-arterial oxygen gradient in young and elderly men during air and oxygen breathing." *Am Rev Respir Dis* 1968;97:376.
4. Gilbert R, Keighley JF. "The arterial/alveolar oxygen tension ratio. An index of gas exchange applicable to varying inspired oxygen concentrations." *Am Rev Respir Dis* 1974;109:142.
5. Lecky JH, Ominsky AJ. "Postoperative respiratory management." *Chest* 1972;62:505.
6. Sganga G, Siegal JH, Coleman W, et al. "The physiologic meaning of the respiratory index in various types of critical illness." *Circ Shock* 1985;17:179.
7. Lilienthal JL, Riley RL, Proemmel DD, et al. "An experimental analysis in man of the oxygen pressure gradient from alveolar air to arterial blood." *Am J Physiol* 1946;147:199.
8. Peris LV, Boix JH, Salom JV, et al. "Clinical use of the arterial/alveolar oxygen tension ratio." *Crit Care Med* 1983;11:888.
9. Ahrens TS, Rutherford KA. "The new pulmonary math: Applying the a/A ratio." *Am J Nurs* 1987; 87:337A.
10. Bone RC, Maunder R, Slotman G, et al. "An early test of survival in patients with the adult respiratory distress syndrome. The Pa_{O_2}/F_{IO_2} ratio and its differential response to conventional therapy. Prostagladin E1 Study Group." *Chest* 1989;96:849.
11. Ahrens TS. "Blood gas assessment of intrapulmonary shunting and deadspace." *Crit Care Nurs Clin N Am* 1989;1:641.
12. Covelli HD, Nessan VJ, Tuttle WK. "Oxygen derived variables in acute respiratory failure." *Crit Care Med* 1983;11:646.
13. Horovitz JH, Carrico CJ, Shires T. "Pulmonary response to major injury." *Arch Surg* 1974;108:349.
14. Cohen A, Taeusch HW Jr, Stanton C. "Usefulness of the arterial/alveolar oxygen tension ratio in the care of infants with respiratory distress syndrome." *Respir Care* 1983;28:169.
15. Maxwell C, Hess D, Shefet D. "Use of the arterial/alveolar oxygen tension ratio to predict the inspired oxygen concentration for a desired arterial oxygen tension." *Respir Care* 1984;29:1135.
16. Herrick IA, Champion LK, Froese AB. "A clinical comparison of indices of pulmonary gas exchange with changes in the inspired oxygen concentration." *Can J Anaesth* 1990;37:69.
17. Viale JP, Percival CJ, Annat G, et al. "Arterial-alveolar oxygen partial pressure ratio: A theoretical reappraisal." *Crit Care Med* 1986;14:153.
18. Cane RD, Shapiro BA, Templin R, et al. "Unreliability of oxygen tension-based indices in reflecting intrapulmonary shunting in critically ill patients." *Crit Care Med* 1988;16:1243.
19. Martyn JAJ, Aikawa N, Wilson RS, et al. "Extrapulmonary factors influencing the ratio of arterial oxygen tension to inspired oxygen concentration in burn patients." *Crit Care Med* 1979;7:492.
20. Giovannini I, Boldrini G, Sganga G, et al. "Quantification of the determination of arterial hypoxemia in critically ill adults." *Crit Care Med* 1983; 11:644.

4

The Influence of Hemoglobin on Oxygen Transport

Catherine I. Vierheller RN, BSN, CCRN

The major role of the cardiorespiratory system is to transport an amount of oxygen adequate to meet tissue demand. This concept is based on the work of Barcroft, who recognized that the circulation system was an oxygen-transport system dependent upon three mechanisms: oxygenation of blood in the lungs, carrying ability of the blood, and cardiac output.[1] In order to assess and identify deficits in oxygenation, it is necessary to understand those factors influencing oxygenation and their importance in oxygen transport.

Hemoglobin (Hgb) has long been identified as the major vehicle in oxygen transport. Even at a time when knowledge of the structure of hemoglobin itself was new, scientists began to study hemoglobin in order to better understand oxygen transport.[2] The purpose of this chapter is to examine the influence of hemoglobin on oxygen transport, thereby providing the clinician with a fundamental tool in assessing oxygenation.

DESCRIPTION OF HEMOGLOBIN (HGB)

A hemoglobin molecule consists of two parts, the globin and the heme portions. The globin is a single protein composed of amino acids. The heme portion comprises four heme molecules. Each molecule of heme contains one iron atom; therefore, a single hemoglobin molecule contains four iron atoms, enabling it to unite with four oxygen molecules (see Figure 4.1). While Hgb synthesis is not the purpose of this chapter, it is worthy to note that the process is complex, beginning in the bone marrow with the production of erythrocytes. Each erythrocyte contains 200 to 300 million molecules of hemoglobin.[3]

FACTORS INFLUENCING HEMOGLOBIN LEVELS

Hemoglobin concentration is expressed in grams per 100 ml of blood, or grams per deciliter (gm/dl). The normal values of Hgb differ with age and sex. Altitude as well will affect the hemoglobin measurement, in that the normal concentration is greater in higher altitudes than at sea level. The normal range for adult women is 12–15 gm/dl and for adult men is 14–16 gm/dl.[4] Along with age, sex, and altitude, other physiological variations influencing Hgb have been documented, such as exercise. Muscular activity, if strenuous, raises the hemoglobin, presumably due to the re-entry into the circulation of cells previously secluded in dormant capillaries or to the loss of circulating plasma.[5] Cigarette smoking, through unspecified effects, also appears to stimulate erythropoiesis; slightly higher hemoglobin values are found in smokers.

There are many different laboratory techniques available to determine hemoglo-

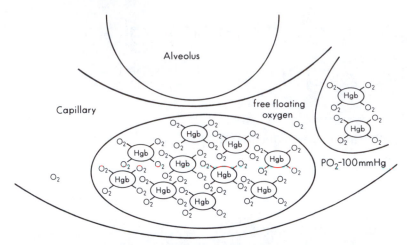

FIGURE 4.1.   Most of the oxygen transported to cells is carried by hemoglobin. This illustration represents only a portion of the hemoglobin in a normal red blood cell but proportionately illustrates oxygen carried on hemoglobin versus that transported by the Pa_{O_2}. Note that most of the oxygen is attached to hemoglobin with only a small amount floating unattached (the Pa_{O_2}).

bin concentration. In most laboratories, automated techniques are used that have several advantages such as accuracy, greater speed, lower cost per test, and greater reproducibility. The equipment requires careful standardization and accurate calibration (Figure 4.2). The methods used in the routine clinical laboratory employ photoelectric colorimetry.[6] In clinical practice, a centrifuged (spun) hematocrit can be quickly obtained. The value of knowing the hematocrit is that the hematocrit is about triple the Hgb level. If, for example, the hematocrit is 30%, the Hgb will be approximately 10 gms/dl.[7]

The centrifuged hematocrit is relatively accurate but should be verified with a colorimetry Hgb determination. The clinician should be cautious in interpreting any Hgb level because of the potential for hemoconcentration (with slow vascular loss) and hemodilution (with administration of IV fluids). Even if normal Hgb levels are present, the clinician must consider the clinical presentation of the patient. For example, in the early phase of acute blood loss the he-

moglobin will remain normal before decreasing. An Hgb determination at the time of acute blood loss may not reflect the extent of the blood loss.

HEMOGLOBIN OXYGEN-CARRYING CAPACITY

Each gram of hemoglobin can potentially carry 1.34 ml of oxygen but doesn't always do so.[8] The hemoglobin saturation (S_{O_2}) represents the difference between the amount of oxygen actually carried versus the potential. Arterial hemoglobin should be loaded to an Sa_{O_2} of .95.[9] There is also a small amount of oxygen dissolved in blood (Pa_{O_2}) unattached to Hgb (Chapter 2). Together, the amount of hemoglobin-bound oxygen and dissolved oxygen equals the arterial oxygen content (Ca_{O_2}). Ca_{O_2} can be measured by the equation below:

$$\text{Arterial } O_2 \text{ content } (Ca_{O_2}) = O_2 \text{ bound to Hgb} + Pa_{O_2}$$
$$= (1.34 \times \text{Hgb} \times Sa_{O_2}) + (.0031 \times Pa_{O_2})$$

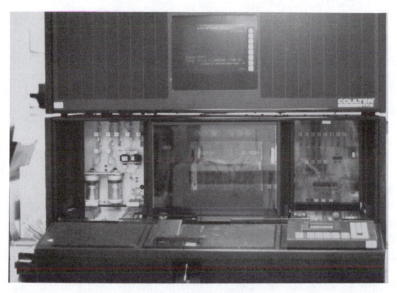

FIGURE 4.2.   Hemoglobin measuring system. Measurement of hemoglobin generally occurs outside the ICU setting, in the clinical laboratory.

Example: If the Hgb is 15 gm/dl, the Sa_{O_2} is .98 and the Pa_{O_2} is 100 mm Hg, then

$$\begin{aligned}
Ca_{O_2} &= (1.34 \times 15 \times .98) + \\
&\quad (.0031 \times 100) \\
&= 19.7 + .31 \\
&= 20 \text{ ml/dl}
\end{aligned}$$

Note, .0031 is the solubility coefficient for oxygen. Because the contribution of Pa_{O_2} to the total arterial content is small, the equation (.0031 Pa_{O_2}) is often omitted from the calculation of Ca_{O_2} in order to simplify the mathematics. However, the Pa_{O_2} is valuable in that it can be used to estimate the Sa_{O_2} because of hemoglobin's binding ability to oxygen at different oxygen pressures. The oxyhemoglobin-dissociation curve illustrates this binding of hemoglobin to oxygen.

It is essential to remember that hemoglobin levels are more important than Pa_{O_2} and Sa_{O_2} for adequate oxygen transport. For example, given a normal cardiac output of 5 l/min, a Sa_{O_2} of .98, Pa_{O_2} of 100 mm Hg, and a normal hemoglobin (12 mg/dl), the O_2 transport (D_{O_2}) will be adequate at 989 ml/min. If the hemoglobin were to drop to 8 gm, the oxygen transport would only be 525 ml/min, despite maintaining the high Sa_{O_2} and Pa_{O_2}.

As previously stated, oxygen transport (D_{O_2}) to tissue depends not only on the carrying ability (arterial oxygen content or Ca_{O_2}), but also on the rate of blood flow or cardiac output (CO). In the resting state, the heart delivers an average about 4–8 l/min of oxygen-carrying blood to the tissues.[10] Cardiac output is determined by stroke volume and heart rate (Chapter 6). Normal resting oxygen transport or delivery (D_{O_2}) can be calculated if both Ca_{O_2} and CO are known.

$$\begin{aligned}
O_2 \text{ delivery} &= \text{cardiac output} \times \text{oxygen} \\
(D_{O_2}) &\quad \text{content} \\
&= CO \times Ca_{O_2} \times 10 \\
&= CO \times (1.34 \times \text{Hgb} \times \\
&\quad Sa_{O_2}) \times 10 \\
&= 5 \times 20 \times 10 \\
&= 1000 \text{ ml/min}
\end{aligned}$$

(Where 10 is a constant to express Ca_{O_2} in ml/min.)

While some components in the mechanisms of oxygen transport remain within "normal" limits, a change of one component can greatly alter the amount of oxygen delivered to tissue.[11] A change in a parameter of D_{O_2} is possibly the result of an imbalance between oxygen supply and demand. With oxygen insufficiency, cell metabolism becomes anaerobic, and the only substrate that can continue without oxygen, glucose, ceases at the level of lactic-acid formation. Should this state of insufficient oxygenation continue, increased anaerobic metabolism leads rapidly to cellular death. Following are some examples of how a decrease in hemoglobin alone can affect oxygen transport. Table 4.1 illustrates how alterations in just one aspect of D_{O_2} can affect oxygen transport.

CO(l/min)	Hgb(g/dl)	Sa_{O_2}	=	D_{O_2} (nl = 1000 ml/min)
5	15	.98	=	1000
5	10	.98	=	656
5	5	.98	=	525
5	6	.98	=	393

In the normal individual, compensatory mechanisms assist when Hgb levels decrease in maintaining adequate oxygen transport to cells. These compensatory mechanisms include an increase in respiratory drive and cardiac output (tachycardia primarily).[12] If hypoxia is present (owing to a decrease in Sa_{O_2}, Hgb, or CO), an increase in red-cell production eventually occurs to maintain adequate circulatory hemoglobin. However, as is often seen in critical illness, an acute increase in red cell production is not possible. Failure of inadequate tissue oxygenation may occur.

Since hemoglobin has been recognized as the major vehicle for oxygen transport to tissues, much research over the past decade has been done to develop an "artificial" blood. Among the synthetic oxygen-carrying compounds are perfluorocarbon emulsions and stroma-free hemoglobin.[13] Unfortunately the detergent used to maintain perfluorocarbon emulsions in a stable form activates complement and may produce respiratory insufficiency.[14] The other synthetic compound, stroma-free hemoglobin, has the advantage that no crossmatch is needed and it can be made from outdated banked blood. More on Hgb treatment is presented in Chapter 13. A major factor controlling the rate of red-cell production is the oxygen content of the blood. Hypoxemia appears to be a strong stimulus, as shown by the compensating red-cell production seen in people living in high altitudes. A lower Sa_{O_2} has the effect of raising the hemoglobin and increasing the number of circulating red cells. Hypoxemia does not have a direct control on the bone marrow because red-cell production is mediated by a hormone (erythropoietin).[15] This hormone is released primarily by the kidneys in response to the decrease in tissue oxygenation.

A feedback control of red-cell production is present: a decrease in arterial oxygen content (Ca_{O_2}) is followed by a decrease in tissue oxygenation. In time, if compensatory mechanisms fail to supply adequate amounts of oxygen to the kidneys, erythropoietin is released and red-cell formation be-

TABLE 4.1. Effects of Different Hgb, Sa_{O_2}, and Pa_{O_2} Levels on Oxygen Transport

	CO(l/min)	Hgb(g/dl)	Pa_{O_2}	Sa_{O_2}	D_{O_2} (nl = 1000 ml/min)
All components of D_{O_2} normal	5	12	100	.98 = 788 ml/min
20% decrease in Hgb	5	9.6	100	.98 = 630 ml/min
20% decrease in Sa_{O_2} and Pa_{O_2}	5	12	80	.94 = 756 ml/min
	5	12	50	.80 = 643

Note: the loss of Hgb has much more of an impact on D_{O_2} than do decreases in Pa_{O_2} and Sa_{O_2}.

gins. However, it is interesting to note that other organs can also produce this hormone-like substance, as demonstrated by patients with renal failure who are still able to maintain red-cell production, albeit at a reduced level.

OPTIMAL HEMOGLOBIN

A controversial question in clinical practice is, "What is the optimal hemoglobin level?" In the case of Hgb, more does not always mean better tissue oxygenation. Increased Hgb can increase the blood viscosity and thereby reduce the flow of blood. The loss of blood flow from increased viscosity offsets an increase in hemoglobin. Examples in clinical practice, research, and exercise settings have demonstrated that Hgb levels above normal do not always offer improvement in tissue oxygenation. Athletes have attempted to improve oxygen transport (and their exercise performance) through the technique of "blood doping."[16-18] In blood doping, the athlete donates blood a few weeks before an athletic event. Then, prior to the event, the blood is retransfused. While in theory the increased Hgb should improve oxygen transport, the actual effect (at least in terms of improving exercise performance) is controversial.

In clinical practice, oxygen delivery to tissue can be diminished with excessively high hematocrit. This is likely due to the increase in the viscosity of blood and the decrease in flow with the increasing hematocrit.

Traditionally, Hgb levels less than 10 gm/dl are thought to be the minimal level for maintaining Ca_{O_2}, although 7–8 gms may be well tolerated.[19] Levels below 7–10 gm/dl cause the heart to increase the CO in an attempt to offset the low Ca_{O_2}. Levels of Hgb near 10 gm/dl may be beneficial, however, because of the reduction in blood viscosity. The reduced blood viscosity may increase blood flow. The increased blood flow can maintain oxygen delivery to cellular areas, despite a lower than normal Hgb. The point where a reduced viscosity and Hgb

actually improve blood flow is, unfortunately, not clear. As a rule, Hgb levels below 10 gm/dl should be considered for treatment.

The role of the Ca_{O_2} on the myocardial work (MV_{O_2}) is an important concept in clinical practice. If the patient has normal myocardial function, a decreased Hgb of about 10 gm/dl will not be a problem. If, however, myocardial disease is present, a Hgb of 10 gm/dl or less can precipitate congestive heart failure or angina because of the increased MV_{O_2}.

Surgeons have attempted for years to find optimal levels of Hgb. Attempts to increase Hgb values have the potential to improve oxygenation and, therefore, tissue recovery. Again, no specific level has been identified, perhaps because of the ability of the CO to help offset changes in Hgb. Due to the influence of elevated hemoglobin on blood viscosity, it is evident that transfusions of whole blood, red blood cells, or other cell-containing components are indicated only when oxygen transport to cells is compromised, that is, when the oxygen supply doesn't meet tissue demand. Perhaps the key point to remember in regard to Hgb levels is that the optimal hemoglobin concentration varies with clinical circumstances and compensating mechanisms. As long as compensating mechanisms, such as an increase in cardiac output, are possible, lower Hgb levels can be tolerated. If the compensating mechanisms are limited, a lower Hgb may not be tolerated.

Increasing Hgb levels through the transfusion of red-cell products should not be thought of as a "cure all" or without risks. Transfusions are almost never indicated to elevate a patient's hemoglobin or hematocrit value to some arbitrary level. Rather, transfusions should be administered until the parameters of oxygen transport are improved, for example, until a compensating tachycardia is decreased. In addition, in the presence of chronic illness such as cancer, leukemia, arthritis, or uremia, where anemia may be present, transfusion will only serve as a temporary supportive measure.

One approach to determining the need for transfusion might be to look at several parameters of oxygen transport: arterial oxygen content, the rate of blood flow (cardiac output), and oxygen consumption.

Few observations have been made on the rate of readjustment of blood volumes after transfusion. Some studies indicate that the hemoglobin concentration is higher in the 24-hour and 48-hour samples than in samples taken minutes after transfusion.[20] In other words, the readjustment or equilibration period following the transfusion varies. It has been observed that some patients may take as long as 24 hours to readjust blood volume. Therefore, it is important for the clinician to closely monitor individuals who require large amounts of blood and who are at risk for volume overload, such as those suffering heart failure.

Since some individuals take as long as 24 hours to readjust blood volume, the effect of large amounts of blood must be closely monitored, especially in the individual whose venous pressure is elevated prior to the transfusion. The rate of transfusion must also be tailored to the individual and should last no longer than 4 hours. Red cells are stored at 4°C (± 1°C). As the cells warm, bacterial growth is increased and cell survival decreases.

The amount of blood to be transfused depends on the improvement of the symptoms that warranted transfusion. Should an individual clinically improve after a single unit of red cells, regardless of hemoglobin or hematocrit levels, the risks versus the benefits should be considered. Each unit of whole blood should raise the hemoglobin, although the exact increase is difficult to predict. For example, in a patient with a pretransfusion hemoglobin of 10 gm/dl and a hematocrit of 30%, one expects a post-transfusion Hgb of 11 to 11.5 and a Hct of 33%, although this increase may not be consistent.

The effect of blood loss on hemoglobin depends on both the rate and the amount of blood loss. With acute blood loss, the changes reflect the loss of blood volume rather than the loss of hemoglobin. With chronic blood loss, hemoglobin, not the circulating blood volume, is affected and the changes seen are reflective of this; for example, iron deficiency anemia may result.[12] In acute blood loss, volume is rapidly restored from the interstitial-fluid compartment, causing hemodilution. Hemoglobin and hematocrit values are less reliable at this time of hemodilution. Although fluid from the interstitial space does not have the oxygen-carrying capacity of whole blood, it does help to stabilize the circulation. At the time of any blood loss, it is imperative to assess oxygenation status, that is, whether supply is meeting demand.

Table 4.2 lists more examples of oxygen supply-and-demand imbalances that can occur in different states and the parameters used to assess them.

SUMMARY

The influence of hemoglobin on adequate oxygen transport to the tissues is critical. However, many variables, including oxygen uptake from the atmosphere, the rate of blood flow, hemoglobin-oxygen binding capacity, and tissue demands make determination of the specific acceptable Hgb difficult to identify. All parameters of oxygenation interact to determine whether oxygen transport is adequate to meet the metabolic demands at the cellular level. Alterations in one or more of these vari-

TABLE 4.2.   Effects of Different Clinical Conditions on D_{O_2}

	CO	Hgb	Sa_{O_2}		Arterial O_2 Supply
Normal	5	15	.98	=	1000
Exercise	20	15	.98	=	3940
Hypoxemia	5	15	.85	=	854
Anemia	5	8	.98	=	525
Pump Failure	1.6	15	.98	=	315
Septic Shock (Early)	15	15	.80	=	2412
Septic Shock (Late)	9	15	.98	=	1773

Note: V_{O_2} refers to O_2 consumption, approximately 3.5 cc/kg.

ables without sufficient compensation can seriously affect the amount of oxygen delivered to the tissue. However, without adequate hemoglobin, cardiac output must increase, and this increase places a strain on myocardial function. In patients without the ability to increase the CO, cellular hypoxia may develop with inadequate Hgb levels.

REFERENCES

1. Barcroft J. "Physiological effects of insufficient oxygen supply." *Nature* 1920;106–125.
2. Bunn, HF, Forget BG. *Hemoglobin: Molecular, Genetics, and Clinical Aspects*. Philadelphia: WB Saunders, 1986.
3. Dickerson RE, Geis I. *Hemoglobin: Structure, Function, Evolution, and Pathology*. Menlo Park: Benjamin/Cummings, 1983.
4. Bauer JD. *Clinical Laboratory Methods*. St. Louis: CV Mosby, 1982, 46.
5. Dacie JV, Lewis SM. *Practical Hematology*. 7th Ed. Edinburgh: Churchill Livingston, 1990, 11.
6. Hall R, Malia RG. *Medical Laboratory Haematology*, 2/e. Oxford: Butterworth, 1991, 101–104.
7. Rutman RC, Miller WV. *Transfusion Therapy Principles and Procedures*, 2/e. Rockville: Aspen, 1985, 35.
8. Shapiro BA, Kacmarek RM, Cane RD, et al. *Clinical Application of Respiratory Care*. 4th Ed. St. Louis: CV Mosby, 1991, 116.
9. Lane EE, Walker JF. *Clinical Arterial Blood Gas Analysis*. St. Louis: CV Mosby, 1990, 49.
10. Ahrens TS, Taylor L. *Hemodynamic Waveform Analysis*. Philadelphia: WB Saunders, 1992, 328.
11. Mims BC. "Physiologic rationale of Sv_{O_2} monitoring." *Crit Care Nurs Clin North Am* 1989;1.
12. Carpenter KD. "Oxygen transport in the blood." *Crit Care Nurse* 1991;11: 20–31.
13. Biro GP, Blais P. "Perfluorocarbon blood substitutes." *CRC Crit Rev Oncol Hematol* 1987;6: 311–74.
14. Hong F, Shastri KA, Logue GL, Spaulding MB. "Complement activation by artificial blood substitute Fluosol: in vitro and in vivo studies." *Transfusion* 1991;31: 642–47.
15. Fleming JS. Drugs and the Delivery of Oxygen to Tissue. Boca Raton: CRC Press Inc., 1990; 3–4.
16. Jones M, Tunstall Pedoe DS. "Blood doping—a literature review." *Br J Sports Med* 1989;23: 84–8.
17. Blood doping. "A statement from the Medical Commission of the International Olympic Committee." *Br J Sports Med* 1989;23: 60.
18. Wagner JC. "Enhancement of athletic performance with drugs." *Sports Med* 1991;12: 250–65.
19. "Perioperative red blood cell transfusion." *JAMA* 1988;260: 2700.
20. Mollison PL, Engelfriet CP, Contreras M. Blood Transfusion in Clinical Medicine. Oxford: Blackwell Scientific Pub, 1987, 117.

5

Hemoglobin Saturation (Sa_{O_2}) and D_{O_2}

Kim Rutherford MSN(r), RN, CCRN

Hemoglobin provides the main carrying capacity for oxygen. Each molecule of hemoglobin has the ability to combine with four oxygen molecules. When hemoglobin is fully saturated with oxygen, oxyhemoglobin is formed. Arterial oxygen saturation (Sa_{O_2}) is the ratio of oxygenated hemoglobin to total hemoglobin:[1]

$$Sa_{O_2} = \frac{Hb_{O_2}}{Hb_{O_2} + Hb}$$

Hemoglobin is unique in its ability to change affinity for oxygen, thus varying oxygen saturation. The high oxygen abundance in the pulmonary capillaries promotes binding of oxygen with hemoglobin resulting in an arterial saturation of over 90%. The low oxygen level at the capillary beds prompts release of oxygen from hemoglobin, thus venous oxygen saturation ($S\bar{v}_{O_2}$) is usually 60–75%.[2,3] The relationship of oxygen tension and oxyhemoglobin saturation is graphically depicted in the oxyhemoglobin-dissociation curve (ODC) (Figure 5.1).

Arterial oxygen saturation is a key component of arterial oxygen content (Ca_{O_2}). The significance of (Ca_{O_2}) to oxygen transport (D_{O_2}) has been discussed in Chapter 4. A low Sa_{O_2} will decrease the Ca_{O_2} (Table 5.1), thus affecting oxygen transport.

Technological advances in oximetry have greatly contributed to the ease of assess-

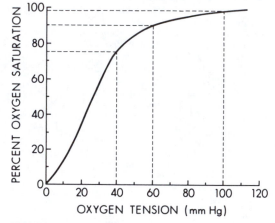

FIGURE 5.1. Oxyhemoglobin dissociation curve.

ment of oxygen saturation. The purpose of this chapter is to discuss the technological methods of oxygen-saturation assessment, the physiologic influences affecting the saturation value, and the clinical implications regarding changes of oxygen saturation.

OXIMETRY
Historical Review

Oximetry measures the saturation of hemoglobin based on light spectral differences between hemoglobin and oxyhemoglobin.[3-10] R. Lower, in 1669, was the first to document the color differences of oxyhemoglobin (bright red) and reduced hemoglobin (blue). Later, Angstrom (1855) described the color differences in relation to light absorption properties (spectrophotometry).[3,6]

TABLE 5.1. Effect of Varying Sa_{O_2} on Ca_{O_2}

Sa_{O_2}	Ca_{O_2}
100	$15 \times 1.34 \times 1.00 = 20.1$
.95	$15 \times 1.34 \times .95 = 19.1$
.90	$15 \times 1.34 \times .90 = 18.1$
.85	$15 \times 1.34 \times .85 = 17.1$
.75	$15 \times 1.34 \times .75 = 15.1$

W.C. Stadie (1919) first attempted to quantify an oxygen saturation value based on spectral differences using the unaided eye. Stadie's correlation of low oxygen-saturation values and visual observance of cyanosis prompted further studies. These studies concluded that cyanosis will become visible when 5 gm of reduced hemoglobin per 100 cc blood is present.[6] These optical properties of hemoglobin form the basis of oximetry. Two technologies of oximetry have developed: those that measure absorption characteristics of hemoglobin (arterial pulse oximeters) and those that measure the reflectance of light by oxyhemoglobin/reduced hemoglobin (mixed-venous fiberoptic catheters). The absorption technique (arterial pulse oximeters) will be discussed here, and reflectance spectrophotometry will be discussed with venous saturation (Chapter 10).

Arterial Pulse Oximeters

The first instrument to measure oxygen saturation was introduced in 1934.[6-7] The cumbersome methods used in the early instruments, although not practical, stimulated development of the modern-day oximeter. Hewlett Packard introduced the first ear oximeter in 1960. Clinical application was limited because of technical difficulties in differentiating tissue, arterial blood, and venous blood.[8] In 1972, a Japanese bioengineer by the name of Takuo Aoyagi noted a problematic pulsatile waveform in his research of noninvasive cardiac-output measurements. He tried to electrically silence the waveform by using infrared wavelengths. This problematic pulsatile waveform led directly to pulse oximetry.[3,11]

The pulsation of arterial blood identified by infrared light absorption allowed the isolation of an oxygen saturation specific to arterial blood. The combination of plethysmographic waveforms and spectrometry forms the technical basis for today's pulse oximeters. Advances in computer technology have resulted in a quick, accurate digital processing of arterial oxygen saturation.

Technical Principles of Pulse Oximetry

Pulse oximeters measure the absorption of specific wavelengths of light by oxyhemoglobin (Hb_{O_2}) as compared to reduced hemoglobin (Hb).[3,5-10] A probe is placed over a finger, nose, or ear. One side of the probe has two light-emitting diodes that transmit light wavelengths through an arterial vascular bed to a photodetector on the opposite side (Figure 5.2). One diode transmits red light and the other infrared light. Arterial blood with high amounts of oxyhemoglobin absorbs most of the infrared light and allows red light to pass. Reduced hemoglobin absorbs the red light and allows the infrared light to pass.[8] Oxygen saturation is derived

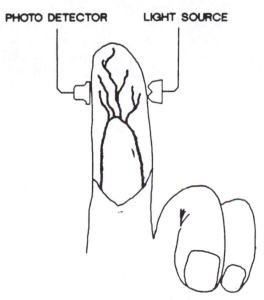

PHOTO DETECTOR   LIGHT SOURCE

FIGURE 5.2. Photo Detector. (Reprinted with permission from W.B. Saunders Co. Brown M, Vender JS. "Noninvasive Oxygen Monitoring." *Crit Care Clinics* 1988;4:493.)

by the Beer–Lambert law. This law states that if hemoglobin concentration and light intensity are held constant, then oxygen saturation becomes a logarithmic function of the intensity of light transmitted through the hemoglobin sample to the photodetector.[6-8] The amount of light transmitted to the photodetector is directly proportional to the absorption of light by the hemoglobin. This absorption is dependent on the type and amount of hemoglobin present.[9] The two light wavelengths of 660 nanometers (nm) (red) and 940 nm (infrared) are used since these represent the maximal absorption differences between oxyhemoglobin and reduced hemoglobin (see Figure 5.3).[1,7,8,12]

The two wavelengths of light pulse through the arterial bed 30 times a second.[12] The light-emitting diodes and the photodetectors each have two components; one for pulsating arterial blood and one for nonpulsatile venous blood, tissue, bone, and skin. The latter becomes a reference signal since it is constant. The pulsatile signals are amplified and converted to a digital signal. The plethysmographic waveform is a graphic display of the critically important pulsatile flow (Figure 5.4). A microprocessor, through complex calculations, converts the spectrometric and plethysmographic principles to a digital display.[12] The micro-

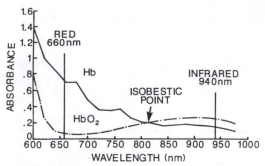

FIGURE 5.3. Spectrum of optical absorption of oxyhemoglobin and reduced hemoglobin in visible and near-infrared wavelength range. (Reprinted with permission from C.V. Mosby Co., Szaflarski NL, Cohen NH. "Use of pulse oximetry in critically ill adults." *Heart Lung* 1989;18:444.)

processor is able to calculate the pulse oximeter arterial-saturation value (Sp_{O_2}) 30 times per second. Thus the saturation is a ratio of oxyhemoglobin as compared to the total oxyhemoglobin and reduced hemoglobin. Differentiating light absorption and transmission properties of pulsating blood versus venous blood allows a value specific to arterial saturation.[3,7,12]

TECHNICAL CONSIDERATIONS OF PULSE OXIMETRY

Despite the ease of use of pulse oximetry, some technical considerations must be acknowledged. These include external light interference, optical shunting, motion arti-

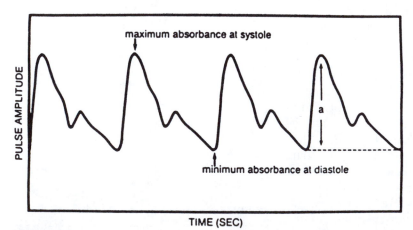

FIGURE 5.4. Plethysmographic waveform. (Reprinted with permission from W.B. Saunders Co., Brown M, Vender JS. "Noninvasive oxygen monitoring." *Crit Care Clinics* 1988;4:493.)

fact, and interference by an intravenous dye.

A common misconception when using pulse oximetry is that nail polish must be removed. Sp_{O_2} is not affected by nail polish, artificial nails, skin pigmentation, or dirty skin. The optical density of the tissue between the light-emitting diodes and the photodetector is not as significant in oximetry operation as is the critical pulsatile flow.[8]

External Light Interference

External light absorbed by the photodetector in significant amounts may alter the Sp_{O_2}. Examples are fluorescent light, bilirubin light, surgical light, sunlight, or light from fiber-optic sources or infrared heating lamps. The photodetector cannot differentiate bright light of an external source from light transmitted through the hemoglobin.[7-8] Correct probe position, with the light-emitting diodes directly across the vascular bed from the photodetector, may decrease the occurrence of external light interference. The probe should be flush with the skin. Covering the probe with an opaque material such as a sheet will eliminate external-light interference.[9]

Optical Shunting

Light wavelengths that reach the photodetector before transversing the arterial bed will distort the Sp_{O_2}. This is known as optical shunting. The resulting Sp_{O_2} will be a combination of the actual arterial saturation and the shunted light.[8-9] The overall effect on the Sp_{O_2} will depend on the patient's arterial saturation. If the patient's Sa_{O_2} is less than 85%, the Sp_{O_2} will be falsely elevated. If the Sa_{O_2} is greater than 81%, the resulting Sp_{O_2} will be falsely low.[8-9] Following the manufacturer's directions for probe placement should prevent optical shunting. For example, some manufacturers use printed dots on the disposable probe surface to indicate the light source and the photodetector. Correct probe placement mandates that these dots be placed directly across from each other with an arterial blood supply in between. Specific disposable probes are manufactured for each possible anatomical application. Ear, finger, toe, and nose probes are made for adult application. Toe or finger probes are usually used for the pediatric population. Nondisposable probes for the ear and finger are available for adults.

Motion Artifact

Excessive movement by the patient may interfere with the signal processing of the Sp_{O_2} and reflect an erroneous value. Motion artifact is usually prevented since the saturation measurements occur 30 times a second. Isolated erratic values caused by movement are discarded and the displayed saturation remains constant.[12] Erratic changes in the heart-rate display and/or Sp_{O_2} that frequently occur with motion artifact may be a warning that the value is erroneous. When an electrocardiogram (ECG) is monitored in conjunction with pulse oximetry, a comparison of the heart-rate displays from each may be helpful. If the heart-rate display on the oximeter does not correlate with the heart-rate display of the monitor, the Sp_{O_2} should not be considered valid. If the signal strength of the pulsatile waveform is weak due to probe placement, hypothermia, vasoconstriction, or poor circulation to the probe site, motion artifact is more likely to cause an erroneous value. Manufacturers are developing improvements in signal processing to further minimize the effects of motion artifact. One such technique is the synchronization of the Sp_{O_2} data with the ECG. The oximeter processes the saturation data at a set number of milliseconds after the R wave of the ECG signal.[8,13] Theoretically, this timed Sp_{O_2} value should correlate to the arterial pulsatile peak. If ECG synchronization is used, comparison of the ECG and the pulse oximeter heart-rate correlations to determine the adequacy of signal strength is no longer valid. With ECG synchronization, the pulse oximeter heart rate is taken from the monitor, so it will always match the monitor heart rate regardless of the adequacy of signal strength.

Intravenously Administered Dyes

Intravenously administered dyes have been found to absorb light wavelengths at 660 nm. This may interfere with the processing of the Sp_{O_2} value, causing a falsely low value.[7,8,14] Examples of such dyes are methylene blue, indigo carmine, and indocyanine green.[14]

Other Technical Considerations

Elevated serum bilirubin and endogenous and exogenous lipids have been shown to interfere with oximetry. Each has significant spectral absorption which causes overestimation of oxyhemoglobin and underestimation of Sp_{O_2}.[8]

Excessive venous pulsations may affect the accuracy of pulse oximeters. Restrictive taping of the sensor, which limits arterial blood flow and potentiates venous pulsations, is the most common cause of excessive venous pulsation. Other situations associated with increased venous pressure, such as right-sided heart failure, tricuspid regurgitation, and use of high positive end expiratory pressure, may cause erroneous Sp_{O_2} values.[8]

PHYSIOLOGIC CONSIDERATIONS OF PULSE OXIMETRY

To use pulse oximetry most effectively, certain physiologic limitations must be recognized. Low pulsatile flow states and large amounts of dysfunctional hemoglobin may alter the Sp_{O_2}. Understanding the relationship of arterial saturation and the partial pressure of oxygen in the arteries (Pa_{O_2}), i.e. the ODC, will enhance recognition of the clinical significance of Sp_{O_2}. Certain factors influence the ODC, causing shifts to the right or left. It is important to recognize that pulse oximetry offers little value in assessment of oxygen transport. Each of these considerations will be discussed in detail.

Low Pulsatile Flow States

The arterial pulsatile flow in oximetry is crucial. When low pulsatile states are present, the oximeter has difficulty differentiating between arterial blood and the background reference of venous blood, tissue, bone, and skin. The resulting Sp_{O_2} may not truely reflect Sa_{O_2}. Low pulsatile states occurring from hypotension (mean blood pressure less than 50 mm Hg) may preclude the use of pulse oximetry.[8,9] Hypoperfusion of the probe surface area caused by hypothermia, vasoconstriction, or peripheral vascular disease produces similar effects and may negate the use of pulse oximetry. Vasopressors commonly used in critical care areas such as norepinephrine, epinephrine, dopamine (at greater than 15 mcg/kg/min), and neo-synephrine hydrochloride cause vasoconstriction, which may limit peripheral blood flow and the accuracy of pulse oximetry. Changing the probe site may result in a stronger pulsatile signal, increasing the success of pulse oximetry. The nasal probe may be best for extreme low perfusion states since the blood flow in the nasal septum anterior ethmoid artery remains greater than the finger pulse in compromised flow states.[10] The ECG synchronization feature (mentioned with motion artifact) has increased the success of pulse oximetry in low perfusion states.

Arterial blood flow to a finger probe surface area may be intermittently occluded by nursing maneuvers. Tourniquet application, for example, on the same arm as the oximeter probe while starting an intravenous line and/or collecting a blood sample will severely limit arterial pulsatile flow. If a blood pressure cuff is inflated on the same arm as the oximeter probe, the arterial blood flow will be occluded, preventing accurate processing of the Sp_{O_2}.

Correct probe application includes avoiding constriction of the probe surface area which may decrease arterial blood supply. Avoid restrictive taping of the probe which may constrict arterial blood flow and alter the Sp_{O_2}.

Dysfunctional Hemoglobin

Pulse oximetry utilizes only two light wavelengths which measure the functional saturation of hemoglobin. Functional saturation of hemoglobin is the amount of oxyhemoglobin as compared to oxyhemoglobin and reduced hemoglobin. Hemoglobin may combine with other substances besides oxygen. If hemoglobin combines with carbon monoxide, for instance, carboxyhemoglobin is formed. A reaction between oxyhemoglobin and hydrogen sulfide produces sulfhemoglobin. Methemoglobin may be formed when the ferrous component of iron in hemoglobin is changed to the ferric form. These are known as dysfunctional hemoglobins, since they can no longer combine with oxygen and/or unload oxygen at the tissues.[1] Fractional hemoglobin saturation represents the percentage of oxyhemoglobin as compared to all types of hemoglobin present. Most laboratories use an eight-wavelength light source so that fractional hemoglobin saturation is reported. Usually the amount of dysfunctional hemoglobins is clinically insignificant, accounting for less than 2%. However, since pulse oximeters do not measure these dysfunctional hemoglobins, it is common to see a 2–3% higher Sp$_{O_2}$ than Sa$_{O_2}$ measured in the laboratory.[1,3,7,8] The greater the amount of dysfunctional hemoglobins in the blood, the greater the degree of Sp$_{O_2}$ error in estimating Sa$_{O_2}$.[8,10]

Dysfunctional hemoglobins may be clinically significant in a few instances. For example, heavy smokers may have a carboxyhemoglobin level greater than 3–4% gm/dl. The Sp$_{O_2}$ will be falsely elevated in these patients. In chronic lung disease in which a patient has an elevated carboxyhemoglobin level, a 3–4% increase in Sp$_{O_2}$ may be clinically significant. The falsely elevated Sp$_{O_2}$ may contribute to a false security and indicated therapy may not be instituted if the effect of dyshemoglobins on Sp$_{O_2}$ is not recognized. Acute increases in carboxyhemoglobin may occur with inhalation injuries caused by fire, smoke from fireplaces, or exhaust from stoves and automobiles. Carbon monoxide will not affect Pa$_{O_2}$ values but will decrease Sa$_{O_2}$. Pulse oximeters will display high Sp$_{O_2}$ values in the presence of carboxyhemoglobin, yet the Sa$_{O_2}$ will be low.[8] Thus use of pulse oximetry with inhalation inju-

ries is misleading and therefore contraindicated.

Methemoglobinemia may occur as an idiosyncratic reaction to oxidant drugs such as lidocaine, nitroprusside, nitroglycerin, and chlorates.[8] Methemoglobin levels higher than 1.5 gm/dl will again cause Sp$_{O_2}$ to overestimate Sa$_{O_2}$. The presence of sulfhemoglobin (0.5 gm/dl) may also falsely elevate Sp$_{O_2}$.[10]

Correlation of Sa$_{O_2}$ and Pa$_{O_2}$

An understanding of the relationship between hemoglobin saturation and Pa$_{O_2}$ is important for clinical application of pulse oximetry. The sigmoidal shape of the ODC (see Figure 5.1) demonstrates that the Pa$_{O_2}$ may decrease from 100–60 mm Hg, yet the arterial saturation decreases only from 99% to 90%. Once saturation decreases below 90%, smaller changes in Pa$_{O_2}$ will be associated with larger percentage changes in Sa$_{O_2}$. For instance, assume that the P$_{O_2}$ decreases from 60 mm Hg to 40 mm Hg. The S$_{O_2}$ will fall from 90% to 75%. At the top portion of the ODC, the P$_{O_2}$ fell 30 mm Hg with a corresponding change in S$_{O_2}$ of 10 mm Hg. Once on the steep portion of the ODC, the P$_{O_2}$ fell only 20 mm Hg, yet this correlated to a decrease in S$_{O_2}$ of 15%. Table 5.2 lists the correlation of several P$_{O_2}$ values to S$_{O_2}$ values assuming normal pH, body temperature, and 2,3 DPG.

Understanding the correlation between Pa$_{O_2}$ and saturation may promote prompt intervention when indicated. As one author points out, a saturation of 85% may be improperly ignored since it is a seemingly high value. Yet this seemingly high Sa$_{O_2}$ represents a Pa$_{O_2}$ in the 50s.[9]

Factors Affecting ODC

Certain influences will shift the ODC. An increased partial pressure of carbon dioxide in the arteries (P$_{CO_2}$), hyperthermia, acidosis, and increased 2,3 DPG will cause the ODC to shift to the right. The hemoglobin affinity for oxygen will decrease so that oxygen unloading will be promoted at the tissue beds. Clinically, a lower Sa$_{O_2}$ will be

TABLE 5.2.   Correlation of S_{O_2} to P_{O_2}

S_{O_2}	P_{O_2}
100	150
.90	60
.85	50
.75	40
.50	27

appreciated for a given Pa_{O_2}. For example, under normal conditions, a Pa_{O_2} of 60 mm Hg correlates with an Sa_{O_2} of 90%. A patient admitted with a fever and respiratory acidosis from pneumonia may have a Pa_{O_2} of 60 mm Hg with a correlating Sa_{O_2} of 87%. Shifts to the right may cause undue anxiety for clinicians and/or unnecessary clinical interventions since the Sa_{O_2} appears lower than under normal conditions.

The ODC may also shift to the left. A decreased P_{CO_2}, hypothermia, alkalosis, and decreased 2,3 DPG will increase the hemoglobin affinity for oxygen. Thus oxygen unloading at the tissues may be decreased, yielding a higher saturation than expected. For example, a surgical patient brought to the postanesthesia care unit (PACU) with a core body temperature of 96°F and alkalotic blood gases from hyperventilation during surgery may have a Pa_{O_2} of 60 mm Hg with a Sa_{O_2} of 93%. Shifts to the left may promote a false security for clinicians since the Sa_{O_2} is higher than anticipated under normal conditions. Necessary interventions may be withheld if the leftward shift in ODC and subsequent affect on Sa_{O_2} is not recognized.

CLINICAL APPLICATION OF Sa_{O_2}

Normal Sa_{O_2} is greater than 90%. Most clinically significant decreases in Sa_{O_2} will correlate with decreases in Pa_{O_2}. Alveolar hypoventilation, anatomical venous shunting, decreased barometric pressure, diffusion defects, and intrapulmonary shunting (from ventilation/perfusion mismatching) will each contribute to a low Pa_{O_2} and, subsequently, to a lower Sa_{O_2}. Ideally the Sa_{O_2} should always be greater than or equal to

90%, correlating to a Pa_{O_2} of greater than or equal to 60 mm Hg. Treatment interventions should be considered when Sa_{O_2} is less than 90%, assuming a normal pH, body temperature, P_{CO_2}, and 2,3 DPG.

Sa_{O_2} and D_{O_2}

The Sa_{O_2} is one component of the arterial oxygen content (Ca_{O_2}). Low Sa_{O_2} values will decrease Ca_{O_2}. A previous list of examples illustrated the impact of Sa_{O_2} on Ca_{O_2} (Table 5.1). Table 5.3 expands on Table 5.1 and illustrates the ultimate effect of altered Sa_{O_2} on oxygen transport (D_{O_2}).

The Sa_{O_2} may decrease in heavy exercise states, prompting the unloading of oxygen in the presence of a high metabolic demand. The Sa_{O_2} may also decrease in low perfusion states to compensate for a low cardiac output. A low hemoglobin concentration may increase the unloading of oxygen at the tissues, resulting in a lower Sa_{O_2}. However, a decrease in Sa_{O_2} due to a low cardiac output and/or low hemoglobin may be so small that it seems insignificant or is unnoticed. For the most part, very little information (if any) regarding oxygen transport may be derived from the Sa_{O_2} value alone.

CLINICAL APPLICATION OF PULSE OXIMETRY

When using pulse oximetry, an initial blood gas is recommended for the following reasons: (1) the correlation of Sa_{O_2} to Sp_{O_2} can be evaluated, (2) the influence of dysfunctional hemoglobins may be noted in any discrepancy between Sa_{O_2} and Sp_{O_2}, and (3) the relationship between the Pa_{O_2} and Sa_{O_2} can be determined to assess for

TABLE 5.3.   Effect of Sa_{O_2} on D_{O_2}

Sa_{O_2}	Ca_{O_2}	CO	D_{O_2}		
100	20.1	× 5	× 10	=	1005
.95	19.1	× 5	× 10	=	955
.90	18.1	× 5	× 10	=	905
.85	17.1	× 5	× 10	=	855
.75	15.1	× 5	× 10	=	755

shifts in the ODC. The value of pulse oximetry lies in its ability to continuously monitor Sp$_{O_2}$. Decreases in Sp$_{O_2}$ may alert clinicians to impending problems so that interventions may prevent further insults in oxygenation. Sp$_{O_2}$ values greater than or equal to 92% should be considered normal. This allows for the small percentage of dysfunctional hemoglobins that may cause an overestimation of Sa$_{O_2}$. It is also a safe guideline in conjunction with factors contributing to a left-sided shift of the ODC.

The ease of use of pulse oximetry, coupled with the attractive qualities of being quick, painless, accurate, noninvasive, and a representation of real time Sa$_{O_2}$, has contributed to its popularity in a variety of clinical settings.[3,5,7–10,13] Pulse oximetry has many beneficial applications in critical care areas. Pulse oximeters are extremely valuable for patients with known ventilation/perfusion abnormalities. For example, patients with pneumonia, emphysema, chronic bronchitis, asthma, pulmonary embolism, or congestive heart failure are ideal candidates for oximetry. Sp$_{O_2}$ may help establish desirable therapeutic modalities and serve as a warning when further intervention(s) may be indicated. Sp$_{O_2}$ monitoring can be used to assure adequate oxygenation during nursing maneuvers such as suctioning, bathing, and turning. The effect on oxygenation of many therapeutic interventions such as chest physiotherapy, bronchodilators, and antibiotics for pneumonia and/or bronchial infections can be evaluated by pulse oximetry. Continuous Sp$_{O_2}$ is a valuable adjunct when weaning the patient's fraction of inspired oxygen (F$_{IO_2}$). The F$_{IO_2}$ may be weaned as long as the Sp$_{O_2}$ remains above 92%, assuming physical assessment parameters are stable. Pulse oximeters are helpful in identifying patient tolerance of common procedures performed in acute care areas. Bronchoscopy, endoscopy, invasive-line insertions, and elective cardioversion are some examples of procedures during which Sp$_{O_2}$ values have guided clinicians to assure adequate oxygenation.[8]

Pulse oximeters have been utilized in emergency departments to evaluate emergent clinical conditions and/or interventions. Oximeters are also used extensively in surgery and postanesthesia care units to evaluate effects of anesthesia and/or mechanical ventilation on oxygenation status. Specialty areas such as cardiac rehabilitation programs, pulmonary rehabilitation programs, sleep laboratories, stress-testing laboratories, and dialysis units have utilized pulse oximeters for endpoints of therapy or exercise and/or diagnostic applications. Continuous Sp$_{O_2}$ is helpful during certain radiologic procedures such as cardiac catheterization, angiography, ventilation/perfusion scans, computerized tomography scans, and magnetic-resonance imaging in which lying supine may have a deleterious effect on the patient's cardiopulmonary status.

Pulse oximeters in the neonatal/pediatric population may help establish oxygen requirements for preterm/full-term neonates and serve as an indicator of potential ventilation/perfusion problems. The Sp$_{O_2}$ may also reflect tolerance of weaning from mechanical ventilation/oxygen therapy.[7,8,10]

CLINICAL REVIEW

The following are several patient examples of Sp$_{O_2}$ in acute care settings.

Example 1

(This case study will present several scenarios regarding pulse oximetry.)

Mr. M was admitted to the respiratory intensive care unit (RICU) with an exacerbation of his chronic obstructive pulmonary disease (COPD). He was acutely short of breath and dyspneic with labored respirations of 45 per minute. Arterial blood gases, drawn on admission without oxygen therapy, showed

pH	7.28
P$_{CO_2}$	57
Pa$_{O_2}$	45
C$_{CO_2}$	25
Sa$_{O_2}$	75%

A pulse oximeter was placed on his left forefinger. The Sp_{O_2} was 78%. He was intubated with initial ventilator settings of tidal volume, 800cc; assist-control ventilation with a back-up rate of 12; and Fl_{O_2} of .90. Once intubated, his Sp_{O_2} was 100%.

1. Does the Pa_{O_2} of 45 correlate with a Sa_{O_2} of 75%, based on a normal ODC?

ANSWER

A Pa_{O_2} of 45 should correlate to a Sa_{O_2} of 78–79%, based on a normal ODC. Mr. M has a lower Sa_{O_2} since he is acidotic with an increased P_{CO_2} and has shifted his ODC to the right. Right-sided shifts result in a lower Sa_{O_2} for a given Pa_{O_2}.

2. What is a likely explanation for the discrepancy between the Sa_{O_2} and the Sp_{O_2}?

ANSWER

Mr. M may have more dysfunctional hemoglobins than normal, thus accounting for the discrepancy between Sa_{O_2} and Sp_{O_2}. With a history of COPD, assess for a smoking history in which a likely reason for the difference is an elevated carboxyhemoglobin.
An infiltrate was noted on Mr. M's chest x-ray in the right lower lobe. Antibiotics, aminophyllin, bronchosol therapy, and chest physiotherapy (CPT) were begun. His F_{lO_2} was decreased to .40 by monitoring Sp_{O_2}, which remained between 93 and 95%. The respiratory therapist noted that the Sp_{O_2} values decreased when Mr. M's head was put in Trendelenburg's position for chest physiotherapy. His head was raised from Trendelenburg's to a flat position, with a resulting increase to the baseline of his Sp_{O_2}. The therapist also noted that when Mr. M was positioned for CPT on his left lower lobe, he again desaturated.

3. Why do you think Mr. M desaturated when positioned for CPT?

ANSWER

Mr. M had a right-lower-lobe infiltrate. When he was positioned with his right lung (bad lung) dependent in order to do CPT on the left lung, his gas exchange decreased, resulting in a lower Sp_{O_2}.
The nurse noted that Mr. M would desaturate when he needed to be suctioned. Mr. M gradually improved and, after reviewing weaning parameters on the third day of admission, his physician ordered that he be placed on a T-tube for a weaning trial. After ten minutes of breathing per T-tube, the Sp_{O_2} decreased to 82% and the audible alarm alerted the nurse to the low value. Mr. M was anxious, restless, dyspneic, and coughing. The nurse attempted to breathe him with a

manual resuscitator bag and noted some resistance. A second attempt was successful, after which the nurse suctioned a large mucous plug. Mr. M's respiratory rate decreased, he relaxed, and his Sp_{O_2} rose to 93%. He was extubated 20 minutes later and Sp_{O_2} values remained 92–93%.

Example 2

Ms. R is a 45-year-old woman admitted to the coronary care unit with angina and to rule-out a myocardial infarction. On arrival to the CCU, she is short of breath, complains of severe chest pain, has an audible S_3 heart sound, and crackles ⅔ of the way up posteriorly. An arterial blood gas is drawn showing:

pH	7.48
P_{CO_2}	30
Pa_{O_2}	55
C_{CO_2}	24
Sa_{O_2}	90%

A pulse oximeter is applied which shows a Sp_{O_2} of 91%. As a 60% high-humidity mask is applied, her Sp_{O_2} rises to 93%.

1. Does the Pa_{O_2} correlate to the Sa_{O_2}, based on a normal ODC?

ANSWER

The Pa_{O_2} does not correlate to the Sa_{O_2}, based on a normal ODC. Because of her hyperventilation and resulting respiratory alkalosis from hypoxemia, the ODC has shifted to the left. Left-sided shifts show a higher saturation than expected with a given Pa_{O_2}. Recognition of left-sided shifts is important so that indicated therapy is not withheld. Some clinicians may not be concerned with a Sa_{O_2} of 90%; yet, with a left-sided shift this represents a Pa_{O_2} in the 50s. A safe practice for Ms. R is to not allow her Sp_{O_2} to drop below 92–93%.

2. Does the Sa_{O_2} correlate to the Sp_{O_2}?

ANSWER

Yes, the Sa_{O_2} of 90% does correlate with the Sp_{O_2} of 91%. Most manufacturers claim a 2% accuracy rate.
Ms. R is treated with Lasix, intravenous nitroglycerin, and morphine sulphate for her chest pain. Her symptoms do not dissipate, so the physician decides to insert a pulmonary-artery catheter. The internal jugular approach is chosen as the site of insertion. The nurse is quick to point out to the physician that the Sp_{O_2} desaturated to 89% when Ms. R's head was placed in Tren-

delenburg's position. The physician raises the head flat and the Sp$_{O_2}$ rises to 92%. The nurse carefully monitors the pulse oximeter during the catheter insertion since Ms. R's head is covered with sterile sheets and she cannot see her face. Hemodynamic data shows that Ms. R has elevated pulmonary-artery pressures, an elevated pulmonary-wedge pressure, and a low cardiac output.

3. What information did the pulse oximeter contribute concerning the low cardiac output?

ANSWER

The Sp$_{O_2}$ gives no information regarding cardiac output (CO). Here, Ms. R has an acceptable Sp$_{O_2}$ with a poor CO. Very little information (if any) can be extrapolated from the Sp$_{O_2}$ regarding variables of oxygen transport.

Example 3

Mr. D is undergoing a bronchoscopy for transbronchial biopsy and cytology of a lung mass. Pulse oximetry is applied to monitor his saturation during the procedure. Prior to the procedure, his Sp$_{O_2}$ was 92%. Despite supplemental oxygen, Mr. D desaturated during the procedure.

How low can you allow the saturation to decrease before becoming concerned?

ANSWER

When the Sp$_{O_2}$ decreases to 85%, the nurse alerts the pulmonologist. The bronchoscope is removed, and Mr. D's Sp$_{O_2}$ subsequently rises to 90–91%. (Keep in mind that a Sp$_{O_2}$ of 85% correlates with a Pa$_{O_2}$ in the low 50s.)

Example 4

Ms. T is on a mechanical ventilator with the following settings:

VT	800 cc
CMV	mode
Back-up rate	= 10
F$_{IO_2}$	60%

Her blood gases showed:

pH	7.44
P$_{CO_2}$	38
Pa$_{O_2}$	145
C$_{CO_2}$	25
Sa$_{O_2}$	= 99%

How can the pulse oximeter assist in weaning her F$_{IO_2}$?

ANSWER

The a/A ratio on the current blood gas is 38%. (Refer to Chapter 3 if not familiar with a/A ratio.) A predicted Pa$_{O_2}$ based on 35% F$_{IO_2}$ (assuming no change in P$_{CO_2}$ or intrapulmonary shunting) is 76 mm Hg. The F$_{IO_2}$ can be weaned safely by monitoring the Sp$_{O_2}$ and assuring that the Sp$_{O_2}$ stays above 92%. Additional blood gases are unnecessary unless the patient's lung status changes.

ECONOMIC IMPACT

Pulse oximetry is a very economical measurement of Sa$_{O_2}$, with vast clinical implications. Results are pain-free and immediate, which is in stark contrast to collection of an arterial blood-gas sample. Patient cost of arterial blood-gas analysis is approximately $50–$100. Information from a blood-gas sample only reflects data at the time of sample collection. In weaning from oxygen therapy and/or decreasing F$_{IO_2}$ with mechanical ventilation, blood gases can frequently be avoided when using pulse oximetry. The economic implications of the avoidance of arterial blood-gas sampling are readily appreciated. Smoker et al. developed a protocol using pulse oximetry to evaluate oxygen therapy. Specific guidelines were established to determine the continued need for oxygen therapy, the potential for less oxygen therapy and the need for increased oxygen therapy. This protocol not only resulted in improved application of oxygen therapy and thus more positive patient outcomes, but also resulted in a substantial dollar savings. The hospital appreciated a 62% savings by assessment of oxygen therapy with oximetry versus arterial blood-gas analysis. Documentation of the protocol also satisfied reimbursement requirements, potentially increasing reimbursement of services rendered.[15] The authors believe a similar protocol would have implications in extended care facilities, home care, and other hospitals.

Other clinicians have evaluated the clinical and economic implications of substituting oximetry for blood-gas analysis in tapering supplemental oxygen. A decreased number of days on oxygen therapy and decreased arterial blood-gas analysis were appreciated in the oximeter-weaned group versus the control group. Avoidance of frequent blood-gas analysis limited patient discomfort. Economic implications were extrapolated from the decreased blood-gas sampling, decreased days of oxygen therapy, reduced medical personnel time, and the decreased use of the blood-gas analyzer.[16]

Vast clinical applications, ease of use, and economic incentives have all contributed to the popularity of pulse oximetry. As long as the technical and physiological limitations are recognized, pulse oximetry can be an excellent way to continuously monitor Sa_{O_2}.

SUMMARY

Pulse oximetry has widespread clinical implications. It is quick, accurate, and easy to use. As illustrated in Chapter 2, strong economic implications lie in the avoidance of arterial blood-gas sampling. Pulse oximetry's immediate and continuous reflection of Sa_{O_2} is advantageous for clinicians in (1) assessment of therapeutic interventions, (2) assessment of intrapulmonary shunting, and (3) as a warning of changes in gas exchange. It is important for clinicians to recognize the limitations of pulse oximetry, especially in its inability to contribute information regarding oxygen transport.

REFERENCES

1. Nellcor Inc. "Measurement of functional and fractional oxygen saturation." *Pulse Oximetry Note Number 2.* USA;1987.
2. Gutierrez G. "Peripheral delivery and utilization of oxygen." *In* Dantzker DR (ed). *Cardiopulmonary Critical Care.* Orlando: Grune & Stratton, 1986, 169.
3. Rutherford KA. "Principles and application of oximetry." *Crit Care Nurs Clin* 1989;1:649.
4. Lysak SZ, Prough DS. "Monitoring for patients receiving airway pressure therapy." *Anes Clin* 1987;5:821.
5. Bland DS. "Pulse oximetry." *Am Oper Room Nurs J* 1987;45:964.
6. Chapman KR, Rebock AS. "Oximetry." *In* Nochomovitz ML, Cherniack NS (eds). *Noninvasive Respiratory Monitoring.* New York: Churchhill Livingstone, 1986, 203.
7. Brown M, Vender JS. "Noninvasive oxygen monitoring." *Crit Care Clin* 1988;4:493.
8. Szaflarski NL, Cohen NH. "Use of pulse oximetry in critically ill adults." *Heart Lung* 1989;18:444.
9. Harris K. "Noninvasive monitoring of gas exchange." *Resp Care* 1987;32:544.
10. Schroeder CH. "Pulse oximetry: A nursing care plan." *Crit Care Nurs* 1988;8:50.
11. Severinghaus JW, Honda Y. "History of blood gas analysis VII. Pulse oximetry." *J Clin Monit* 1987;3:135.
12. Ohmeda Inc. *Operating/Service Manual.* "Principles of operation." 1986;22.
13. Nellcor Inc. "Hemoglobin and the principles of pulse oximetry." *Pulse Oximetry Note Number 1.* USA;1987.
14. Scheller MS, Unger RJ. "The influence of intravenously administered dyes on pulse oximetry readings." *Anes* 1986;65:A161.
15. Smoker JM, Hess DR, Frey-Zeiler VL et al. "A protocol to assess oxygen therapy." *Resp Care* 1986; 31:35.
16. King T, Simon RH. "Pulse oximetry for tapering supplemental oxygen in hospitalized patients." *Chest* 1987;92:713.

6
Role of Cardiac Output in Oxygen Transport

Ann Padwosjki MSN, RN, CCRN

Four components contribute to the function of oxygen transport. These include cardiac output, hemoglobin, oxygen saturation (Sa_{O_2}), and the Pa_{O_2}. The hemoglobin, oxygen saturation and the Pa_{O_2} are the most easily obtained parameters, whereas measurement of the cardiac output may require invasive monitoring or special equipment. However, the cardiac output is the most important component to transport. Cardiac output provides the flow that transports oxygen. Because of the importance of cardiac output to oxygen transport, an in-depth assessment of this parameter will be presented in this chapter.

The cardiac output is the mechanism that delivers oxygenated blood to the tissues. One analogy that emphasizes the importance of cardiac output to oxygen content is the mail system. One can think of oxygen content as the mail and cardiac output as the mail carrier. Mail can contain much information that people need to work and meet their needs. Yet, mail is of no use if it does not get delivered. In fact, people may be adversely affected by undelivered mail. Cardiac output is the mail carrier delivering the mail. Without this mail carrier, oxygen does not get delivered. By this simple analogy, one can see that cardiac output is essential to oxygen delivery and survival.

DEFINITION OF CARDIAC OUTPUT

Cardiac output can be defined as the volume of blood pumped by the heart over one minute.[1] The determinants of cardiac output are heart rate and stroke volume. Heart rate is defined as contractions or beats per minute, and stroke volume is defined as milliliters ejected per contraction or beat. Either parameter can influence cardiac output. Normal stroke volume ranges from 60–100 milliliters per beat. The normal range for heart rate is usually 60–100 beats per minute (bpm).

COMPONENTS OF CARDIAC OUTPUT

Heart Rate

A person with a heart rate of 75 bpm and a stroke volume of 70 ml would have a cardiac output of 5,250 milliliters or 5.25 liters/minute (75×70). In a patient with heart failure and a low stroke volume, the heart rate can compensate to maintain a normal cardiac output. For example, a patient with a stroke volume of 35 ml and a heart rate of 150 bpm will also have a cardiac output of 5.25 l/min. Heart rate changes respond to neurochemical factors that aid to maintain normal cardiac output and respond to stress situations.[2]

Stroke Volume

Stroke volume is influenced by the components of preload, afterload, and contractility. Preload is the degree of muscle stretching that occurs in the ventricle just before the next ejection (or end diastole). Preload is influenced by the volume and pressure of blood in the ventricle and the compliance or stiffness of the ventricle.[1] Afterload is the resistance to ejection that the heart must overcome to eject blood. High resistance can impede flow, whereas a lower resistance can enhance flow. Contractility refers to the contractile force of the heart, or the strength of the contraction or beat. Weak or strong contractions can influence flow. Contractility is usually influenced by neurochemical factors associated with the sympathetic nervous system.[2-3]

All three factors can influence stroke volume, which directly influences cardiac output. A low preload can reduce cardiac output due to reduced volume. A high preload can overstretch the ventricle over time and affect output by reducing the ability of the ventricle to contract. The Frank–Starling law conceptualizes this preload effect on cardiac output (see Figure 6.1). This concept, presented by Starling in 1918, envisions the muscle-fiber length as determining the work of the cardiac muscle and the force of contraction.[4] Since muscle-fiber length is difficult to measure, it is represented by the intraventricular filling pressure or preload.

The more the cardiac muscle is stretched with blood, the higher the pressure and the stronger the contraction, which results in a better stroke volume. Stronger contractions increase stroke volume until the cardiac muscle fiber is stretched beyond its limits. At this point, the force of contraction and stroke-volume output begins to decline, as is seen in cardiac failure. (See Figure 6.1).

Challengers to the Frank–Starling law have pointed out that other factors affect cardiac output more than the Frank–Starling effect. Nervous, vasomotor, and metabolic influences may have more control over the contractility of cardiac muscle than just preload. These components negate the Frank–Starling effect. Studies suggest neurogenic responses need to be eliminated in order to see the Frank–Starling effect on cardiac contraction and stroke volume.[4]

Despite the controversy over the mechanisms that affect the components of stroke volume, certain facts remain. A strong contraction can enhance stroke volume; a weak contraction can reduce stroke volume. The higher the resistance to outflow of the blood from the ventricle, the more adversely flow is affected. Thus, all three factors; preload, afterload, and contractility, influence stroke volume, which ultimately affects cardiac output.

The influence of heart rate and stroke volume on cardiac output is an extensive topic in itself. A brief review of the influences on these parameters has been presented to enhance understanding of cardiac output and its major influence on oxygen transport.

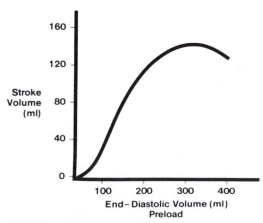

FIGURE 6.1. Frank-Starling's law illustrated in pressure-volume curve.

MEASURING CARDIAC OUTPUT

There are several methods available to measure cardiac output. Three clinically useful methods will be reviewed here.

Fick Equation

The first method to be discussed is the direct Fick method, which was developed by Adolph Fick in the 1880s.[5] The Fick method has been referred to as the gold standard for measuring cardiac output. This method is based on the concept that the amount of a substance taken up or released by an organ is the product of the flow of blood through that organ and the arterial and venous difference of this same substance. The direct Fick method utilizes the lungs as the organ and oxygen as the substance. The Fick formula is

$$CO = \frac{V_{O_2} \text{ (in ml/min)}}{(Ca_{O_2} - Cv_{O_2}) \times 10}$$

where 10 is the conversion factor per 100 ml.[6] Measurement of oxygen consumption commonly uses exhaled gas analysis (see Chapter 10).

The conditions under which O_2 consumption is determined need to be consistent in estimating subsequent cardiac-output measurements. Oxygen-consumption measurements in critically ill patients may be labile due to changing oxygen requirements. If the O_2-consumption measurement is assumed, cardiac-output measurements arrived at with the Fick equation may not be accurate.

Thermodilution Method

Thermodilution is another method for calculating cardiac outputs. It was not consistently utilized until the development of the Swan–Ganz catheter in the early 1970s.[6] With this method, a known amount of solution at a known temperature is injected into the proximal port of a thermodilution catheter (Figure 6.2). The change in temperature from the time of injection to the time the mixed injectate reaches the thermistor at the end of the catheter is plotted on a time-and-temperature curve. The area under the curve determines the cardiac output and is inversely proportional. Thus,

a small area under the curve indicates a higher cardiac output, and a large area under the curve indicates a lower cardiac output (see Figure 6.3).

The accuracy of this method is fairly good, except with conditions where there is retrograde flow on the right side of the heart, as in tricuspid or pulmonic-valve regurgitation, and atrial or ventricular septal defects.[6] Timing can also affect thermodilution cardiac outputs. Injection time should occur within four seconds or inaccurate results can occur.[7] Reproducibility is achieved if the solution is injected at the same point in the respiratory cycle, that is, end expiration.[8]

Injectate temperatures should be stable, and readings should be within 5–10% of each other. Usually 10 ml is used for an injectate volume, however 5 ml can be used if fluid restriction is a necessity. Research suggests that room temperature injectate is accurate as compared with iced injectate, although some authorities suggest using iced injectate for high or low cardiac-output states.[1,7,9–12] Positioning is not a problem as long as the head of the bed is less than 20 degrees and lateral rotation is less than 45 degrees.[7,9,13,14] (See Table 6.1)

Doppler Method

A third method of measuring cardiac output is the Doppler technique. The Doppler technique for determining cardiac outputs is a fairly new technique. The Doppler technique allows for the measurement of the average velocity of flow through a large vessel, which can allow estimation of the cardiac output. Usually the velocity of blood flow in the aortic arch is measured with a continuous-wave Doppler ultrasound apparatus using a transducer held in the suprasternal notch.[15,16] The cross-sectional area of the vessel also needs to be determined.

The Doppler ultrasound apparatus measures the volume of blood ejected over a period of time. This number is multiplied by a known area of the artery to determine

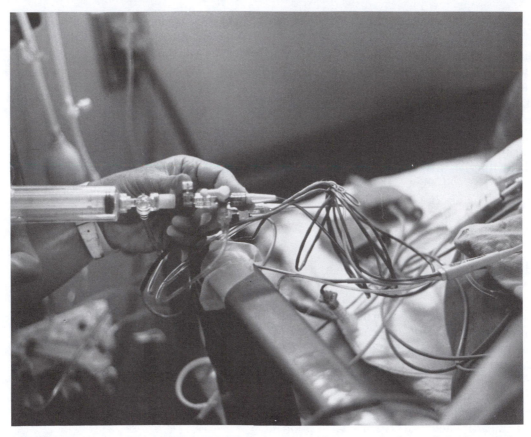

FIGURE 6.2. Thermodilution measurement. Measurement of cardiac outputs by thermodilution is generally performed by injecting a known solution (saline) at a known temperature into the proximal (blue) port of the pulmonary artery catheter. The pulmonary artery catheter is attached to the cardiac output computer near the proximal port.

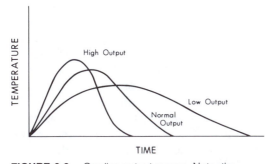

FIGURE 6.3. Cardiac-output curves. Note, the higher the cardiac output, the smaller the area under the curve. When measuring cardiac outputs, the configuration of the curve can be used to detect variations of cardiac output, from both physiological and technical causes.

stroke volume. The volume is measured times the heart rate to determine cardiac output. The velocity of flow and the vessel area can be determined from the ascending aorta.[16]

The Doppler technique for measuring cardiac output has been shown to be fairly accurate in stable clinical studies.[17] The advantage to this technique is low patient risk owing to its noninvasive approach. The potential of this technique is substantial since measuring cardiac output without invasive equipment would greatly increase the number of patients benefiting from cardiac-output measurement. The disadvantage is that the measurement obtained cannot be easily

TABLE 6.1.   Achieving Reproducibility in Cardiac Outputs

Factor	Normal	Effect on CO Value
Injection time	Less than 4 seconds	If greater than 4 seconds, falsely low values obtained.
Injectate volume	5–10 ml adults 1–5 ml children	Falsely elevated CO if volume less.
Temperature of injectate volume	Iced or room	Falsely elevated CO measurement injectate warmer than measured. Thermal loss starts when injectate removed from ice bath. Room temperature may be less accurate in low or high CO states.
Timing of injection	End-expiration	Variability in measurements if CO not performed at end expiration.
Patient position	HOB < 20 degrees Supine with lateral rotation < 45 degrees	May develop clinically significant changes in CO measurement if HOB or lateral rotation is greater than normal. Check patient for reproducibility with position changes.

verified if results are abnormal, as with the Fick equation. Verification would need to be done by thermodilution measurement or another precise method. Any noninvasive approach to determining cardiac output potentially has a significant impact, especially in patients in whom hemodynamic monitoring is technically difficult or a clinical risk.[17] Noninvasive methods such as the Doppler method as well as more recent techniques such as transthoracic electrical bioimpedance show promise as accurate methods of determining cardiac output.

OXYGEN DELIVERY
AND CARDIAC OUTPUT

In most circumstances, oxygen transport increases to meet increasing metabolic needs. However, there are circumstances in which transport is decreased in spite of normal or increasing oxygen consumption. This is usually in disease states and is caused by a failure of one of the components responsible for an adequate oxygen transport. In disease states, transport can be limited by pulmonary failure, cardiac failure, diminished oxygen-carrying capacity of blood, or by vascular diseases that limit the delivery of blood to certain regions of the body.[18] As previously stated, cardiac output is the most important component in oxygen delivery and it responds to compensate for increased demands on oxygen delivery.

The components of cardiac output can help to explain its important role in oxygen delivery. The main components have been identified as stroke volume and heart rate. Heart rate is primarily a compensatory mechanism and responds as such to increases in oxygen consumption. Heart rate compensates by increasing when stroke volume is low or when oxygen delivery demands are increased due to increased oxygen consumption.

Heart rate also compensates when stroke volume is decreased. A deficit in blood volume, as in a traumatic injury that results in acute blood loss, can impair oxygen delivery by decreasing the mean circulatory volume. There is decreased venous return, and thus stroke volume may be decreased.[2] The reduced stroke volume results in a lower cardiac output and less oxygen available to the tissues. Stroke volume is reduced when the pulmonary-capillary wedge pressure (PCWP) is reduced, as in hypovolemia, or when the PCWP is increased, as in left-ventricular failure. Stroke-volume reduction, with its subsequent reduced oxygen delivery, causes compensatory mechanisms to come into play.

Role of Cardiac Output in Oxygen Delivery

Cardiac output plays a major role in the body's physiologic response to an increased oxygen demand, as in exercise, by increasing heart rate. An increase in oxygen demand can occur during exercise or increased metabolic states such as with infection or fever states. The cardiac output can compensate for a substantial increase in oxygen utilization.[19]

For example, during exercise the cardiac output can increase to five times normal to meet the increased demand and keep pace with an increased metabolic activity. An accelerated heart rate increases blood flow, which increases oxygen transport and venous return. Oxygen also diffuses from the smaller arterioles, which lowers oxygen tension and causes vasodilation. This allows an increased availability of oxygen at the tissue level. Blood flow is also distributed to areas of increased demand.[20]

Some clinical examples can help to explain the importance of cardiac output to oxygen delivery. As previously stated, normal oxygen transport is about 1000 ml of oxygen per minute.[21] A patient with a normal cardiac output and a normal oxygen content should present with a normal oxygen transport. For example, a person with a cardiac output of 5 l/min, a Pa_{O_2} of 100, a Sa_{O_2} of 98%, and a hemoglobin of 15 gm/dl would have an oxygen transport of 985 ml per minute (see Table 6.2).

If we take the same person in the example above, and exercise him enough to in-

TABLE 6.2. Importance of Cardiac Output to Oxygen

Formula for oxygen delivery = oxygen content × cardiac output

Oxygen content = (1.34 × Hgb × Sa_{O_2})

Oxygen content × cardiac output x 10 (where 10 converts deciliters to milliliters)

Patient 1, At Rest
CO   = 5 l/min
Pa_{O_2} = 100 mm Hg
Sa_{O_2} = 98%
Hgb = 15 gm/dl

Oxygen delivery = (1.34 × .98 × 15) × 5 × 10 = 985 ml/min

Patient 1, With Exercise
CO = 15 l/min

Oxygen delivery = (1.34 × .98 × 15) × 15 × 10 = 3000 ml/min

Patient 1, With Cardiac Failure
CO = 2.5 l/min

Oxygen delivery = (1.34 × .98 × 15) × 2.5 × 10 = 492 ml/min

---

crease his cardiac output to 15 l/min, his oxygen transport will increase to almost 3000 ml of oxygen per minute (see Table 6.2). Therefore, his oxygen transport has increased to meet the increased oxygen requirements in exercise.

If the cardiac output decreases, sympathetic stimulation increases. Tachycardia occurs to try to enhance blood flow to the tissues.[2] The sympathetic response increases the force of contraction, which tries to distribute a larger flow of blood.

In low cardiac-output states (e.g., left-ventricular failure), oxygen is not adequately delivered to tissues owing to loss of the pump mechanism. Stroke volume is decreased and less oxygen is delivered. As cardiac output decreases and oxygen delivery decreases, more oxygen is given up by hemoglobin for use at the tissue level. This mechanism serves to maintain oxygen consumption.

The importance of cardiac output to oxygen transport can be shown graphically if we take the same person in our first example with a normal oxygen content but decrease the cardiac output by half, as in cardiac failure. The oxygen transport will now decrease to about 492 ml of oxygen per minute, an extremely low oxygen transport. The impact of a decreased cardiac output on oxygen transport is very evident in this example and shows the importance of cardiac output to oxygen delivery (see Table 6.2).

Cardiac Output Compensation for Decreased Oxygen Content

The importance of cardiac output to oxygen transport is evident not only in instances of changes in cardiac output but also when changes in oxygen content occur. The Pa_{O_2}, hemoglobin, or Sa_{O_2} may be decreased, yet transport can be maintained by a normal cardiac output. Cardiac output can compensate for a decreased oxygen content, but oxygen content cannot immediately compensate to increase oxygen delivery if the cardiac output is decreased. Some clinical examples can make this statement more evident.

Cardiac Output Compensation in Decreased Pa_{O_2} and Sa_{O_2}

Changes in available oxygen also affect oxygen transport. Oxygen is transported to tissues in two manners: dissolved in plasma (Pa_{O_2}) or attached to hemoglobin (Sa_{O_2}).[21] The Pa_{O_2} is utilized by many clinicians to estimate the Sa_{O_2}. In low Pa_{O_2} and Sa_{O_2} states, the cardiac output serves as the compensatory mechanism. Cardiac output will start to increase as the Pa_{O_2} approaches 50 mm Hg.[2] The heart rate will begin to increase to try to maintain transport of oxygen to the tissues.

A person with a Pa_{O_2} of 100 mm Hg, a Sa_{O_2} of 98%, a Hgb of 15 gm/dl, and a cardiac output of 5 l/min has a transport of 985 ml of oxygen per minute. As stated above, changes in cardiac output often do not occur unless the Pa_{O_2} drops to 50 mm Hg.[2] Even in this instance, the cardiac output

can compensate to provide an adequate oxygen transport.

For example, if the person in this example dropped her Pa_{O_2} to 50 mm Hg with an oxygen saturation of 80%, and the cardiac output increased to 8 l/min, the oxygen transport would be 1286 ml of oxygen per minute. The ability of cardiac output to maintain a normal oxygen transport in the face of low Pa_{O_2} and Sa_{O_2} is apparent. Therefore, in circumstances in which the Pa_{O_2} is compromised, attention should be given to overall oxygen transport and not only to the Pa_{O_2}, since oxygen transport may be normal. (See Table 6.3.)

Cardiac Output Compensation and Hemoglobin Level

The cardiac output can compensate to adjust for changes in hemoglobin. In fact, the cardiac output increases in response to low amounts of hematocrit.[2] Blood viscosity is the key to changes in cardiac output as far as transport is concerned. For example, if half the blood capacity is replaced with methemoglobin, cardiac output may not change as much as when there is a dilutional effect from fluids.[2] Thus, cardiac output increases with decreases in blood viscosity, as with a low hematocrit. In anemia, the oxygen-carrying capacity of blood decreases and viscosity is decreased. With a lower

TABLE 6.3. Cardiac Output Compensation for Decreased Pa_{O_2} and Sa_{O_2}

Patient 2, Normal Pa_{O_2}
CO = 5 l/min
Pa_{O_2} = 100 mm Hg
Sa_{O_2} = 98%
Hgb = 15 gm/dl

Oxygen delivery = (1.34 × .98 × 15) × 5 × 10 = 985 ml/min

Patient 2, Low Pa_{O_2}
CO = 8 l/min
Pa_{O_2} = 50 mm Hg
Sa_{O_2} = 80%
Hgb = 15 gm/dl

Oxygen delivery = (1.34 × .80 × 15) × 8 × 10 = 1286 ml/min

Oxygen delivery 985 ml/min versus 1286 ml/min of oxygen.

blood viscosity, cardiac output is increased because of a lower resistance, and venous return increases. The cardiac output increases to compensate for the lower oxygen content present in anemia.

Acute blood loss can also lower the hemoglobin level and decrease oxygen content. With a lower hemoglobin level, there is less hemoglobin available to carry oxygen. Cardiac output increases to increase oxygen transport and compensate for the lower hemoglobin level.

Clinical examples can show the compensatory mechanism of the cardiac output in times of decreased hemoglobin levels to maintain oxygen transport. If we take two examples of a person with a normal and a low hemoglobin, the compensation by cardiac output can be shown to have a dramatic effect on oxygen transport.

A person with a hemoglobin of 15 gm/dl, a cardiac output of 5 l/min, and a Pa_{O_2} of 100 has a normal transport of around 985 ml of oxygen per minute (see Table 6.4). If this same person were in an automobile accident in which he fractured his femur and lost two thirds of his hemoglobin to 5 gm/dl, and the cardiac output increased to 15 l/min, the oxygen transport would still be 985 ml of oxygen per minute (see Table 6.4). Thus, changes in hemoglobin can be compensated for by changes in cardiac output.

Problems arise if the cardiac output cannot increase as a compensatory mechanism.

For example, a patient with a low cardiac output at 3 l/min, a hemoglobin of 5 gm/dl, a Pa_{O_2} of 100 mm Hg, and a Sa_{O_2} of 98% has an oxygen delivery of only 200 ml of oxygen per minute. This is inadequate to sustain adequate oxygen delivery to tissues. This example demonstrates that a low cardiac output and hemoglobin may be catastrophic to a patient even if the Sa_{O_2} and Pa_{O_2} are within normal limits (see Table 6.5).

The above examples have demonstrated that even though changes in oxygenation parameters occur, the cardiac output can compensate to maintain a normal oxygen transport. The parameters of Pa_{O_2}, Sa_{O_2}, and hemoglobin are usually assessed to determine if oxygenation is adequate. However, these parameters only give information about the amount of oxygen in the blood. The cardiac output is necessary to determine the amount of oxygen available to the tissue, or the amount of oxygen that is actually transported to the tissues.

Compensatory mechanisms develop when oxygen delivery is threatened by changes in either oxygen content or stroke volume. In circumstances in which cardiac output is impaired due to failure, threats to tissue oxygenation exist. These examples show the importance of cardiac output to transport and the dependence that oxygen delivery has on cardiac output.

The use of the Pa_{O_2}, Sa_{O_2}, and hemoglobin in clinical practice to determine if a patient has adequate oxygenation only tells part of the story. The use of these parameters alone may give false information as to the actual state of oxygenation. The cardiac

TABLE 6.4. Cardiac Output Compensation for Low Hemoglobin

Patient 4, With Normal Hemoglobin
CO = 5 l/min
Pa_{O_2} = 100 mm Hg
Sa_{O_2} = 98%
Hgb = 15 gm/dl

Oxygen delivery = $(1.34 \times .98 \times 15) \times 5 \times 10 = 985$ ml/min

Patient 4, With Low Hemoglobin
CO = 15 l/min
Hgb = 5 gm/dl

Oxygen delivery = $(1.34 \times .98 \times 5) \times 15 \times 10 = 985$ ml/min

TABLE 6.5. Effects of Both Low Hemoglobin and Low Cardiac Output on Oxygen Delivery

Patient with Low Hgb and Low Cardiac Output
CO = 3 l/min
Pa_{O_2} = 100 mm Hg
Sa_{O_2} = 98%
Hgb = 5 gm/dl

Oxygen delivery = $(1.34 \times .98 \times 5) \times 3 \times 10 = 200$ ml/min output is an essential piece of information that may show an adequate oxygenation even though these other measures of oxygenation may be low. Treating these other parameters may be unnecessary in the face of a compensatory response by the cardiac output.

However, it should be noted that cardiac output is still only one component of oxygen delivery. Although it is the component with the most significant effect on oxygen delivery and it can compensate where oxygen content cannot, it should not be assessed by itself. Many clinicians do assess cardiac output by itself and assume that if cardiac output is adequate that transport is adequate. This is partially acceptable if oxygen content is normal. It may not be true when oxygen consumption is increased or if hemoglobin is decreased. All components of oxygen delivery must be included for a complete assessment.

ECONOMIC IMPLICATIONS

Proper assessment is essential to deliver appropriate therapy to patients with oxygen-delivery problems. Appropriate treatment will hopefully result in positive patient outcomes as well as economically efficient care. During these times of cost consciousness in healthcare, it is essential that treatment be effective economically as well as clinically. Knowledge of the components of oxygen delivery will be of benefit in delivering care that serves both needs. Since cardiac output is the most important component to oxygen delivery, particular attention to this parameter can result in appropriate care and the avoidance of overtreatment. Clinical examples should bring this point into better focus.

As previously stated, cardiac output is the parameter that is most important in oxygen delivery. However, it was also stated that this parameter is more difficult to obtain than the parameters of oxygen content (hemoglobin and Pa_{O_2}). Clinical examples explained that even when oxygenation is

lower than normal, a normal cardiac output can ensure adequate oxygen delivery.

For example, a change in the Pa_{O_2} from 100 mm Hg to 60 mm Hg only impacts the delivery of oxygen from 15 ml of oxygen per minute to 9 ml. This changes oxygen delivery from 1000 ml per minute to 905 ml per minute if one assumes that hemoglobin is 90% saturated and cardiac output is measured at 5 l/min. Oxygen delivery is still adequate. Treatment with oxygen therapy to improve the Pa_{O_2} will do little to enhance delivery of oxygen to the tissues.

In another example, a postsurgical patient has dropped her hemoglobin from 15 gm/dl to 10 gm/dl. If we assume that hemoglobin is still 98% saturated and the cardiac output is 5 l/min, the change in transport is from 985 ml per minute to 657 ml per minute. Oxygen delivery may still be adequate. Treatment with additional transfusions may improve transport, but oxygenation is stable because of the normal cardiac output. Avoidance of transfusion therapy will not adversely affect the patient and will result in cost savings for this patient.

These two examples are only a sample of the ways in which knowledge of oxygen delivery and the role of cardiac output in delivery of oxygen can result in appropriate treatment and cost savings. Overtreatment can be costly and will not significantly affect the outcome any more than would nontreatment. With a knowledge of oxygen delivery and its components, and by knowing when treatment is necessary, a nurse can provide treatment that is effective both clinically and economically.

Clinical Application

Several clinical examples can show the importance of cardiac output by showing the effect on all components, including oxygen delivery and oxygen consumption.

In the first example, assume a patient has a decreased Pa_{O_2} caused by pneumonia. The Pa_{O_2} is 50 mm Hg with a Sa_{O_2} of 80%. The cardiac output is normal at 6 l/min, and the hemoglobin is 15 gm/dl. Oxygen consumption is also normal at 250 ml of oxygen per minute. This patient's oxygen delivery would be 965 ml of oxygen per minute, which is adequate. Oxygen extraction would be approximately 26%, which is also within a normal range. Cardiac output helped to maintain a normal oxygen delivery and a normal oxygen extraction rate in the face of a decreased Pa_{O_2}. This example points out that clinical assessment of the Pa_{O_2} alone is not adequate when making an assessment of oxygen delivery. (See Table 6.6.)

In the second example, assume a patient with pernicious anemia has a hemoglobin of 8 gm/dl. The Pa_{O_2} is 95 mm Hg with a Sa_{O_2} of 98%. The cardiac output is normal at 8 l/min. Oxygen consumption is within normal limits at 200 ml per minute. This patient's oxygen delivery would be 840 ml per minute, resulting in an oxygen extraction rate of 24%, which is within the normal range. Again, oxygen delivery and oxygen extraction remain within an acceptable range (see Table 6.7).

To further illustrate the impact of cardiac output, the next examples will show what happens when cardiac output is compromised. For example, a patient is admitted to the coronary care unit with a severe anterior myocardial infarction. The Pa_{O_2} is 90 mm Hg with a Sa_{O_2} of 95%. The hemoglobin is normal at 15 gm/dl, and the cardiac output is 3 l/min owing to the myocardial infarction. The oxygen delivery in this

TABLE 6.7. Example of Cardiac Output Compensation for Low Hemoglobin with Adequate Delivery and Extraction Rate

Patient with Pernicious Anemia and Low Hgb
Pa_{O_2} = 95 mm Hg
Sa_{O_2} = 98%
Hgb = 8 gm/dl
CO = 8 l/min
V_{O_2} = 200 ml/min

Oxygen delivery = (1.34 × .98 × 8) × 8 × 10 = 840 ml/min

Oxygen extraction = $\frac{200}{840}$ = 24%

patient would be 573 ml of oxygen per minute, which is lower than normal. Oxygen delivery is low due to the low cardiac output, even though oxygen content is normal. If oxygen consumption is normal at 250 ml of oxygen per minute, the extraction rate will have to increase to 44%. This example illustrates the importance of cardiac output to oxygen delivery. With a decreased delivery, the extraction rate needs to increase to maintain a normal oxygen consumption (see Table 6.8).

Finally, assume a patient is admitted with a urinary tract infection and has a history of heart failure. The patient's Pa_{O_2} is normal at 90 mm Hg with a Sa_{O_2} of 95%. The hemoglobin is normal at 15 gm/dl, but the cardiac output is decreased at 3 l/min due to the history of heart failure. This results in an oxygen delivery for this patient at 573 ml of oxygen per minute. Owing to the urinary

TABLE 6.6. Example of Cardiac Output Compensation for Low Pa_{O_2} and Sa_{O_2} with Adequate Delivery and Extraction Rate

Patient with Pneumonia and a Low Pa_{O_2}
Pa_{O_2} = 50 mm Hg
Sa_{O_2} = 80%
Hgb = 15 gm/dl
CO = 6 l/min
V_{O_2} = 250 ml/min

Oxygen delivery = (1.34 × .80 × 15) × 6 × 10 = 965 ml/min

Oxygen extraction = $\frac{250}{965}$ = 26%

TABLE 6.8. Example of Decreased Oxygen Delivery and Increased Extraction from Low Cardiac Output

Patient with Anterior Myocardial Infarction and Low CO
Pa_{O_2} = 90 mm Hg
Sa_{O_2} = 95%
Hgb = 15 gm/dl
CO = 3 l/min
V_{O_2} = 250 ml/min

Oxygen delivery = (1.34 × .95 × 15) × 3 × 10 = 573 ml/min

Oxygen extraction = $\frac{250}{573}$ = 44%

tract infection, the patient has a temperature, and this has increased his oxygen consumption to 350 ml of oxygen per minute. Thus, his oxygen extraction rate will increase to meet the increased consumption needs. Oxygen extraction will increase to 61%, which is more than double the normal extraction rate.

The low cardiac output has forced the extraction rate to increase to compensate for an increased oxygen demand. The impact of a lower cardiac output on oxygen delivery is clearly evident in this example. Low oxygen delivery, complicated by an increased oxygen consumption, results in a need for oxygen extraction to increase. The increased extraction rate can lead to anaerobic metabolism, which may result in acidosis and cell death (see Table 6.9).

These clinical examples have shown the importance of cardiac output to oxygen delivery and the consequences of a low cardiac output on oxygen delivery. Even though oxygen content may be normal, a low cardiac output may severely compromise oxygen delivery and cause oxygen extraction to increase, which may have severe adverse consequences to oxygen utilization by the tissues.

CONCLUSION

Knowledge of the role of cardiac output in oxygen delivery is essential to the delivery of appropriate care for patients in whom oxygen delivery may be compromised. The ability of cardiac output to maintain an adequate delivery in the face of a compromised oxygenation status has been shown by the use of clinical examples.

Knowledge of the role of cardiac output in oxygen delivery is important for the healthcare team so that treatment will be appropriate and provide positive patient outcomes. The ability of cardiac output to compensate for changes in oxygenation gives further evidence of its importance in assessing a patient's oxygenation status.

REFERENCES

1. Barcelona M, Patague L, Bunoy M, Gloriani M, Justice B, Robinson L. "Cardiac output determination by the thermodilution method: Comparison of ice-temperature injectate versus room-temperature injectate contained in pre-filled syringes or a closed-injectate delivery system." *Heart Lung* 1985; 14:232–235.
2. Bryan-Brown C. "Oxygen transport and the oxyhemoglobin dissociation curve." In Beck JL, Sampliner JE (eds). *Handbook of Critical Care*. Boston: Little, Brown, and Company, 1982, 557–578.
3. Dennison RD. "Understanding the four determinants of cardiac output." *Nursing '90* 1990;35–41.
4. Altschule M. "Invalidity of using so-called Starling curves in clinical medicine." *Perspectives in Biology and Medicine* 1983;26:444–445.
5. Shoemaker WC. "Physiologic monitoring of the critically ill patient." In Shoemaker WC, Ayres S, Grenvik A, Holbrook PR, Thompson WL (eds). *Textbook of Critical Care*. Philadelphia: WB Saunders Company, 1989, 145–159.
6. Headley JM. *Invasive Hemodynamic Monitoring: Physiological Principles and Clinical Applications*. Baxter: Edwards Critical Care Division, 33–38.
7. Newton KM. "Cardiac catheterization." *In* Underhill SL, Woods SL, Sivarajan-Froelicher ES, Halpenny CJ (eds). *Cardiac Nursing*. Philadelphia: JB Lippincott, 1989, 440.
8. Armengol J, Godfrey CW, Bolsys AJ. "Effects of the respiratory cycle on cardiac output measurements: Reproducibility of data enhanced by timing the thermodilution injections in dogs." *Crit Care Med.* 1981;9:852–854.
9. Gardner PE, Woods SL. "Hemodynamic monitoring." *In* Underhill SL, Woods SL, Sivarajan-Froelicher ES, Halpenny CJ (eds). *Cardiac Nursing*. Philadelphia: JB Lippincott, 1989, 451–477.
10. Richard C, Thuillez C, Pezzano M, Bottineau G, Giudecelli JF, Auzepy P. "Relationship between mixed venous oxygen saturation and cardiac index in patients with chronic congestive heart failure." *Chest* 1989;95:1289–1294.

TABLE 6.9. Example of Decreased Oxygen Delivery and Increased Extraction Owing to Low Cardiac Output and Increased Oxygen Demands

Patient with History of Heart Failure with UTI

Pa_{O_2} = 90 mm Hg
Sa_{O_2} = 95%
Hgb = 15 gm/dl
CO = 3 l/min
V_{O_2} = 350 ml/min

Oxygen delivery = (1.34 × .95 × 15) × 3 × 10 = 573 ml/min

Oxygen extraction = $\frac{350}{573}$ = 61%

11. Riedinger MS, Shellock FG. "Technical aspects of the thermodilution method for measuring cardiac output." *Heart Lung* 1984;13:215–221.
12. Hruby IM, Woods SL. "Effect of injectate temperature in measurement of thermodilution cardiac output in cardiac surgical patients." *Circulation. Part II* 1983;68:III–222.
13. Ciaccio JM. "Measurement of hemodynamics in side-lying positions: A review of the literature." *Focus on Critical Care* 1990;17:250–254.
14. Doering L, Dracup K. "Comparisons of cardiac output in supine and lateral positions." *Nurs Res* 1988;37:114–118.
15. Daniel MK, Bennett B, Dawson A, Rawles JM. "Haemoglobin concentration and linear cardiac output, peripheral resistance, and oxygen transport." *Br Med J* 1986;292:923–926.
16. Nishimura RA, Miller FA, Callahan MJ, Benassi RC, Seward JB, Tajik JA. "Doppler echocardiography: Theory, instrumentation, technique, and application." *Mayo Clin Proc* 1985;60:321–343.
17. Trang TTH, Tibballs J, Mercier J-C, Beaufils, F. "Optimization of oxygen transport in mechanically ventilated newborns using oximetry and pulsed Doppler-derived cardiac output." *Critical Care Medicine.* 1988, 16: 1094–1097.
18. Schumacker PT, Cain SM. "The concept of a critical oxygen delivery." *Intensive Care Medicine.* 1987, 13: 223–229.
19. Finch CA, Lenfant C. "Oxygen transport in man." *New Engl J Med* 1972;286:407–415.
20. Chappell T, Rubin LJ, Markham Jr.R, Firth BG. "Independence of oxygen consumption and systematic oxygen transport in patients with either stable pulmonary hypertension or refractory left ventricular failure." *Am Rev Respir Dis* 1983;128: 30–33.
21. Ahrens TS. "Concepts in the assessment of oxygenation." *Focus* 1987;14:36–44.

Oxygen Transport

Individual oxygen-transport (or delivery, D_{O_2}) components have been the focus of the preceding chapters. In order to assess oxygen transport correctly, however, all the components must be combined. One common problem currently present in many ICUs is the tendency to use only a single component of oxygen transport, such as, Pa_{O_2} or Sa_{O_2}, to assess overall oxygen transport. The use of a single component of D_{O_2} will be a potential source of error in the overall assessment of D_{O_2}. The focus of this chapter will be to illustrate the integration of all aspects of D_{O_2} in order to make an appropriate assessment.

PRIORITIZING OXYGEN TRANSPORT COMPONENTS

As a general principle, cardiac output (CO) is the most important aspect in oxygen transport. Hemoglobin (Hgb) is the next parameter of importance, with arterial hemoglobin saturation (Sa_{O_2}) and oxygen pressure (Pa_{O_2}) the third and fourth parameters of importance. In any assessment of D_{O_2}, the cardiac output and Hgb play the largest roles in delivering oxygen. If cardiac output and Hgb levels are normal, a large tolerance of abnormal Sa_{O_2} and Pa_{O_2} values is possible (Table 7.1). On the other hand, if the CO and Hgb levels are both abnormal, no change in the Sa_{O_2} or Pa_{O_2} will be able to bring D_{O_2} to within normal values (Table 7.2).

TABLE 7.1. Tolerance of Abnormal Sa_{O_2} and Pa_{O_2} When Cardiac Output and Hemoglobin Levels are Normal

Sample Values	Sa_{O_2}	Pa_{O_2}	Total Oxygen Transport (D_{O_2})
CO 4 Hgb 14	.80	50	600
	.88	56	660
	.92	70	690
CO 5 Hgb 12	.80	50	643
	.88	56	708
	.92	70	740
CO 6 Hgb 12	.80	50	772
	.88	56	849
	.92	70	888

If the cardiac output and hemoglobin levels are normal, maintenance of normal oxygen transport levels is still likely despite very low Sa_{O_2} and Pa_{O_2} levels. Minimal normal D_{O_2} is about 600 cc/min.

The value of the cardiac output in D_{O_2} is the ability of the CO to offset problems in abnormal oxygen content (Ca_{O_2}). For example, if any of the Hgb, Sa_{O_2}, or Pa_{O_2} levels decrease, the CO can increase to maintain D_{O_2}. As long as a person has adequate cardiac function, normal D_{O_2} is likely (Table 7.3).

Unfortunately, the Ca_{O_2} cannot increase to any appreciable extent to offset a loss of cardiac output. The only parameters that can acutely increase the Ca_{O_2} are the Pa_{O_2} and Sa_{O_2}. However, since under normal circumstances the Pa_{O_2} and Sa_{O_2} are already near maximal value, the increase is only slight and cannot increase Ca_{O_2} appreciably (Table 7.4).

TABLE 7.2. Low Cardiac Output (CO) and Hemoglobin (Hgb) Levels Uncompensated by Normal or Elevated Sa_{O_2} and Pa_{O_2} Levels

Sample Values	Sa_{O_2}	Pa_{O_2}	Total Oxygen Transport (D_{O_2})
CO 3 Hgb 10	.96	90	394
	1.00	150	415
CO 3.5 Hgb 11	.96	90	505
CO 3.5 Hgb 11	1.00	150	532

Note, if both CO and Hgb levels are abnormally low, normal (and even above normal) values of Pa_{O_2} and Sa_{O_2} cannot compensate to attain minimal normal D_{O_2} (about 600 cc/min).

TABLE 7.3. Cardiac Output Compensates for Decreases in Oxygen Content (Ca_{O_2})

CO	Hgb	Sa_{O_2}	Pa_{O_2}	Ca_{O_2}	Oxygen Transport (D_{O_2})
5	11	.90	60	13.3	663
6	10	.87	55	11.7	700
7	8	.89	58	9.54	668
9	6	.88	56	7.1	637

Normal Ca_{O_2}, 15–20 cc/dl
Normal D_{O_2}, > 600 cc/min

A normal Ca_{O_2} is important in maintaining D_{O_2}, although an increased CO can compensate to a degree to offset abnormally low Ca_{O_2} levels.

TABLE 7.4. Inability of Increasing Sa_{O_2} and Pa_{O_2} Levels to Significantly Raise Oxygen Content

Patient A starts with the following parameters:

Time	CO	Hgb	Sa_{O_2}	Pa_{O_2}	Ca_{O_2}	Oxygen Transport (D_{O_2})
1200	3.5	12	.88	59	14.3	501

If the Sa_{O_2} and Pa_{O_2} are increased through oxygen therapy:

1300	3.5	12	.96	88	15.7	550

(49 cc increase in D_{O_2})

If the Pa_{O_2} and Sa_{O_2} are further increased through PEEP:

1400	3.5	12	1.00	130	16.5	577

(27 cc increase in D_{O_2})

Further increasing the Pa_{O_2} by maximally increasing the F_{IO_2}:

1500	3.5	12	1.00	200	16.68	585

(7 cc increase in D_{O_2})

Note how increasing the Ca_{O_2} is limited as a compensatory mechanism for a low CO unless the Sa_{O_2} and Pa_{O_2} levels start abnormally low (time 1200 to 1300).

GUIDELINES FOR INDIVIDUAL PARAMETERS

When the clinician is presented with individual components of oxygen transport, care must be taken to avoid making erroneous assessments. This section will attempt to put into a working order how individual parameters should be interpreted relative to total D_{O_2}.

Pa_{O_2}

The Pa_{O_2} should be kept over 60 mm Hg in order to avoid problems in hemoglobin saturation. As long as the Pa_{O_2} is greater than 60 mm Hg, no major clinical decrease in oxygen transport will exist. Somewhat surprisingly, however, Pa_{O_2} levels in excess of 60 mm Hg are frequently desired by clinicians. Despite this tendency, unless a problem with Hgb or CO exists, a Pa_{O_2} level greater than 60 mm Hg generally will not increase D_{O_2} in clinically significant degrees.

A potential value in maintaining Pa_{O_2} levels greater than 60 mm Hg may be in the patient with decreased Hgb, increased dysfunctional Hgb, or a decrease in cardiac output. The small improvement in D_{O_2} with large increases in the Pa_{O_2} may help slightly in the treatment of a low D_{O_2}, at least until more definitive treatment can be employed. If, however, a parameter were to be viewed as minimally helpful in the D_{O_2} assessment, the Pa_{O_2} could be such a parameter.

Sa_{O_2}

Sa_{O_2} provides several useful pieces of information when assessing D_{O_2}. Most importantly, the Sa_{O_2} reveals the amount of oxygen attached to Hgb (oxyhemoglobin levels). Changes in Sa_{O_2} can reflect important changes in D_{O_2}. As a rule, however, as long as the Sa_{O_2} is kept within clinically normal levels (>90%), the Sa_{O_2} does not reveal much information regarding D_{O_2}. For example, a decrease in Sa_{O_2} from .98 to .92 would cause approximately a 6% decrease in D_{O_2}, assuming no change in the cardiac output occurred.

The Sa_{O_2} is also potentially useful from the perspective of generating an approximate Pa_{O_2}, from use of the oxyhemoglobin-dissociation curve. If the clinician wants to know a Pa_{O_2} level, the Sa_{O_2} (or Sp_{O_2}) can give this information. When the clinician has Sa_{O_2} (and Sp_{O_2}) information, less value is obtained from a blood-gas sampling and the Pa_{O_2} levels.

Hemoglobin (Hgb)

Hgb is a key parameter in the assessment of D_{O_2} because it comprises most of the Ca_{O_2}. Normal Hgb levels can act to protect the heart against excessive work and can also allow for variations in Pa_{O_2} and Sa_{O_2} levels without lowering Ca_{O_2} levels to clinically significant levels.

Due to the value of Hgb, a D_{O_2} assessment should include an Hgb analysis as one of the first stages. When the Hgb is low, Ca_{O_2} will be reduced regardless of Sa_{O_2} or Pa_{O_2} levels. On the other hand, if Hgb levels are normal, the patient is protected against changes in Pa_{O_2} and Sa_{O_2} levels.

Cardiac Output

The cardiac output plays the most important role in D_{O_2} owing to the movement of blood containing Hgb. No D_{O_2} measurement should occur without an assessment of cardiac output. However, one of the major limitations in the assessment of oxygenation is the frequent inability to obtain CO values. Currently, CO values are practical only in patients with pulmonary-artery catheters in place. This limitation markedly decreases the clinical availability of CO information.

Without CO data, a complete assessment of D_{O_2} is not possible. The use of physical assessment data, such as blood pressure and heart rate (Chapter 11), are not consistently reliable in estimating CO. The clinician must be aware of the lack of D_{O_2} information if the CO is unavailable. If the D_{O_2} is possibly threatened by clinical conditions that may cause an abnormal CO, a pulmonary-artery catheter is helpful. Because of the importance of the CO in D_{O_2}, the clinician should be familiar with incorporating CO in oxygenation assessment.

CONSUMABLE OXYGEN

The individual concepts involved in oxygen transport have been presented in the preceding chapters. The concept of oxygen transport needs to be further refined from the point of view that not all oxygen apparent in transport is actually available for cellular utilization. Several factors exist that limit how much oxygen is actually available to the cells. These factors exist despite the amount of oxygen that may be indicated by the computation of the forementioned values contributing to oxygen transport, that is, cardiac output, hemoglobin, hemoglobin saturation, and the Pa_{O_2} level. A brief review of these oxygen-limiting factors will be helpful in placing the total oxygen transport in perspective. Two key terms will emerge in this presentation: consumable oxygen and oxygen-extraction rate.

The concept of consumable oxygen refers to hemoglobin's inability to release all the oxygen attached to hemoglobin. The affinity for oxygen by hemoglobin is such that hemoglobin could release, in a maximal setting, only about 80% of the oxygen attached to it.[1] Since hemoglobin can release only some of the attached oxygen, the total oxygen transport calculation does not accurately reflect the amount of oxygen available to the tissues. For example, if the total oxygen transport calculation reveals an oxygen transport of 800 cc, the maximum amount of oxygen that is actually available to the tissues is only 80% of this figure, 640 cc. The clinician needs to be aware that there is not 800 cc of oxygen available to the tissues but only about 640 cc. The concept of consumable oxygen refers to how much oxygen is actually available to be released by hemoglobin.[2]

OXYGEN EXTRACTION

The ability of the tissues to take oxygen from hemoglobin is referred to as oxygen extraction.[3] Oxygen extraction is used as a clinical indicator of how much the tissues are tapping into the reserve of oxygen attached to hemoglobin. The reserve of oxygen on hemoglobin is crucial when one considers that the only true oxygen reserve in the body is that provided by hemoglobin's ability to release more oxygen. Under normal circumstances, hemoglobin releases approximately one fourth of its oxygen (see Chapter 4). Since hemoglobin normally releases one fourth of the available oxygen, but has the ability to release up to 80% of that oxygen, one can readily see that the tissues may extract approximately 50% more oxygen from hemoglobin. The ability for hemoglobin to allow increased oxygen extraction provides the only buffer present in the body to adjust to alterations in oxygen transport or increases in oxygen consumption (V_{O_2}).

Measurement of O_2 Extraction

To obtain the O_2-extraction value, divide V_{O_2} by D_{O_2}.[4] Normal O_2 extractions are between 25 and 30%.[5] While maximal extractions of up to 80% can occur, cellular hypoxia is likely occurring at much lower levels.[6] The O_2-extraction level that is associated with cellular hypoxia is unknown.[7] However, if the O_2-extraction rate is increasing over normal, the potential exists for a worsening cellular oxygenation. The higher the extraction rate, the lower the reserve of oxygen.

The role of oxygen extraction and its application to the clinical setting can be illustrated in the following example. A 54-year-old man is admitted into the ICU with a diagnosis of an acute myocardial infarction. Laboratory data reveal the following information:

Cardiac output	4.1
Cardiac index	2.0
Pa_{O_2}	78
Hemoglobin	12.5
Hemoglobin saturation (Sa_{O_2})	.94
Oxygen consumption	280/cc

Based on this information, the oxygen transport can be calculated at 646 cc/min. Oxygen extraction is obtained by dividing the oxygen transport into the oxygen consumption. Oxygen extraction on this patient is 280/646, yielding a value of approximately .43. From this information, one can see that the oxygen-extraction rate is above the normal 25%, or one fourth, of the oxygen on the hemoglobin. But it is clearly much less than the maximal extraction rates of about 80%. As the oxygen-extraction rate increases, an increased likelihood for cellular hypoxia exists. Since there is no clear indicator of when an O_2-extraction rate becomes clinically threatening, an O_2 extraction of .43 simply serves as a warning to the clinician that an increasing cellular threat to oxygenation is developing. If one is to use a guideline for O_2-extraction rates, one empirical guideline is that as O_2-extraction rates climb in excess of 50%, the potential exists for cellular hypoxia to be present. No research studies, however, have consistently confirmed this level.

Limitations of the O_2 Extraction

The key limitation in using O_2 extraction is in situations where cellular dysoxia or the inability to properly process oxygen is present. This process is discussed in more depth in Chapter 9. In cellular dysoxia, the inability of the cells to consume oxygen through expected mechanisms exists. Reasons for problems in oxygen utilization can be multiple, including such problems as microembolization, decreasing capillary density in the tissue area, increased capillary permeability, and changes in ion concentrations. Regardless of the reason, the oxygen-extraction rate may not accurately reflect cellular oxygenation.[8] For example, the lack of perfusion to an area caused by microembolization will cause oxygenated blood to bypass the tissues and re-enter the venous circulation without having oxygen substantially withdrawn. The bypassing of blood past tissues causes an apparent decrease in the oxygen consumption. When one computes the oxygen-extraction ratio, the decreased oxygen consumption is reflected in the numerator of the oxygen extraction equation. This decreased numerator generates an apparently low oxygen-extraction rate. Several clinical studies have described examples of near-normal or slightly elevated extraction rates existing while cellular hypoxia was likely to have been demonstrated.[9–10]. The clinical condition most commonly associated with this situation is sepsis. When cellular dysoxia may be present, the oxygen-extraction rate will be limited in its effectiveness as a warning sign of cellular hypoxia.

SUMMARY

The concept of oxygen transport is the basis for assessing many clinical interventions. Each individual component in D_{O_2} is important, but the clinician should keep in mind the factors which most likely impact D_{O_2}: cardiac output and Hgb. In addition, use of any single component, without assessing total D_{O_2}, increases the likelihood of misinterpreting D_{O_2}.

The clinician must be aware that oxygen transport is calculated from the standard oxygen-transport equation and does not take into account key factors such as the limited amount of oxygen that hemoglobin can release. The term "consumable oxygen" should be applied whenever doing an oxygen-transport computation.

In addition, the concept of oxygen extraction can be applied to estimate the degree of cellular hypoxia that may be developing. Although no specific number correlation is present between oxygen extraction and the degree of cellular hypoxia, the clinician can be aware that if cellular hypoxia develops, the oxygen-extraction rate usually will increase. The primary exception to this guideline is in the example of sepsis. For the patient who develops sepsis or some other dysoxia problem, the oxygen extraction rate will no longer accurately reflect cellular oxygenation status. The following examples help illustrate the clinical application of oxygen delivery concepts presented in this chapter.

Example 1

A 71-year-old woman with the diagnosis of chronic bronchitis is admitted to the ICU with complaints of shortness of breath, although no orthopnea exists. A pulmonary-artery catheter is inserted to differentiate cardiac versus pulmonary origin of the shortness of breath. Lung sounds reveal scattered crackles that are independent of position change. She has slight circumoral cyanosis. The following laboratory and clinical information is available:

BP	134/84
P	104
CO	4.9
CI	2.6
Pa_{O_2}	57 mm Hg
Sa_{O_2}	.88
Hgb	16 gm/dl

Based on the above information, does this person have an adequate oxygen transport?

ANSWER

The oxygen content and transport can be calculated as follows:

$$Ca_{O_2} = 1.34 \times 16 \times .88 = 18.9 \text{ cc/dl}$$
$$\text{(normal 15–20 cc/dl)}$$

$$D_{O_2} = 18.9 \times 10 \times 4.9 = 926 \text{ cc/dl}$$

Based on the above calculations, her oxygen content and transport are both within normal limits. The cyanosis, crackles, and shortness of breath do not reflect oxygen transport, potentially misleading the clinician into assuming that the patient has abnormal oxygenation. For example, the shortness of breath may be caused by intrapulmonary factors or a hypoxemia drive to breathe, not by a low oxygen transport. The origin of the shortness of breath does not appear related to cardiac limitations, based on the normal oxygen transport and cardiac output. The cyanosis does not interfere with oxygen content because of the high hemoglobin level.

Example 2

A 34-year-old man is admitted to the ICU for observaton following potential chest injury from a motor-vehicle accident. The x-rays are negative for head, neck, or rib fractures. A pulmonary-artery catheter is inserted to aid in the observation. Initial readings are obtained at 0200. At 0300, he complains of increased chest discomfort. Lung sounds remain clear and the pulse oximeter remains constant at 100%. Repeat readings reveal the following:

	0200	0300
BP	118/72	100/58 (decrease on inspiration)
P	104	112
RR	18	28
Pa_{O_2}	100	104
FI_{O_2}	.40	.40
Sp_{O_2}	1.00	1.00
Hgb	13	13
CO	5.1	3.4
CI	2.6	1.7

Based on the above information, what is occurring regarding oxygen transport?

ANSWER

The oxygen transport has markedly decreased from 0200 (D_{O_2} 888 cc/min) to 0300 (592 cc/min). The reason for this decrease is a decreased cardiac output, which appears unassociated with blood loss (stable hemoglobin). The patient may be developing a pericardial tamponade and needs to be aggressively assessed and treated. The stable Sp_{O_2} and Pa_{O_2} reflect a stable intrapulmonary shunt. Since lung function has not been altered, no change in parameters reflecting pulmonary gas exchange should be expected.

Example 3

A 78-year-old woman with the diagnosis of acute myocardial infarction is in her second day in ICU. She develops mild orthopnea at 1500 and complains of shortness of breath. Analyses of her hemodynamics and blood gases reveal the following:

Pa_{O_2}	65 mm Hg
Sp_{O_2}	.94 (Assume Sp_{O_2} = Sa_{O_2})
Hgb	12.1 gm/dl
CO	3.7 l/min
CI	2.1 l/m²
PA	36/20
PCWP	18 mm Hg
CVP	9 mm Hg

The physician requests that the FI_{O_2} be increased from the current 2 l/min to 6 l/min. Assuming no other parameters change, how much will the D_{O_2}

improve if the Pa_{O_2} increases to 81 mm Hg and the Sp_{O_2} to .97?

ANSWER

Calculating the D_{O_2} reveals a change from 571 cc/min to 591 cc/min. The increase in the FI_{O_2} would be considered a minor improvement in oxygen transport. A more important therapy is in the improvement of the cardiac output. For comparison purposes, assume the cardiac output increases from 3.7 to 4.7 l/min. The change in D_{O_2} would be from 571 cc/min to 726 cc/min. This is a much more substantial improvement in oxygen transport and is more likely to improve her current symptoms.

REFERENCES

1. Miller MJ. "Tissue oxygenation in clinical medicine: An historical review." *Anes Anal* 1982;61:527.
2. Bryan-Brown C, Baek S, Makabali G, Shoemaker W. "Consumable oxygen: Availability of oxygen in relation to oxyhemoglobin dissociation." *Crit Care Med* 1973;1:17.
3. Veremakis C. "Hemodynamic monitoring." *In* Kirby RR, Taylor RW (eds). *Respiratory Failure.* Chicago: Year Book Medical Pubs, 1986,563.
4. Downs JB. "Monitoring oxygen delivery in acute respiratory failure." *Resp Care* 1983;28:608.
5. Ahrens, TS. "Concepts in the assessment of oxygenation." *Focus on Crit Care* 1987;14:36.
6. Bryan-Brown WC. "Gas transport and delivery." *In* Shoemaker WC, Thompson WL, Holbrook RR (eds). *Textbook of Critical Care.* Philadelphia: WB Saunders, 1984,212.
7. Bryan-Brown CW, Gutierrez G. "Gas transport and delivery." *In* Shoemaker WC, Ayres S, Grenvik A, et al. (eds). *Textbook of Critical Care.* Philadelphia: WB Saunders, 1989,491.
8. Snyder JV. "Assessment of systemic oxygen transport." *In* Snyder JV, Pinsky MR (eds). *Oxygen Transport in the Critically Ill.* Chicago: Year Book Medical Pubs, 1987,179.
9. Shoemaker WC, Appel PL, Kram HB. "Tissue oxygen debt as a determinant of lethal and non lethal postoperative organ failure." *Crit Care Med* 1988; 16:1117.
10. Weg JG. "Oxygen transport in adult respiratory distress syndrome and other acute circulatory problems: Relationship of oxygen delivery and oxygen consumption." *Crit Care Med* 1991;19:650–57.

Part III

Oxygen Consumption (V_{O_2}) and Cellular Assessment of Oxygenation

8
Oxygen Consumption (V_{O_2})

The concept of oxygen consumption (V_{O_2}) addresses the cellular requirements for oxygen. How much oxygen is utilized by the cells is one of the key determining factors in the adequacy of oxygenation. Oxygen transport has to be present in sufficient quantities to supply the amounts of oxygen required by the cells. Normally, V_{O_2} is independent of oxygen transport and varies according to the cellular need for oxygen. In critically ill patients with specific disease entities such as ARDS and sepsis, evidence exists that indicates oxygen consumption may become dependent upon oxygen transport. When V_{O_2} becomes dependent on oxygen transport, research suggests cellular hypoxia may be developing. Due to the importance of understanding how much oxygen is being consumed in order to determine the adequacy of oxygenation, the concept of oxygen consumption is a major component in the assessment of oxygenation, particularly in the critically ill patient.

Clinical measurement of oxygen consumption is not always available on patients in critical care settings. V_{O_2} is the type of concept with which many clinicians are unfamiliar, despite the importance of V_{O_2} in understanding oxygenation. The lack of readily available measurements in V_{O_2} may be a major reason why clinicians are unfamiliar with the V_{O_2} concept. In order to address the potential unfamiliarity with V_{O_2}, techniques for measuring oxygen consump-

tion are presented first in this chapter. Then, clinical use of V_{O_2} will be the focus in the second part of this chapter. Through this presentation, the application and value of V_{O_2} will be better appreciated.

MEASUREMENT OF OXYGEN CONSUMPTION

Normal oxygen consumption levels are generally about 3.5 cc/kg/min, or can be defined as 150–300 cc/m²/min.[1-2] Oxygen consumption values are a function of the body size of a person; a larger body size requires a higher O_2 consumption. Measurement of oxygen consumption is typically done by one of three methods: (1) estimation, (2) measurement of exhaled gases, and (3) use of the Fick equation.

The first method is not actually a direct measurement but an estimation of V_{O_2}. It is based on the general concept that most people require about 3.5 cc of oxygen per kilogram of body weight.[3] A 70-kilo person has an estimated oxygen consumption of 245 cc/min (3.5 cc × 70 kg = 245 cc). This method is, however, simply an estimation and is not considered adequate when trying to determine the adequacy of a patient's oxygenation status. This estimation is useful as a ballpark figure in regard to a general concept of oxygenation. Its primary use is in a stable population that is not at risk for oxygenation disturbances.

Direct measurement of oxygen consumption typically occurs by one of two methods. The first method is the most accurate, that is, the direct measurement of oxygen consumption through the use of exhaled gas analysis. The formula for measuring oxygen consumption is given in Table 8.1.

The measurement of oxygen consumption through exhaled gases is technically not difficult but has many clinical and technical exceptions that make its application less than easy. In order to measure V_{O_2}, one needs to be able to measure the volume of air that is inspired or expired by the patient and multiply it by the difference between the inspired and expired gas concentrations, specifically inspired and expired oxygen concentration ($V_{O_2} = V_E (F_{IO_2} - F_{EO_2})$). The formula that is given here is a simplified formula that is clinically accurate but is not ideal because it does not take into account other gas changes and gas compositions, such as nitrogen. A more specific formula is included in Table 8.1. In addition, V_E must be converted from the measurement obtained via a spirometer (or flow transducer) to a standard V_E, which compensates for varying atmospheric pressures and temperatures. The formula for this conversion is listed in Table 8.2.

For clinical purposes, this simple exhaled gas equation is adequate. To perform this measurement one needs a relatively simple piece of equipment such as a spirometer (to

measure the volume of air inspired or expired) and a relatively complicated piece of equipment, a gas analyzer (to measure the expired and inspired gases). Many techniques exist for collecting and measuring the gas, ranging from direct collection of the gas, through a collection system such as a Douglas bag, to the end-line sampling of inspired and expired gases through various types of metabolic systems (Figures 8.1 and 8.2).

The collection of the inspired volume and the measurement of the gases have several technical difficulties that limit the ease of use of this technique. Technical problems of gas measurement include the limited accuracy of direct gas measurement with oxygen concentrations in excess of 50% and the difficulty in getting a sample gas that is free of any contamination with atmospheric air.[4-6] Measurement of exhaled gases requires very careful collection in order to prevent any contamination with

TABLE 8.2.   Adjustment of Minute Ventilation (V_E)

V_E is normally converted from
$V_{E_{ATPS}}$ Atmospheric temperature and pressure of a gas

to

$V_{E_{STPO}}$ standard temperature and pressure of a dry gas by the following formula:

$$V_{E_{STPO}} = V_{E_{ATPS}} \times \left(\frac{273}{273 + T°C}\right) \times \left(\frac{P_B - P_{H_2O}}{760}\right)$$

TABLE 8.1.   Measurement of Oxygen Consumption Through Exhaled Gas

Simplest Formula

Oxygen consumption = minute ventilation (V_E) $\times$ $F_{IO_2} - F_{EO_2}$)
Where F_{IO_2} = fraction of inspired oxygen
Where F_{EO_2} = fraction of expired oxygen
V_E = amount of air expired in one minute

More Accurate Formula

$$V_{O_2} = V_E(\frac{F_{IN_2} - F_{IO_2}}{F_{EN_2} - F_{EO_2}} - F_{EO_2}) - F_{EO_2}$$

Where F_{IN_2} = Fraction of inspired nitrogen
F_{EN_2} = Fraction of expired nitrogen

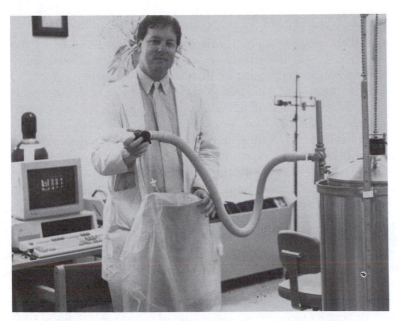

FIGURE 8.1. Measurement of oxygen consumption with exhaled gas bags. Collection of exhaled air via large (50-l) gas bags is cumbersone but accurate.

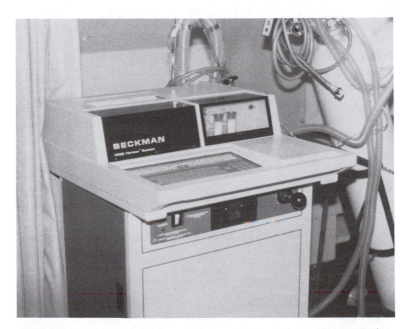

FIGURE 8.2. Use of metabolic carts for measurement of oxygen consumption. The use of metabolic carts has improved the ease of measurement of oxygen consumption and carbon-dioxide production. These systems are useful but are considered relatively expensive and still labor intensive.

atmospheric air. If atmospheric air is entrained, V$_{O_2}$ is quickly rendered inaccurate owing to the change in inspired (or expired) gas concentrations.

An example of oxygen-consumption gas analysis can be illustrated in the following data: Assume a patient has a ventilation of 6 l/min, a F$_{IO_2}$ (fraction of inspired oxygen) of 40%, and a F$_{EO_2}$ (fraction of expired oxygen) of 35%. Multiplying the 6 l/min (or 6,000 cc) by 40% and subtracting 35% gives the value of 300 cc/min.

Another method for measuring oxygen consumption is through an application of the Fick equation given in Table 8.3. Applying the indirect Fick equation is not as accurate as actually measuring the exhaled gas.[7-8] However, measurement of oxygen consumption through the Fick equation allows the approximate measurement of oxygen consumption.[9-10] To measure oxygen consumption through this method, one needs simultaneous measurements of cardiac output, arterial and mixed-venous oxygen saturations, and hemoglobin levels. The Fick equation allows more practical clinical applications of V$_{O_2}$. V$_{O_2}$ can be performed via the Fick equation without exhaled gas collection and simply requires a pulmonary catheter to be in place. An example of the Fick equation for calculating O$_2$ consumption follows:

1. CO = 5 l/min
2. Hgb = 15 gm/dl
3. Sa$_{O_2}$ (arterial hemoglobin saturation) = 100%
4. S$\bar{v}_{O_2}$ (venous hemoglobin saturation) = 75%

These values yield an arterial oxygen content of 20.1 and a venous oxygen content of 15.1, to give a net arterial venous content difference of 5 (20.1 − 15.1 = 5). The cardiac output of 5, multiplied by the arterial venous content of 5 and then multiplied by 10, gives an O$_2$ consumption of 250 cc/min (5 × 5 × 10 = 250). Measurement of oxygen consumption by the Fick equation is not difficult, particularly since its measurement is incorporated automatically in many newer bedside monitoring systems. With the advent of continuous arterial and venous oximetry and cardiac outputs, the frequent measurement of oxygen consumption becomes possible without laboratory data. See Table 8.4 and Figure 8.3.

OXYGEN CONSUMPTION AND OXYGEN DELIVERY

Oxygen consumption is normally independent of oxygen transport. Under normal circumstances, oxygen consumption is dependent on cellular levels of ADP. Changes in oxygen consumption based on changing

TABLE 8.4. Use of S$\bar{v}_{O_2}$, Sp$_{O_2}$, and Cardiac Output (10) to Measure V$_{O_2}$ Without Laboratory Blood Samples

	0600	0900	0800	0900
Measured Values				
Sp$_{O_2}$	.96	.94	.98	.98
S$\bar{v}_{O_2}$	.64	.65	.58	.62
CO	4.3	5.0	3.9	4.2
Hgb	9.5	9.5	9.5	9.5
Calculated Values				
Ca$_{O_2}$	12.2	12	12.5	12.5
C$\bar{v}_{O_2}$	8.15	8.3	7.4	7.9
V$_{O_2}$	166	185	199	193

Assume Sp$_{O_2}$ = Sa$_{O_2}$

Ca$_{O_2}$ = 1.34 × Hgb × Sa$_{O_2}$
C$\bar{v}_{O_2}$ = 1.34 × Hgb × S$\bar{v}_{O_2}$

$$V_{O_2} = (Ca_{O_2} - C\bar{v}_{O_2}) \times 10 \times CO$$

TABLE 8.3. Measurement of O$_2$ Consumption by Fick Equation

Oxygen consumption = cardiac output × (Ca$_{O_2}$ − C$\bar{v}_{O_2}$) × 10
Where Ca$_{O_2}$ = arterial oxygen content
C$\bar{v}_{O_2}$ = venous oxygen content

The 10 represents a constant to correct for the difference between the cardiac output, which is measured in liters, and the O$_2$ content, which is measured in deciliters.

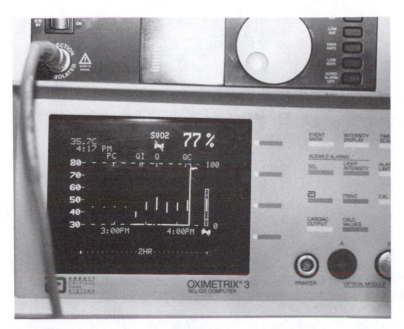

FIGURE 8.3. Simultaneous use of pulse and mixed-venous oximetry. The use of dual pulse and venous oximetry allows several computations to be possible, including those for intrapulmonary shunt, cardiac output, and oxygen consumption analysis. These functions can be manual or automated.

levels of cellular ADP may dictate the need for oxygen transport to adapt. For example, as the need for oxygen increases, as with exercise, oxygen transport will need to increase to keep pace with the increased need for oxygen. Normally this would be accomplished by an increase in cardiac output.

If oxygen transport changes, oxygen consumption normally will be unaffected. For example, if oxygen transport decreases, oxygen consumption will be unchanged. Normally if the oxygen transport falls, the oxygen consumption is maintained by extracting more oxygen off hemoglobin (resulting in a reduced venous-hemoglobin oxygen saturation, $S\bar{v}_{O_2}$). The same situation applies during times of increased requirements for oxygen. Again using exercise as an example, as oxygen consumption increases, oxygen transport increases in an attempt to match the increase in consumption. As the increase in consumption is unable to be matched by an increase in transport, the Sv_{O_2} level starts to decrease. Eventually the exercise must stop due to

the increasing imbalance between oxygen transport and consumption.

There is developing research evidence that supports the independence of oxygen consumption from oxygen transport as a normal adaptive response. An abnormal response is when oxygen consumption becomes dependent on oxygen transport.[11-13] Oxygen consumption has been identified in several disease states, specifically ARDS and sepsis, as related to O_2 transport at a point where cellular hypoxia is likely to occur.[14-15] The point of hypoxia is often referred to as a critical O_2 point (Figure 8.4).

This critical O_2 point has been estimated at an oxygen delivery (D_{O_2}) of about 330 ml/ m^2/min in anesthetized patients.[16] This estimate was obtained in a relatively small number of patients but can serve as a warning point. For nurses, the clinical significance of the potential V_{O_2} dependence on oxygen transport is that oxygenation assessment must not take place without always considering the relationship between oxygen transport and consumption. The rela-

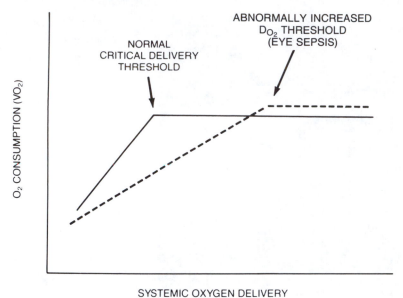

FIGURE 8.4.   Critical oxygenation point. When oxygen consumption becomes dependent on oxygen transport, cellular hypoxia is likely. Normally, V_{O_2} is independent of oxygen transport (horizontal line). At locations on the angled line, oxygen consumption is dependent on oxygen transport and potentially represents cellular hypoxia.

tionship between O_2 transport and O_2 consumption may indicate the point where cellular hypoxia is present. This relationship is not assessed with most traditional methods of monitoring oxygenation. For example, oxygen transport is primarily influenced by the cardiac output and hemoglobin. If these levels are adequate, the clinician may assume oxygenation is acceptable. However, when applying oxygen consumption simultaneously with oxygen transport, the clinician might find that despite normal oxygen transport levels, oxygenation may be threatened if a dependence of O_2 consumption on O_2 transport can be identified. In patients with sepsis, for example, high oxygen transports are associated with critical O_2 points. From a practical point of view, clinicians must be aware that management of oxygen consumption in conjunction with oxygen transport is a necessary component of the oxygenation assessment.[17]

Some controversy exists over the relationship between V_{O_2} and D_{O_2}. Some authors have questioned the measurement of V_{O_2} by the Fick equation as not accurate enough to establish a V_{O_2}/D_{O_2} relationship.[18-19] Others have defended the use of the Fick equation as opposed to exhaled gas analysis as acceptable.[20-21] Regardless of the V_{O_2}/D_{O_2} relationship, the clinician must be aware of the importance of including V_{O_2} in combination with D_{O_2} in an oxygenation assessment.

In clinical practice, O_2 consumption measurements are frequently unavailable. Spot measurements of O_2 consumption can help identify a relationship between oxygen transport and O_2 consumption, but this is not necessarily easy to do. Only with continuous measurements of O_2 consumption is one likely to establish a dependence on transport. One of the clinical problems that must be addressed is what to do when making an assessment of oxygenation if O_2 consumption is unavailable.

If oxygen consumption data is unavailable, the clinician must make an assessment of oxygenation incorporating as many other parameters as possible. In patients with sepsis or ARDS, oxygen transport should be kept as high as possible.[22-23] The clinician can help protect the patient from cellular hypoxia by ensuring high oxygen transport. The clinician can also encourage or perform V_{O_2} measurements, particularly if the data is available. Maintaining trends of V_{O_2} and D_{O_2} can also help identify the V_{O_2}/D_{O_2} relationship. Tables 8.5 and 8.6 illustrate a dependent and independent V_{O_2}/D_{O_2} relationship based on trend analysis.

Oxygen consumption's relationship with oxygen transport is difficult to predict despite the use of other available methods. For example, $S\bar{v}_{O_2}$ levels are one of the better indicators of the balance of oxygenation. $S\bar{v}_{O_2}$, however, may not accurately indicate when O_2 consumption becomes dependent on oxygen transport. While $S\bar{v}_{O_2}$ can be used to help calculate oxygen consumption, $S\bar{v}_{O_2}$ changes by themselves have not been shown through research to mirror the critical oxygen point.[24] $S\bar{v}_{O_2}$ values should be used, however, whenever possible to allow for measurement of oxygen consumption (via Fick equation) in the absence of exhaled gas analysis.

One point that is also important to keep in mind is that oxygenation may not be adequately reflected even when measuring

TABLE 8.6. Independence of Oxygen Consumption on Oxygen Transport Identified Through Trend Analysis

	1000	1100	1200	1300	1400
Pa_{O_2}	64	71	84	76	80
Sa_{O_2}	91%	92%	95%	93%	94%
$S\bar{v}_{O_2}$	64%	61%	53%	53%	62%
Hgb	10	10.2	10.2	10.2	10.6
CO	4.5	4.1	3.4	3.5	4.7
CI	2.5	2.3	1.9	1.9	2.6
D_{O_2}	549	516	441	445	628
D_{O_2}/m^2	305	287	245	247	349
V_{O_2}	163	174	195	191	214
V_{O_2}/m^2	91	97	108	106	118

In this trend, notice how oxygen consumption changes independently (usually in the opposite direction) of oxygen transport. This is a normal response of the oxygen consumption/transport relationship.

both oxygen transport and oxygen consumption. The possibility of dysoxia or the inability to properly utilize oxygen should be considered. Whether dysoxia is due to mitochondria dysfunction, increased distance between the capillaries and the cell, or other reasons, an inability to properly process oxygen may exist despite adequate levels of oxygen transport and consumption. Cellular inability to utilize oxygen reminds us of the difficulty in making assessments of oxygenation, particularly without examining cellular functions. Understanding oxygen consumption and its relation to oxygen transport may improve our assessment of oxygenation. However, it is still important to keep in mind that our current knowledge of oxygenation assessment is limited without an assessment of cellular oxygenation.

CLINICAL EXAMPLES

TABLE 8.5. Dependence of Oxygen Consumption on Oxygen Transport Identified Through Trend Analysis

	0100	0200	0300	0400	0500
Pa_{O_2}	87	91	76	81	100
Pa_{CO_2}	37	32	39	41	38
Sa_{O_2}	96%	96%	93%	94%	98%
$S\bar{v}_{O_2}$	57%	51%	49%	50%	52%
Hgb	11	11.5	11.5	11.1	10.9
CO	3.9	5.1	6.1	8.1	7.2
CI	2.3	3.0	3.6	4.8	4.2
D_{O_2}	552	754	874	1132	1031
D_{O_2}/m^2	324	443	514	666	606
V_{O_2}	224	354	414	530	484
V_{O_2}/m^2	132	208	244	312	285

In this example, notice how the oxygen consumption tracks the changes in oxygen transport. This dependence indicates a potential pathological relationship between consumption and transport and may indicate cellular hypoxia despite high oxygen transport levels.

Example 1

A 43-year-old man, 78 kg, is admitted into the ICU following a right colectomy. Initial postoperative course was unremarkable until a fever developed on the third postoperative day. He became short of breath and within about 12 hours felt marked respiratory distress. He was transferred to the ICU with the following blood gases: pH 7.27, Pa_{CO_2} 28, Pa_{O_2} 63, Sa_{O_2} .91, $F_{I_{O_2}}$ 50%, bicarbonate (HCO_3) 17, hemoglobin 13, lactate 5.3 mmol. Vital signs indicated blood pressure of 86/52, pulse 123, respiratory rate 38, temperature 39.9°C. A pulmonary catheter was inserted and revealed the following information: pulmonary-artery pressure was 42/25, pulmonary-capillary wedge pressure 11, CVP 6, cardiac output 11.2, cardiac index 6.9, $S\bar{v}_{O_2}$ .73. Based on this information, answer the following questions:

(1) What is this person's oxygen transport and oxygen consumption?
(2) Does the estimated oxygen consumption approximate the measured oxygen consumption?
(3) Does an oxygenation imbalance exist?

ANSWERS

1) The oxygen transport is obtained by computing the following data:

$$Ca_{O_2} \times CO \times 10 = D_{O_2}$$

$(1.34 \times 13 \times .91) \times 11.2 \times 10 = 1775$ cc/min

The oxygen consumption is obtained by computing the following data:

$$(Ca_{O_2} - Cv_{O_2}) \times CO \times 10 = V_{O_2}$$

$[(1.34 \times 13 \times .91) - (1.34 \times 13 \times .73)] \times 11.2$
$\times 10 = 351$ cc

2) Estimated oxygen consumption is obtained by the following computation:

Body weight (in kgs) $\times$ 3.5 cc/min

78 kg $\times$ 3.5 = 273 cc/min

In this case, the estimated oxygen consumption is markedly dissimilar from the measured oxygen consumption (273 cc estimated V_{O_2}, 351 cc measured V_{O_2}). Keep in mind, the measured oxygen consumption is preferred in clinical situations. Estimations are utilized only in the absence of measured V_{O_2}.
3) Despite high D_{O_2} levels, a metabolic acidosis and high lactate level exists. The high D_{O_2} level may not be adequate for this V_{O_2}. When a high D_{O_2} exists in the face of a higher than expected V_{O_2}, the D_{O_2} may not be adequate.

Example 2

A 33-year-old woman is admitted to the ICU with complaints of dyspnea on exertion and a history of cardiomyopathy. You do not want to estimate oxygen consumption, but you need to determine if the cardiac output is adequate. A measured O_2 consumption measurement is requested. The

F_{IO_2} is 30%, the F_{EO_2} is 27%, and the minute ventilation is 15 liters. Based on this information, what is this patient's oxygen consumption?

ANSWER

396 cc. This answer was obtained by subtracting F_{EO_2} (27% oxygen) from the F_{IO_2} 30% oxygen and multiplying the difference times the Vestro of 13.2 LPM. (.30 − .27) × 15 = 396 cc.

Example 3

A 63-year-old man with the diagnosis of recurring colon cancer is admitted into the ICU with symptoms of acute shortness of breath. A pulmonary catheter is inserted and reveals the following information. Based on this information, does a dependent or independent relationship exist between V_{O_2} and D_{O_2}?

			Time		
	0600	0700	0800	0900	1000
Arterial hemoglobin saturation Sa_{O_2}	91%	88%	92%	93%	98%
$S\bar{v}_{O_2}$ level	58%	54%	59%	62%	48%
Hemoglobin	10	10	10	9.5	9.5
Cardiac output	4.2	5	6	6.5	6.5
D_{O_2}	512	590	740	770	811
V_{O_2}	186	228	265	257	414

ANSWER

Based on the above information, an apparent dependent relationship exists between D_{O_2} and V_{O_2}. While at 0900 V_{O_2} and D_{O_2} change independently, the change is within measurement error; that is, very little change has occurred. The overall consistency in the change in V_{O_2} and D_{O_2} lends evidence of a potential pathologic relationship between V_{O_2} and D_{O_2}.

ECONOMIC IMPLICATIONS OF OXYGEN CONSUMPTION MEASUREMENT

The measurement of oxygen consumption has some practically difficult clinical questions. If V_{O_2} is measured continuously with exhaled gas analysis, a rather expensive and labor-intensive operation will be necessary. Cost justification of this type of set-up has not been demonstrated. This does not mean the system is without value, but no overt evidence suggests continuous measurement of oxygen consumption will change patient outcome. Studies could be performed which may actually show that continuous oxygen consumption is very useful, but, at this point in time, these studies remain to be performed.

Fortunately, use of V_{O_2} is getting easier. Oxygen consumption can be calculated relatively easily if nurses have at their disposal new types of bedside monitoring that have the ability to do computations of oxygenation data. The most that would be required of the nurse at this point would be to enter the data for the computations. Some computer systems already allow for automatic data entry with communications through laboratory systems. In any event, if the monitoring equipment can perform computations, O_2 consumption does not become a difficult task, except it will require the measurement of a $S\bar{v}_{O_2}$ blood-gas sample. A $S\bar{v}_{O_2}$ blood-gas sample has its own inherent cost unless the patient has a continuous $S\bar{v}_{O_2}$ reading available from a pulmonary catheter. Continuous $S\bar{v}_{O_2}$ catheter has increased expense associated with it, but it is still a relatively inexpensive method of continuous oxygen-consumption measurement. At this point in time, the best method is a pulmonary catheter that has continuous $S\bar{v}_{O_2}$-monitoring capabilities and allows for continuous assessment of oxygen consumption. All this is more expensive than a normal pulmonary catheter, but it also provides information unavailable from the normal pulmonary catheter. Through use of the Fick equation utilizing the $S\bar{v}_{O_2}$ value, V_{O_2} information may make an important contribution to oxygenation through the establishment of critical O_2 points.

OXYGEN CONSUMPTION AND ENERGY MEASUREMENT

Oxygen consumption has been used for most of this century as a mechanism to estimate how many Calories (kcal) are being consumed.[25] The use of oxygen consumption measurements and the measurements

of Caloric requirements (energy expenditure) add to the assessment of oxygen consumption. These measurements can be of substantial use in the critically ill patient. Through measuring oxygen consumption, the appropriate kcal needs can be provided. Nutritional support services and unit dietitians can utilize oxygen consumption to help determine their kcal regimes for the critically ill patient.

Oxygen consumption was first identified as the mechanism to measure energy expenditure in the early 20th century.[26] This concept of measuring kcal expenditure through oxygen consumption is called indirect calorimetry.[27] Direct calorimetry, or the measurement of kcal expenditure through measurement of heat loss, is and has been considered the best mechanism by which to measure energy expenditure.[28] Unfortunately, the measurement of heat loss in a person is difficult to perform in the environment of the critically ill. Direct calorimetry requires specially constructed rooms or suites to measure heat production in the body. The equipment involved in direct calorimetry is both complex and expensive.

Heat loss as the basis for assessing Caloric needs can be understood through the definition of Calorie. Calorie is defined as the amount of heat necessary to raise one kilogram of water one degree centigrade (from 14.5 to 15.5°C).[29] The term kilocalorie is used when the measure of heat that is raising water is measured by one kilogram of water, as is the case when measuring the energy value of food. The term "kilocalorie" (kcal) is more appropriate than "Calorie" when discussing the body's nutritional needs, and so will henceforth be used in this text.

Direct calorimetry chambers have been constructed for the measurement of energy expenditure, but the elaborateness of these chambers or the body-encircling measurement systems that are necessary, make this method of assessing energy expenditure impractical in the critical care setting (Figure 8.5).

Indirect calorimetry, or the measurement

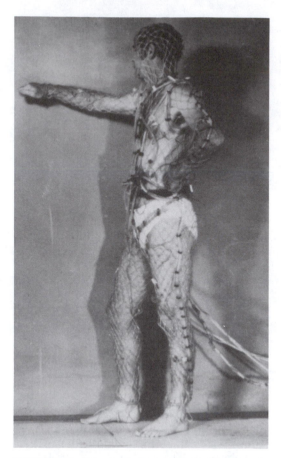

FIGURE 8.5. Direct calorimetry. Direct calorimetry is the ideal form of measurement of caloric expenditure. However, the systems that require measurement of heat loss, as illustrated in this body suit, are frequently impractical. From Webb P. *Human Calorimeters*. New York: Praeger, 1985.

of oxygen consumption, can be used in place of direct calorimetry to estimate energy expenditure through the following principles. Through direct calorimetry measurements, the amount of kilocalories consumed during catabolism can be extrapolated to oxygen consumption. For example, for every 1,000 cc of oxygen consumed, 4.8 kilocalories will be utilized.[30] The 4.8 kilocalories varies slightly depending on the substrate utilized for energy (i.e., fats, carbohydrates, or proteins), but is a good approximation of the number of kilocalories used as oxygen is consumed. Subsequently, if oxygen consumption is known and multiplied by 4.8, one can determine how many

kilocalories will be used in a given period of time. If 1000 cc of oxygen are consumed, then approximately 4.8 kilocalories have been spent. The measurement of oxygen consumption multiplied by 4.8, in conjunction with the length of the activity measured, can generate how many kilocalories will be consumed during a given period of time.

If a person consumes 250 cc of oxygen for one minute, then the number of kilocalories consumed in that time can be computed by multiplying .250 (or one fourth of 1000 cc) by 4.8, yielding a total number of kilocalories consumed in that 1 minute of about 1.2 kcal (.250 × 1 × 4.8 = 1.2).

In the critical care population the interest is in measuring how many kilocalories a person needs over a given period of time, specifically, one day. The correct number of kilocalories is helpful to avoid problems with either under- or overfeeding patients. If a person has an O_2 consumption of 200 cc per minute for an entire 24-hour time period, the total number of kilocalories necessary for that patient is obtained by multiplying .200 by the number of minutes in a day (1,440) by 4.8. This patient uses approximately 1,440 kilocalories per day (.200 × 1,440 × 4.8). Controversy exists over the use of a single measurement of V_{O_2} to determine daily Caloric needs, particularly considering the changing metabolic needs of the critically ill patient.[31-33] The single measurement of V_{O_2} is best analyzed as a rough estimate of daily energy needs, rather than as a precise indicator of daily Caloric needs.

The use of single measurements in the use of energy estimation has led to questioning the cost benefit of the measurements, since other estimates, such as the Harris–Benedict equation, are possible based on physical characteristics.[34-35] However, no estimation method is consistently accurate. The V_{O_2} measurement does give an accurate picture of what is occurring at the time of measurement. From this perspective, V_{O_2} is more accurate than other estimates of caloric need. Whether it is cost effective in changing patient outcome is yet to be demonstrated.

Weight Loss
as a Nutritional Tool

Measurement of oxygen consumption has several clinical applications. The most obvious one is the understanding of the caloric need of the patient in a critical care setting. It also helps to point to an observation that helps allow for better nutritional assessments of patients in ICU settings. For example, the concept of weight loss in both a critical care and normal population setting can be easily measured through the principle of oxygen consumption. If, for example, one is making an assessment of nutritional status, the principle of weight loss as a nutritional tool becomes clearly inadequate. Weight loss in the ICU setting is not an appropriate tool for determining nutrition because of the limited amount of tissue that can be lost or gained in a day.[36] As an example of this, consider the following situation. A person who weighs approximately 65 kilos and has a measured O_2 consumption of 225 cc per minute, has a caloric expenditure over a day's period of time of $.225 \times 1440 \times 4.8$, yielding a value of approximately 1,600 kilocalories per day. If this person is NPO during an entire day's time period, he will lose approximately 1,600 kilocalories. When assessing how this reflects in total body weight, consider how many kilocalories exist in a pound of substrate. For example, one pound of fat contains approximately 3,500 kilocalories.[37] There are approximately 1,600 kilocalories in a pound of glucose or protein. Assuming this patient uses a normal mixture of fats and carbohydrates and few proteins during catabolism, he may have seen a one-half-pound weight loss. A scale has difficulty measuring a half-pound weight loss; however, the loss of water can much more markedly affect weight than the loss of kilocalories. For example, one pound of water is approximately equal to 454 cc of fluid (2.2 lb

$$= 1 \text{ kg} = 1 \text{ liter} = 1000 \text{ cc}, \frac{1000}{2.2} = 454).$$

A patient in a critical care setting is commonly given either parenteral or enteral fluid volumes that exceed a 500-cc output. A diuretic resulting in fluid loss is much more likely to be reflected in a weight measurement than in nutritional status. To give an example of the scale not properly accessing nutritional status, consider what would happen if one were to take a diuretic and lose approximately 2 kilos of water. Loss of 2 kilos of water results in a loss of approximately 4 pounds. This would reflect very quickly on a scale but would have very little affect on nutritional status. Weight changes are much more likely to reflect fluid changes than they are nutrition changes.

USE OF THE RESPIRATORY
QUOTIENT

The value of oxygen consumption in nutrition can be further extended if combined with another gas, that is, carbon dioxide. Measurement of carbon-dioxide production (V_{CO_2}) in conjunction with oxygen consumption yields the respiratory quotient, or RQ. RQ is obtained by dividing carbon-dioxide production (V_{CO_2}) by oxygen consumption (V_{O_2}). The value of the respiratory quotient is that it reflects the substrate being catabolized for energy.

Each substrate that the body uses for energy produces carbon dioxide in specific quantities relative to the amount of oxygen consumed. Fats, for example, produce 7 molecules of carbon dioxide while consuming 10 of oxygen (RQ = 7/10 = .7). Carbohydrates produce 10 molecules of carbon dioxide when consuming 10 molecules of oxygen (RQ = 10/10 = 1). Proteins produce 8 molecules of carbon dioxide when consuming 10 molecules of oxygen (RQ = 8/10 = .8). This gives the respiratory quotient values that range anywhere from .7 for fat up to 1 for carbohydrates (Figure 8.6). Normal catabolism yields a respiratory quotient near .8, which reflects the use of approximately 60% fats and 40% carbohydrates.[38] The respiratory quotient, when

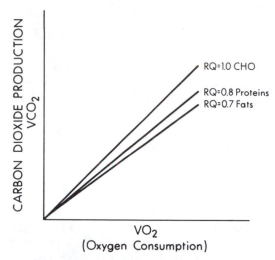

FIGURE 8.6. Different respiratory quotients with each substrate. CHO (carbohydrates) produce equal amounts of carbon dioxide (CO_2) relative to oxygen (O_2) consumed. Fats produce 7 molecules of CO_2 for every 10 oxygen molecules consumed. Proteins produce 8 molecules of CO_2 for every 10 oxygen molecules consumed.

used in conjunction with the oxygen-consumption measurement, provides a potentially powerful nutritional assessment tool. While V_{O_2} provides the number of kilocalories that are being used, the respiratory quotient provides information regarding the type of substrate being used for food.

Under normal circumstances, fats and carbohydrates provide virtually all the substrate necessary for oxidative phosphorylation. Under conditions of stress, proteins will provide the increased amount of energy.[39] When using the respiratory quotient, the clinician is provided information regarding substrate utilization patterns. One key use of the RQ is in the determination of the adequacy of supplemental feedings. For example, if a respiratory quotient drops below .8, this reflects an increase in reliance on fat for energy. The increased reliance on fat may potentially indicate a lack of adequate nutritional sources. If a patient has a respiratory quotient of .75, approximately 80% of his or her energy is coming from fat sources. This is a greater-than-normal reliance on fat stores. Potential indications of

increased fat utilization can be that the nutritional sources either are (1) incomplete or (2) not being adequately utilized. For example, in a patient receiving enteral preparations, one of the most common side effects is that of diarrhea. If the diarrhea is marked and does not allow for absorption of nutrients in the enteral feeding, the patient may not be absorbing the kilocalories despite being given an apparent adequate number of kilocalories. If malabsorption is present, inadequate nutritional support may exist. The respiratory quotient below .8 could aid in identification of this problem. Adequate nutritional status is more likely when the respiratory quotient is maintained at .8 or higher. As a rule, the respiratory quotient should be no greater than 1, since values in excess of 1 indicate a potential conversion of substrates, such as carbohydrates, into fat stores.[40] Under these circumstances the patient actually could gain weight.

Use of RQ to Assess Work of Breathing

The RQ can be employed as an aid in the assessment of V_{CO_2} and its role in breathing. Several studies have suggested increased V_{CO_2} can interfere with weaning from mechanical ventilation.[41-43] Increased V_{CO_2} can increase breathing, due to carbon dioxide's role in regulating breathing. Diets high in carbohydrates (CHO) have the potential to increase V_{CO_2}. Since CHO have an RQ at 1, reflecting that more CO_2 is being produced in comparison to other substrates such as fat and protein, an increased respiratory stimulus may be generated.

Identifying difficult-to-wean patients is the first step in the use of the RQ for assessing excessive breathing stimulation. These patients typically include those who are on mechanical ventilation for prolonged periods, are nutritionally depleted, or have large metabolic requirements. When this type of patient has been identified, the second step is to increase the fat percent of the diet.[44] The third step is to follow the RQ to monitor which substrates are being utilized.

The goal is to keep the RQ near .8 and avoid any increased CO_2 loads.

Use of the respiratory quotient is easily applied to noncritical care settings as well. If a patient, for example, is placed on a kilocalorie-restricted diet with weight loss as a goal, the use of a scale is not the best measurement of how much weight is being lost (due to the potential influence of water). One would be much more successful in determining the adequacy of the diet through measurement of the respiratory quotient. The RQ would be used in identifying how long a period of time fat catabolism was the predominant method of energy use. For example, if the RQ is measured at a level greater than .8, weight loss is unlikely. The RQ would need to decrease below .8 for increased fat utilization to be occurring.

If one wants to gain weight, measuring the RQ and noting values in excess of 1 is a better indicator of weight gain.

CLINICAL EXAMPLES

Example 4

Given a female patient with a V_{O_2} of 325 cc/min and a V_{CO_2} of 280 cc/min, determine the daily kilocaloric need and the respiratory quotient.

ANSWER

Her daily kilocaloric need is determined by: V_{O_2} × 1440 (minutes in day) × 4.8 (kilocalories burned per liter of O_2 consumed).

.325 × 1440 × 4.8 = 2246 kcal/day

Respiratory quotient is obtained by:

$$\frac{V_{CO_2}}{V_{O_2}}$$

$$\frac{280}{325} = .86$$

Example 5

A 32-year-old, 80-kg man is in the ICU following a motor-vehicle accident. He currently is receiving mechanical ventilation and is hemodynamically stable. This is the third ICU day and nutritional support is to be initiated. His V_{O_2} is 350 cc/min and V_{CO_2} is 310 cc/min. Based on this information, answer the following two questions:
1. What is his daily kilocaloric need?
2. What substrate is primarily being utilized?

ANSWER

1. The daily caloric need is: 351 × 1440 × 4.8 = 2419 kcal
2. The substrate being utilized is based on the respiratory quotient. The respiratory quotient is: 310/350 = .89. Based on the RQ of .89, the primary substrate being utilized is CHO. The origin of the increased CHO catabolism could be an adequate nutritional intake over the past few days.

Example 6

A 68-year-old, 60-kg woman is in her sixth postoperative day following coronary-artery-bypass surgery. She has been unable to wean from mechanical ventilation. The physician orders V_{O_2} and V_{CO_2} measurement to assess the adequacy of current nutritional support. V_{O_2} is 198 cc and V_{CO_2} is 155 cc. The nutritional support consists of 50 cc/hour (about 1,200 kcal/day). Based on this information, (1) is the kilocalorie regime adequate, and (2) is the RQ suggestive of a problem with excessive V_{CO_2} load?

ANSWER

The calorie intake of 1,200 is less than required, based on the V_{O_2}. Kilocalorie need, based on V_{O_2}, is 1,369 (.198 × 1,440 × 4.8). The RQ is .78.

$$RQ = (\frac{V_{CO_2}}{V_{O_2}} = \frac{155}{198}) = .78$$

The RQ less than .8 indicates increased use of fat, supporting the inadequacy of the current enteral feeding program. In addition, the RQ of .78 indicates that the diet is not excessively loaded with carbohydrates. No dietary alteration would help in the weaning of this patient from mechanical ventilation.

SUMMARY

Oxygen consumption (V_{O_2}) is an essential parameter in the assessment of oxygenation. In addition, V_{O_2} data can be applied to the assessment of energy (kilocalorie) requirements of the critically ill. Unfamiliarity by clinicians with the concept of V_{O_2} is attributable partially to the difficulty associated with measuring oxygen consumption. Methods to measure V_{O_2} have been presented, which should improve the ease of understanding how to obtain V_{O_2} data. Without a measure of oxygen consumption, the nurse can estimate V_{O_2}; however, the accuracy of V_{O_2} is much improved with direct measurement.

Application of V_{O_2} to oxygenation has two primary values: the assessment of the adequacy of oxygen transport (D_{O_2}) and the determination of whether V_{O_2} is pathologically dependent on D_{O_2}. Normally V_{O_2} is independent of D_{O_2}, a situation that indicates a normal response to changing D_{O_2}. If V_{O_2} is dependent on D_{O_2}, a critically low level of cellular oxygen may exist. When V_{O_2} and D_{O_2} are related, the nurse must realize that a dangerously low level of oxygen may be present at the cellular level.

Measurement of oxygen consumption is increasing in its importance to overall oxygenation. Research such as that which indicated a potential for a V_{O_2}/D_{O_2} relationship only increases the importance of understanding the role of V_{O_2} in oxygenation. If V_{O_2} is not included in the overall oxygenation assessment, an adequate oxygenation assessment is not possible.

REFERENCES

1. Shoemaker WC. "Physiologic monitoring of the critically ill patient." *In* Shoemaker WC, Ayres S, Grenvik A, Holbrook PR, Thompson WL (eds). *Textbook of Critical Care.* Philadelphia: WB Saunders, 1989, 145.
2. Buran MJ. "Oxygen Consumption." *In* Snyder JV, Pinsky MR (eds). *Oxygen Transport in the Critically Ill.* Chicago: Year Book Medical Pubs, 1987, 16.
3. Damask MC, Schwarz Y, Weissman C. "Energy measurements and requirement of critically ill patients." *Crit Care Clin* 1987;3:71.
4. Ultman JS, Burszstein S. "Analyses error in the determination of respiratory gas exchange at varying FI_{O_2}." *J Appl Physiol* 1981;50:210.
5. Browning JA, Linber SE, Turney SZ, et al. "The effects of a fluctuating FI_{O_2} on metabolic measurement in mechanically ventilated patients." *Crit Care Med* 1982;10:82.
6. Damask MC, Askanazi J, Weissman C, et al. "Artifacts in measurement of resting energy expenditure." *Crit Care Med* 1983;11:750.
7. Levinson MR, Groeger JS, Miodownik S, et al. "Indirect calorimetry in the mechanically ventilated patient." *Crit Care Med* 1987;15:144.
8. Westenskow DR, Cutler CA, Wallace WD. "Instrumentation for monitoring gas exchange and metabolic rate in critically ill patients." *Crit Care Med* 1984;12:183.
9. Liggett SB, St. John RE, Lefrak SS. "Determination of resting energy expenditure utilizing the thermodilution pulmonary artery catheter." *Chest* 1986;91:562.
10. Pomes Iparraguirre H, Giniger R, Garber VA, et al. "Comparison between measured and Fick derived values of hemodynamic and oxymetric variables in patients with acute myocardial infarction." *Am J Med* 1988;85:349.
11. Gutierrez G, Pohil R. "Oxygen consumption is linearly related to O_2 supply in critically ill patients." *J Crit Care* 1986;1:45.
12. Mohsenifar A, Goldbach P, Tashkin DP, et al. "Relationship between O_2 delivery and O_2 consumption in the adult respiratory distress syndrome." *Chest* 1983;84:267.
13. Danek SJ, Lynch JP, Weg JD, Dantzker DR. "The dependence of oxygen uptake on oxygen delivery in the adult respiratory distress syndrome." *Am Rev Respr Dis* 1980;122:387.
14. Schumaker PT, Cain SM. "The concept of a critical oxygen delivery." *Int Care Med* 1987;13:223.
15. Mohsenifar A, Amin D, Jasper AC, et al. "Dependence of oxygen consumption on oxygen delivery in patients with chronic congestive heart failure." *Chest* 1987;92:447.
16. Shibutani K, Komatsu T, Kubal K, et al. "Critical level of oxygen delivery in anesthetized man." *Crit Care Med* 1983;11:640.
17. Snyder JV, Carrol GC. "Tissue oxygenation: A physiologic approach to a clinical problem, Part I." *Current Problems in Surgery* 1982;19:650.
18. Archie JP. "Mathematical coupling of data may produce invalid results and unjustified conclusions (abstract)." *Crit Care Med* 1980;8:252.
19. Chappell TR, Rubin LJ, Markham RV Jr, et al. "Independence of oxygen consumption and systemic oxygen transport in patients with either stable pulmonary hypertension or refractory left ventricular failure." *Am Rev Respir Dis* 1980;122:30.
20. Cain SM. "Review: Supply dependency of oxygen uptake in ARDS: Myth or reality." *Am J Med Sci* 1984;288:119.
21. Russell JA, Ronco JJ, Lockhat D, et al. "Oxygen delivery and consumption and ventricular preload are greater in survivors than in nonsurvivors of the adult respiratory distress syndrome." *Am Rev Respir Dis* 1990;141:659.
22. Bland RD, Shoemaker WC, Abraham E, et al. "Hemodynamic and oxygen transport patterns in surviving and non surviving post operative patients." *Crit Care Med* 1985;13:85.
23. Astiz ME, Rackow EC, Kaufman B, Falk JL, Weil MH. "Relationship of oxygen delivery and mixed

venous oxygenation to lactic acidosis in patients with sepsis and acute myocardial infarction." *Crit Care Med* 1988;16:655.

24. Dahn MS, Lange MP, Jacobs LA. "Central mixed and splanchnic venous oxygen saturation monitoring." *Intensive Care Medicine* 1988;14:373.

25. Atwater WO, Benedict FG. "A respiration calorimeter with appliances for the direct determination of oxygen." Carnegie Institute of Washington, Wash DC, Pub 42, 1905, 193.

26. Benedict FG. "A portable respiration apparatus for clinical use." *Boston Med Surg J* 1918;178:667.

27. Ferrannini E. "The theoretical bases of indirect calorimetry: A review." *Metabolism* 1988;37:287.

28. Linder MC. "Energy metabolism, intake and expenditure." *In* Linder MC (ed). *Nutrition, Biochemistry and Metabolism* New York: Elsevier, 1985, 199.

29. McArdle WD, Katch FI, Katch VL. *Exercise Physiology.* Philadelphia: Lea & Febiger, 1981, 50.

30. Kleiber M. *The Fire of Life.* New York: John Wiley & Sons, 1964, 126.

31. Lanschot JJ, Feenstra BW, Vermeij CG, Bruining HA. "Calculation versus measurement of total energy expenditure." *Crit Care Med* 1986;14:981.

32. Weissman C, Kemper M, Askanazi J, et al. "Resting metabolic rate of the critically ill: Measured versus predicted." *Anesthesiology* 1986;64:673.

33. Swinamer DL, Phang PT, Jones RL, et al. "Twenty four hour energy expenditure in critically ill patients." *Crit Care Med* 1987;15:637.

34. Harris JA, Benedict FG. *Standard Basal Metabolism Constants for Physiologist and Clinicians: A Biometric Study of Basal Metabolism in Man.* Philadelphia: JB Lippincott, 1919.

35. Quebbeman EJ, Ausman RK, Schecter TC. "A reevaluation of energy expenditure during parenteral nutrition." *Ann Surg* 1982;195:282.

36. Parsa MH, Shoemaker WC. "Nutritional failure." *In* Shoemaker WC, Ayres S, Grenvik A, Holbrook PR, Thompson WL (eds). *Textbook of Critical Care.* Philadelphia: WB Saunders, 1989, 1080.

37. Pike RL, Brown ML. *Nutrition: An Interpretive Approach.* New York: John Wiley & Sons, 1988;770.

38. Jones NL, Campbell EJM. *Clinical Exercise Testing.* Philadelphia: WB Saunders, 1982, 20.

39. Elwyn DH. "Protein metabolism and requirements in the critically ill patient." *Crit Care Clin* 1987;3:57.

40. Cerra, FB. "Nutrition in trauma, stress and sepsis." *In* Shoemaker WC, Ayres S, Grenvik A, Holbrook PR, Thompson WL (eds). *Textbook of Critical Care.* Philadelphia: WB Saunders, 1989, 1118.

41. Laaban JP. "Influence of caloric intake on the respiratory mode during mandatory minute volume ventilation." *Chest* 1985;87:67.

42. Askanasi J, Rosenbaum SH, Hymen AI. "Respiratory changes induced by the large glucose loads of total parenteral nutrition." *J Am Med Assn* 1980;243:1444.

43. Bartlett RH, Dechert RE, Mault JR, Clark SF. "Metabolic studies in chest trauma." *J Thor Cardio Surg* 1984;87:503.

44. Weissman C, Hyman AI. "Nutritional care of the critically ill patient with respiratory failure." *Crit Care Clin* 1987;3:185.

9
Cellular Assessment of Oxygenation

INTRODUCTION

Integration of all concepts involved with tissue oxygenation can be difficult to assess, even with some of the most advanced techniques available. However, it is this assessment of overall tissue oxygenation that is at the heart of accurate assessments of clinical oxygenation. In this chapter, a review of mechanisms will be presented by which the assessment of both oxygen transport and oxygen consumption, together with cellular utilization of oxygen, can be assessed in an integrative manner. This integrative manner requires methods that may not be common in clinical practice but are necessary for the actual assessment of oxygenation. The components that are mentioned in this chapter should serve as examples of the end points when analyzing whether an oxygenation status is appropriate or tolerable. Also keep in mind during the presentation of concepts in this chapter that some of this information may not be readily available. Due to unavailability, these data may not be part of the routine oxygenation assessment. However, to assess cellular oxygenation, the clinician must rely as much as possible on the concepts presented in this chapter and avoid the singular use of individual components of oxygen transport or consumption. Even using the techniques presented in this section, there will be exceptions to the rules, and a clear understanding of oxygen-

ation may not be present in many patient situations.

In this section, the assessment of cellular oxygenation will be analyzed through the concepts of (1) lactate production, (2) transcutaneous P_{O_2} levels, (3) gastric pH, (4) $S\bar{v}_{O_2}$ monitoring, and some methods that are in the research phase and not readily available. These include magnetic-resonance imaging with phosphate and positron-emission tomography. Owing to the common use of $S\bar{v}_{O_2}$ monitoring, $S\bar{v}_{O_2}$ analysis is presented in a chapter by itself.

LACTATE PRODUCTION

The measurement of lactate levels has been of interest as a reflector of oxygenation problems for many decades.[1] Lactate reflects an oxygen imbalance through the failure to utilize oxygen at the cellular level. Lactate metabolism is a normal byproduct of glucose degradation for energy. Normally at the end of the breakdown of glucose, both pyruvate and lactate are generated. In the presence of adequate oxygen levels, pyruvate is combined with coenzyme A (acetic acid) into acetyl-CoA. Acetyl-CoA enters the Krebs cycle at this point to proceed with oxidative phosphorylation (Figure 9.1). If oxygen levels are not adequate for oxidative phosphorylation, increased amounts of lactate will be produced. As mentioned in Chapter 1, lactate by itself is not a problem.

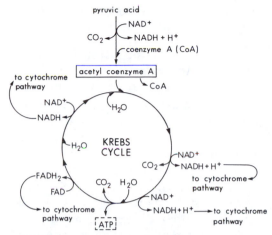

FIGURE 9.1. Acetyl CO-A initiates the Krebs cycle and oxidative phosphorylation. From this pathway, ATP is generated during electron transfer. The pathway terminates when oxygen accepts the hydrogen electron (oxidative phosphorylation). Adapted from McArdle D, Katch Fl, Katch V. *Exercise Physiology*, 3rd ed. Philadelphia: Lea & Febiger, 1991.

Unfortunately, in the utilization of lactate for energy, both ATP and hydrogen are generated. The hydrogen produced will eventually cause an acidosis to develop and create a situation referred to as lactic acidosis. Lactic acid is the anionic base of lactate (Figure 9.2) and is produced when lactate is utilized for energy. The anionic form of lactate is produced when hydrogen is released from lactate. The actual breakdown of lactate into lactic acid to create energy is a beneficial process in many organs, but when occurring systemically reflects an inability to proceed with pyruvate formation. The lack of pyruvate formation is due to the lack of

oxygen. Subsequently, with increased lactate production, the eventual production of an acidosis creates a situation which the increased hydrogen-ion concentration impairs mitochondrial function.[2] From this basis, an increased amount of lactate produced in the serum can reflect an overall problem with oxygenation (Figure 9.3).

Lactate has been identified as a potentially good indicator of both oxygenation difficulties in the acute phase and as a prognostic indicator of problems with overall oxygenation.[3-6] Lactate levels over 4 mmol have been identified as indicative of problems with overall oxygenation and survival.[7] It is not the sudden accumulation of lactate that is a problem; postseizure lactate levels can rise as high as 12 mmol,[8] and in sudden anaerobic activity, lactate will increase sharply. However, lactate levels will quickly return to normal in the absence of a chronic oxygen debt and with normal renal function. The persistence of lactate in the blood is a significant indicator of problems with tissue oxygenation. If lactate levels increase for more than several hours and remain elevated, the clinician should view this elevation as ominous.

Measurement of lactate levels ideally is from a mixed venous or an arterial source in order to avoid the potential problems associated with regional hypoperfusion or oxygenation.[9] Arterial or mixed-venous serum lactate levels will not project regional distur-

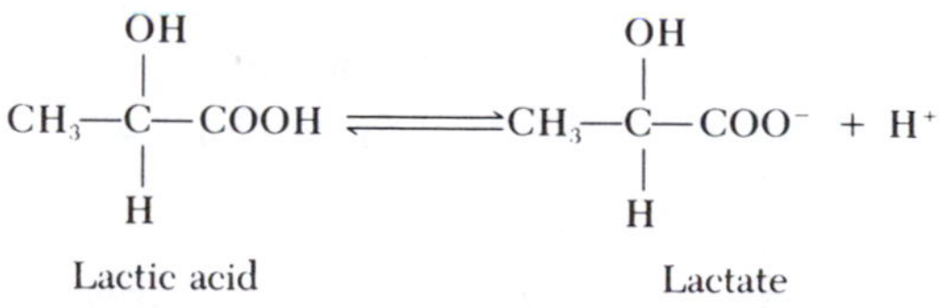

$$
\underset{\text{Lactic acid}}{\overset{\overset{\displaystyle OH}{\mid}}{CH_3-\underset{\underset{\displaystyle H}{\mid}}{C}-COOH}} \; \rightleftharpoons \; \underset{\text{Lactate}}{\overset{\overset{\displaystyle OH}{\mid}}{CH_3-\underset{\underset{\displaystyle H}{\mid}}{C}-COO^-}} \;+\; H^+
$$

FIGURE 9.2. Relationship of the molecular forms of lactate and lactic acid. Lactic acid is the anionic base of lactate. Adapted from Kruse JA, Carlson RW. "Lactate metabolism" *Crit Care Clin* 1987;727.

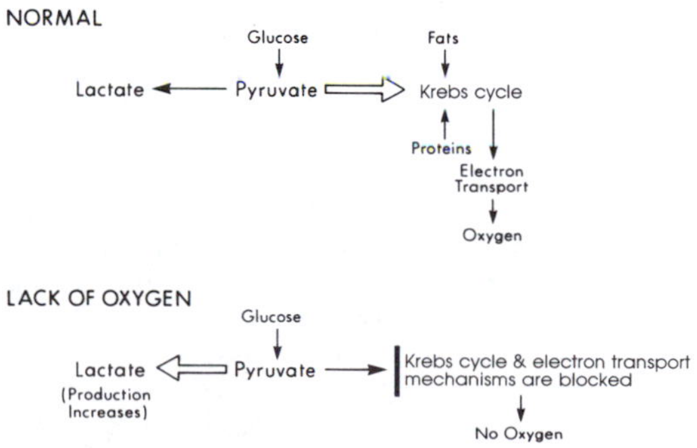

NORMAL

Lactate ← Pyruvate ⇌ Krebs cycle

Glucose ↓   Fats ↓
Pyruvate   Krebs cycle
            Proteins ↓
            Electron Transport ↓
            Oxygen

LACK OF OXYGEN

Glucose ↓
Lactate ⇐ Pyruvate → Krebs cycle & electron transport mechanisms are blocked
(Production Increases)
                        No Oxygen

FIGURE 9.3. Increased lactate production with oxygen deprivation.

bances but will reflect an overall tissue imbalance. How important the serum lactate level is in the routine determination of oxygenation is unclear at this time. Research literature seems to support lactate as an indicator of cellular oxygenation disturbances.[10,11] At this point, a lactate determination may be as good an indicator of overall oxygenation, or failure of oxygenation at the cellular level, as any other single indicator. Based on this evidence, potential oxygenation disturbances should include lactate determination.

One problem with lactate analysis is that the change in lactate level from cellular to vascular space is not instantaneous.[12] (See Figure 9.4.) The delay can range anywhere from seconds to minutes before cellular levels equilibrate with serum levels. Owing to this delay, lactate assessment is not an instantaneous measure of overall oxygen-

Normal Blood Flow

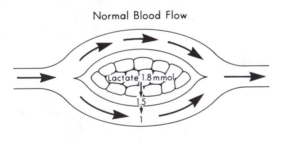

Decreased Blood Flow

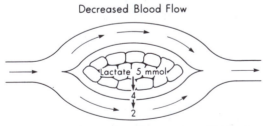

FIGURE 9.4. Lactate transfer may vary with blood-flow states. As long as blood flow and cellular oxygenation are normal, lactate levels in the cells and serum are relatively close. When blood flow decreases or cellular oxygenation worsens, a discrepancy develops between lactate levels in the cells and serum. The degree of lactate discrepancy and the time it takes to equilibrate levels between serum and cells vary. Equilibration may take many minutes.

ation. Lactate levels should be obtained in a series to establish trends in oxygenation.

Use of Lactic Acidosis as an Indicator of the Cause of an Oxygenation Problem

The assessment of oxygenation requires essentially the assessment of three potential types of problem: reduced oxygen transport, increased oxygen consumption, or inability of cellular (mitochondrial) processes to incorporate oxygen. The advantage of measurements such as lactic acidosis or lactate levels is that they allow the clinician to attempt to differentiate between these problems. For example, in a patient with normal oxygen transport and normal oxygen consumption but elevated lactate levels, the problem is likely an inability to adequately process oxygen. In other words, a mitochondrial or extracellular problem in utilization of oxygen is likely present. When overtly decreased oxygen transport or increased O_2 consumption exists, then the problem can be identified as stemming from one of those two. This is an important point to keep in mind since identifying where the problem exists is the focus for early intervention.[13–14]

Lactate/Pyruvate Ratio

Measurement of lactate in isolation can be misleading in terms of clinical application.[15] Since lactate production can be affected by many factors, interpretation of the absolute lactate level needs to proceed with caution. One factor which can help the interpretation of the lactate level is to also measure the pyruvate level. Under normal circumstances, pyruvate is only about $1/10$ the level of lactate.[16] If lactate levels increase in the same proportion as pyruvate, then an increase in glucose metabolism may be taking place without the presence of hypoxia. On the other hand, if lactate increases disproportionately to a change in pyruvate, then the change is more likely reflective of hypoxia. In order to avoid misinterpretation of the lactate level, the lactate/pyruvate ratio may be a more valuable clinical parameter than lactate alone.

TRANSCUTANEOUS OXYGEN (Ptc$_{O_2}$)

The concept of transcutaneous oxygen has been present since the early 1950s.[17-18] Other methods to estimate oxygen pressures beneath the mucous membrane, such as conjunctival oxygen pressures, exist; but only Ptc$_{O_2}$ levels will be presented here. Neonates have been assessed through transcutaneous-oxygen levels more than adults, primarily because there is a smaller distance between the skin in the neonate. The major advantage of transcutaneous oxygen is that it has the potential of assessing cellular imbalances. Cellular oxygenation assessment is possible since oxygen in the tissue, not just the blood vessels, is measured (Figure 9.5).

The Ptc$_{O_2}$ has been proposed as a measure to estimate Pa$_{O_2}$ (oxygen tension in the artery) levels. The correlation between Ptc$_{O_2}$ and Pa$_{O_2}$ varies with local perfusion. However, the Pa$_{O_2}$ is limited in assessing tissue oxygenation. Ptc$_{O_2}$ may not be as limited as the Pa$_{O_2}$, since Ptc$_{O_2}$ can be an indicator of oxygenation through reflecting cellular oxygen levels. Pa$_{O_2}$ levels simply reflect the oxygen pressure in the artery, not the cells. If the transcutaneous P$_{O_2}$ level falls below normal (less than 60 mm), then the potential exists for loss of cellular oxygen (Figure 9.6). Normal Ptc$_{O_2}$ levels are near

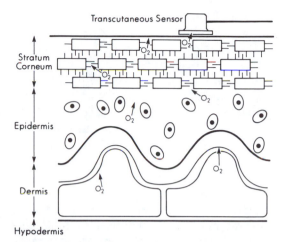

FIGURE 9.5. Transcutaneous oxygen measurement. Transcutaneous oxygen sensors work by detecting the amount of oxygen that diffuses from the cells to the surface. Normally, the oxygen levels of the stratum corneum are very low. For transcutaneous sensors to be effective, they must heat the region to improve local blood flow and increase the oxygen level in the stratum corneum. Adapted from Brown M, Vender JS. "Noninvasive oxygen monitoring." *Crit Care Clin* 1990;4:500.

(slightly lower than) arterial P$_{O_2}$ levels. When oxygenation decreases, the Ptc$_{O_2}$ correlates more closely with tissue P$_{O_2}$ than does Pa$_{O_2}$. For this reason, Ptc$_{O_2}$ is more likely to be of value in an oxygenation assessment than are Pa$_{O_2}$ levels.

The loss of cellular oxygen may reflect a poor local blood supply, a failure to utilize oxygen properly, or an increase in oxygen

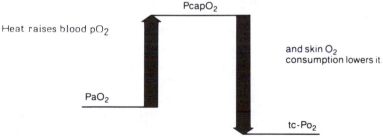

FIGURE 9.6. Correlation with transcutaneous oxygen and oxygen in other tissues. Normally, transcutaneous oxygen does not correlate well with arterial oxygen until the area is heated and blood flow increases. Fortunately, transcutaneous-oxygen levels can track tissue oxygen requirements: as local areas increase oxygen need (or a reduction in supply occurs), the transcutaneous-oxygen level will decrease to reflect the change. Adapted from Novametrix 1986.

consumption. Advocates of transcutaneous-oxygen levels in adults believe that if the transcutaneous P_{O_2} level is low, the oxygen supply to the area underneath the transcutaneous sensor is at risk for problems in oxygenation.[19-21] As such, transcutaneous oxygenation has the potential to reflect changes in cellular metabolism as opposed to reflecting only partial pressures of oxygen in the blood.

In adults, the use of transcutaneous oxygen has had mixed results.[22-23] The use of transcutaneous-oxygen measurement has several practical limitations, such as the need for a heated probe, the distance that is between the probe and the vascular supply, and the warm-up time (probe stabilization) before accurate readings are obtainable (Figure 9.7). Studies exist that support the use of transcutaneous P_{O_2} as an indicator of oxygenation of the regional level, but little evidence exists of transcutaneous oxygen being successfully applied to reflect an overall oxygenation balance. This is both a strength and a weakness of transcutaneous-oxygenation use. For example, if one wants to know about regional oxygenation, transcutanous-oxygen measurements may reflect this as well as any currently available technique. If one wants to assess overall oxygenation, then transcutaneous oxygen may not be as useful. Transcutaneous-oxygen measurement is not yet a primary tool in the application and assessment of oxygenation. However, it does have potential value and this value should be investigated through further research. At this point, if indications of regional oxygenation are desired, transcutaneous-oxygen levels may be useful.

GASTRIC MUCOSAL pH
AS A MEASURE OF HYPOXIA

During periods of hypoxia, preferential shunting of blood flow may take place to the heart and brain. During such periods, blood flow may be diverted from other organs, particularly the gastrointestinal system. Due to this diversion of blood flow, a change in the gastric mucosal pH may occur. The pH

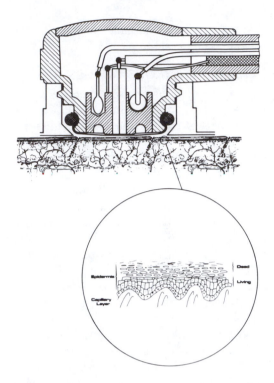

FIGURE 9.7. Limitations of transcutaneous-oxygen application. For transcutaneous-oxygen measurements to be useful, the probe has to be rotated frequently (due to the heat produced by the probe). In addition, the probe measures the area immediately under the skin, increasing the chances of disruptions in local blood supply altering the interpretation of the oxygen reading. Adapted from Novametrix, 1986.

change is of an acidic nature, reflecting a potential hypoxia of the gastric region secondary to loss of blood flow. Because of this loss of blood flow, the gastric mucosal pH may reflect early compensation for systemic hypoxia.

Measurement of gastric pH can take place with a water filled balloon equipped with pH sensors. The balloon is placed into the stomach and is filled in order for the balloon to come into contact with the gastric mucosa. As the pH of the gastric mucosa changes, the change will be measured by the pH sensors in the balloon.

The use of gastric mucosal pH measurements offers promise as an early indicator of systemic hypoxia. Clinical studies are continuing at this time attempting to assess it's application although initial results are promising that gastric pH may be an improved tool for the assessment of systemic oxygenation.[24]

FUTURE TECHNIQUES

Techniques that may be available in the coming decade to assess oxygenation include radiologic studies such as magnetic-resonance imaging (MRI) and positron-emission tomography (PET). Each of these techniques and its potential use and application will be briefly presented. Other measurement techniques are also being developed; however, the presentation of MRI and PET analysis will illustrate the coming changes in the assessment of oxygenation.

MAGNETIC-RESONANCE IMAGING (MRI)

Magnetic-resonance imaging holds a promise of accurately measuring oxygen use at the cellular level. MRI does not actually measure oxygen but rather types of phosphates. Phosphates are necessary in the formation of ADP, ATP, and PCr (Chapter 1). MRI functions by identifying specific molecules such as phosphate. MRI isolates the molecule of interest by generating a magnetic field that initially produces a uniform alignment of the molecular orbit (Figure 9.8).[25] A radio-frequency pulse specific to the molecule of interest is passed through the magnetic field, causing a slight "tilt" off the magnetic center. This tilt is detectable by the MRI scanner. When the pulse is removed, the molecule returns to the prior alignment. The movement is measurable and allows for detection of specific quantities of molecular concentrations (Figure 9.9). The decay orbit of any molecule with the specific radio frequency employed, not just phosphate, can be tracked and imaged.

In energy assessment, the primary element of interest is phosphate, owing to the presence of phosphate in ADP, ATP, and PCr. The MRI is capable of identifying each of these elements (Figure 9.10).

As oxygen stores decrease, ATP levels are maintained by utilizing PCr. This causes a reduction in PCr levels. A decrease in PCr

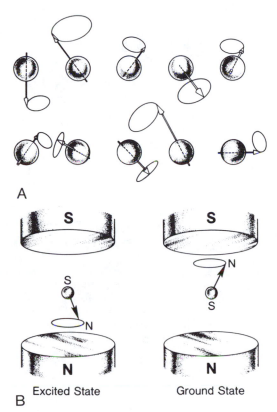

FIGURE 9.8.   Magnetic resonance imaging principles. Normal molecular alignment is random (A). With the pulsation of a magnetic field, the molecules will align in an excited state (B). Adapted from Harms SE, Morgan TJ, Yamanaski WS, et al. "Principles of nuclear magnetic resonance imaging." *Radiograpics* 1984;4:28–31.

levels is an early indication of hypoxia. ATP stores do not decrease until near-terminal stages, partially due to the utilization of PCr.

The limitations of using MRI include the difficulty in placing a critically ill patient in the magnetic environment. MRI is presently not available for practical use in the ICU. In the future, measurements of ADP, ATP, and PCr levels may become a common clinical practice based on techniques such as magnetic-resonance imaging.

POSITRON EMISSION TOMOGRAPHY (PET)

Magnetic-resonance imaging is only one of the newer advanced techniques in the assessment of oxygenation. Positron-emission tomography is another example of an

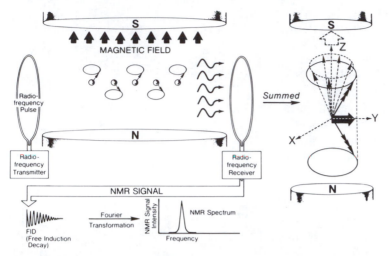

FIGURE 9.9. Detection of molecular activity with magnetic-resonance imaging. As the radiofrequency pulse corresponding to the molecule of interest passes through the magnetic field, the molecules are "knocked off" their magnetic orientation. As they realign, their movement is detectable and measured as a spectrum. Adapted from Harms SE, Morgan TJ, Yamanaski WS, et al. "Principles of nuclear magnetic resonance imaging." *Radiograpics* 1984;4:28–31.

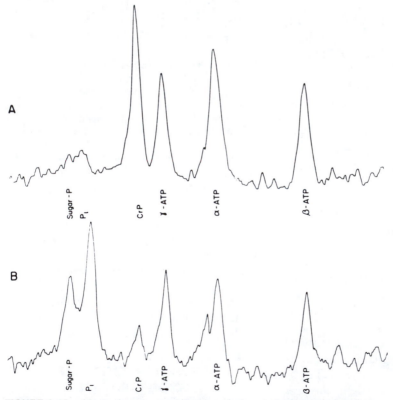

FIGURE 9.10. Magnetic-resonance imaging of phosphate. Normal phosphate levels (A) differ under conditions of hypoxia (B). During hypoxia, creatine phosphate (CrP) levels fall, indicating a depletion of cellular energy. Adapted from Ingwall JS. "Phosphorus nuclear magnetic resonance spectroscopy of cardiac and skeletal muscles." *Am J Physiology* 1982;242:H729–744.

assessment method. At this point in time, positron-emission tomography, like magnetic-resonance imaging, is limited in its ability to assess critically ill patients primarily due to the limitations of the equipment required (Figure 9.11). The assessment of oxygenation through positron-emission tomography can be understood as PET scanning is explained.

Positron-emission tomography works through the injection of a radioisotope of the molecule of interest.[26] For example, in the assessment of oxygenation, one isotope that could be created and injected into the human body is oxygen. Whereas other isotopes, such as carbon derivatives, can and frequently are used instead of oxygen, oxygen serves for the most simple explanation of positron-emission tomography application.

Positron-emission tomography works,

then, through the measurements of a specific radioisotope injected into the body via the blood. The advantage of PET scanning is that the isotope injected is utilized inside the body, and the radiation that is emitted comes from inside the body. This differs from traditional radioactive analysis of human function in that the body is analyzed from the outside. The emitting isotope can be traced to the tissue active in the metabolism of the isotope. This tissue utilization allows for great specificity in the isolation of both how and where the isotope is used. The radioisotope that is injected has the chemical properties of an unstable nucleus. A positron is emitted from the nucleus and collides with one of the circulating electrons outside the molecule's nucleus. The resulting collision of the positron and the electron causes the annihilation of both particles and the subsequent release of two photons.

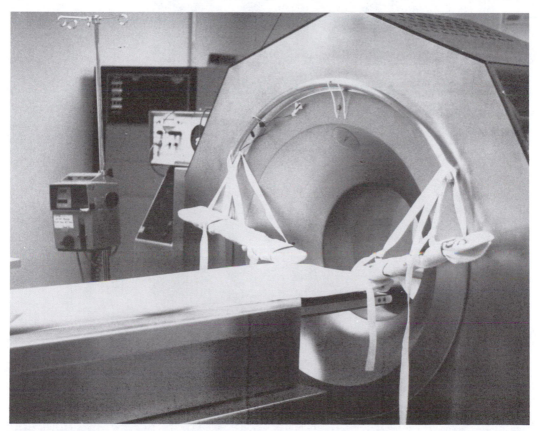

FIGURE 9.11. Positron-emission tomography unit.

These photons are released simultaneously at a 180° angle (Figure 9.12). These two photons, which are released at exactly a 180° angle, can be detected through a mechanism that encircles the body part being studied (simultaneous detection system). For example, if the brain is to be assessed for areas of regional or general oxy-genation deficits, then the brain (the head) is placed in a PET scanner that detects the utilization of oxygen isotopes. Any tissue that normally uses oxygen will take up these oxygen isotopes. Tissue that takes up oxy-gen isotopes is identified through the pho-ton release. The sensing mechanisms placed around the body, in this case the head, mea-

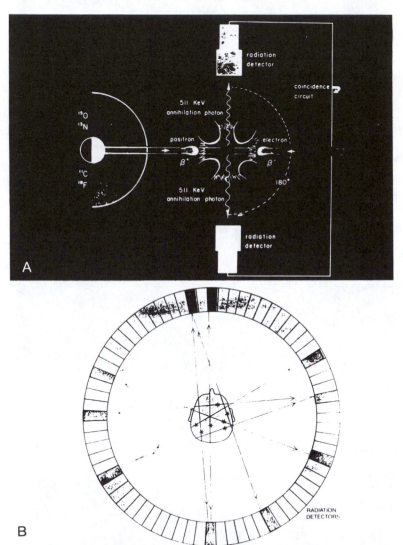

FIGURE 9.12. Positron-emission tomography principles. The release from the nucleus (of the radioisotope of interest) of a positron is the basis for positron-emission tomography. The positron collides with an orbiting electron, resulting in a collision which destroys both particles. During the destruction, photons are released in 180-degree angles. The simultaneous sensing of photons in 180-degree direc-tions allows isolation of the origin of the collision. In this manner, utilization by living tissue of the molecule of interest can be located and quantified. Adapted from Ter-Pogossian M, Raichle M, Sobel B. "Positron emission tomography." *Scientific American* 1980;243:173A.

sure only photons that are released at exactly 180° angles to each other. This tends to eliminate artifacts that may be generated through isolated photon generation for other reasons. The advantage of positron-emission tomography, is its ability to isolate a particular body part and measure that part's utilization of any substrate of interest, such as oxygen. If the isotope oxygen is injected, any tissue that metabolizes oxygen can be identified through the PET scanner. Any part of the body that is not able to process oxygen will not generate the simultaneous photon release, and subsequently will not be detected with the PET scans. The tissues undetectable by the PET scan are not actively utilizing oxygen. These tissues are either very low in metabolism or are dead. In myocardial injury patterns, for example, the exact part of the heart that is being threatened by loss of oxygen could be identified. If a medication or treatment were to be assessed for efficacy or adequacy, the PET scanner would pick up change in tissue function. In many treatments, for example coronary bypass grafting, an improvement in blood flow to a region may occur, but if the tissue cannot utilize oxygen, the improved blood flow will only serve to flow past areas of the heart that no longer have function. The PET scanner offers the ability to generate much more sophisticated assessments of tissues that are viable or that may be threatened. Through this assessment, PET scanning is much more likely to identify the adequacy of treatment modalities. Positron-emission tomography offers an exciting potential and increased sophistication of assessments of oxygenation. The use of techniques such as positron-emission tomography, however, again are limited primarily due to the tremendously sophisticated equipment and the cost associated with such equipment. Positron-emission tomography is a technology that will be increasing its clinical application primarily through increased use and refinement of the technology.

Other types of measurement systems for oxygenation will undoubtedly occur in the relatively near future. Measurements, for example, of NADH levels, which are necessary for electron transfer and are integral in the process of oxidative phosphorylation, will likely be an example of a measurement tool that will improve our assessment of tissue oxygenation. All of these tools, however, at this point in time, are not practical for the clinician. The practicing clinician can look to these types of measurement devices in the future for help in making better assessments of oxygenation and understanding the effectiveness of current treatments. Unfortunately, for the time being clinicians must rely on the assessment of global concepts of oxygen transport and consumption, and the cellular assessment techniques that are currently available, such as serum-lactate levels, transcutaneous-oxygen measures, and $S\bar{v}_{O_2}$ monitoring. While the future for assessment of oxygenation is tremendously exciting, the present reality is much more limited.

LACTATE UTILIZATION (CLINICAL EXAMPLES)

Example 1

A 68-year-old woman with a diagnosis of acute respiratory failure is admitted to the unit with severe shortness of breath, tachypnea (respiratory rate 38), tachycardia (heart rate 130), and hypotension (blood pressure 86/54). Arterial blood gases reveal P_{O_2} of 69, F_{IO_2} 50%, P_{CO_2} 33, pH 7.38, hemoglobin 13, and hemoglobin saturation 92%. Serum-lactate levels are 3.1. From this data, what is the status of this patient's overall oxygenation?

ANSWER

Based on the information presented, the patient has a relatively normal oxygen content but potentially decreased cardiac output as indicated by the tachycardia and hypotension, and a possible increase in oxygen consumption based on increased respiratory rate. Due to the potential combination of increased O_2 consumption and decreased O_2 transport, the woman has a threat to overall oxygenation, but how great a threat is unknown. Standard treatment indicates that she be treated to increase the blood pressure, improve the cardiac output, and decrease the heart rate by increasing the stroke volume. In addition, attempting to reduce the work of breathing may be useful. The serum-lactate level of 3.1 indicates that the overall oxygenation problem actually does exist and that this woman should be aggressively treated. If the lactate level were lower or within normal levels, then the patient's oxygenation status might not be as much of a problem as it appears. The use of the lactate level helps the clinician determine the severity of the oxygenation problem without the use of invasive techniques such as pulmonary-artery monitoring. The use of serum-lactate levels may aid in the assessment of the severity of oxygenation problems and the need for intervention.

Example 2

A 53-year-old man is admitted to the unit post-operatively for repair of an aortic aneurysm. After 8 hours in the ICU, he begins to complain of mild shortness of breath. Vital signs and hemodynamic data are listed below:

	Time	
	0600	0700
Blood Pressure	112/74	110/70
Heart Rate	98	110
Respiratory Rate	22	28
F_{IO_2}	40%	40%
Pa_{O_2}	98	96
Hemoglobin Saturation (Sa_{O_2})	.98	.97
Hemoglobin	10.2	10.1
Cardiac Output	4.8	5
Cardiac Index	2.5	2.6
Lactate	2.0	2.5

At 0800, the patient becomes confused and the question arises, is the confusion secondary to medications, metabolism difficulty, or changes in oxygenation? A repeat of hemodynamic analysis and pulmonary status reveal:

	Time: 0800
Blood Pressure	114/70
Heart Rate	112
Respiratory Rate	30
Pa_{O_2}	98
Hemoglobin Saturation (Sa_{O_2})	98
Pa_{CO_2}	40
pH	7.35
F_{IO_2}	50%
Cardiac Output	5.1
Cardiac Index	2.65
Lactate Level	3.2

Based on this information, could a change in oxygenation be the cause of behavior change?

ANSWER

Yes. Based on the data presented, overall oxygen transport has remained constant and overall oxygen consumption may be increased. Increased V_{O_2} may be reflected in the changes, although slight, in respiratory rate. In this scenario, the change in respiratory rate may be a clinically significant clue to the increase of oxygen consumption. The lactate level, which is increasing, may reflect an imbalance between transport and consumption or the failure to adequately utilize oxygen. Under this circumstance, the patient's overall oxygenation status appears to be worsening. The use of lactate level in this case seems more beneficial in asessing oxygenation status than other techniques.

Example 3. Transcutaneous Oxygen (Clinical Examples)

A patient has a transcutaneous-oxygen probe in place which reveals the following:

	Time 1200
Blood Pressure	110/70
Heart Rate	68
Respiratory Rate	20
Hemoglobin	11.1
Pa_{O_2}	96
Pa_{CO_2}	41
Sp_{O_2}	98%
pH	7.4
Ptc_{O_2}	78

The patient has a diagnosis of GI bleed and is in the unit for observation. An endoscopy revealed a 2-cm gastric bleed, which has been cauterized. The patient receives a transfusion. Two hours later the following data is taken:

	Time 1400
Blood Pressure	110/70
Heart Rate	82
Hemoglobin	9
Respiratory Rate	20
Sp_{O_2}	98%
Transcutaneous Oxygen	42

What may be occurring based on the above information?

ANSWER

Based on the transcutaneous-oxygen level, the overall tissue oxygenation, at least locally, may be deteriorating. As indicated by a decrease in Ptc_{O_2}, the deterioration may be due to a loss of hemoglobin, whereas the increase in heart rate may be an attempt to try and offset the loss of oxygen transport. At this point, the transcutaneous-oxygen level serves as a potential warning sign that a problem in oxygenation at the tissue level may be developing, even though no overt clinical signs are present. A potential for tissue oxygen to be reflected quickly by transcutaneous O_2 levels is one of the primary benefits of transcutaneous-oxygen analysis.

REFERENCES

1. Cournand A, Riley RL, Bardley SF, et al. "Studies of circulation in clinical shock." *Surgery* 1943; 13:964.
2. Kraig RP, Petito CK, Plum F, Pulsinelli WA. "Hydrogen ions kill brain at concentrations reached in ischemia." *J Cereb Blood Flow and Metab* 1987;7:379.
3. Cowan BN, Burns HJG, Boyle P, et al. "The relative prognosic value of lactate and hemodynamic measurement in early shock." *Anaesthesia* 1984;39:750.
4. Mizock BA. "Controversies in lactic acidosis. Implications in critically ill patients." *JAMA* 1987; 258:497.
5. Rashkin M, Boxkin C, Baughman R. "Oxygen delivery in critically ill patients. Relationship to blood lactate and survival." *Chest* 1985;87:580.
6. Peretz D, Scott H, Duff J, et al. "The significance of lactacidemia in the shock syndrome." *Ann NY Acad Sci* 1965;119:1133.
7. Broder G, Weil MH. "Excess lactate: An index of reversibility of shock in human patients." *Science* 1964;143:1457.
8. Orringer CE, Eustace JC, Wunsch CD, et al. "Natural history of lactic acidosis after grand mal seizure." *N Engl J Med* 1977;297:796.
9. Kruse JA, Carlson RW. "Lactate Metabolism." *Crit Care Clin* 1987;5:725.
10. Astiz ME, Rackow EC, Kaufman B, et al. "Relationship of oxygen delivery and mixed venous oxygenation to lactic acidosis in patients with sepsis and acute myocardial infarction." *Crit Care Med* 1988;16:655.
11. Weil MH, Afifi A. "Experimental and clinical studies on lactate and pyruvate as indicators of the severity of acute circulatory failure." *Circulation* 1970;61:989.
12. Snider GL, Fairley HB, Fulmer JD, Weg JG. "Scientific basis of oxygen therapy." *Chest* 1984; 86:236.
13. Bryan-Brown CW. "Gas transport." *In Textbook of Critical Care.* Shoemaker WC, Thompson WL, Holbrook PR (eds). Philadelphia: WB Saunders, 1989, 492–497.
14. Ahrens TS. "Changing perspectives in oxygenation." *Crit Care Nurse* (in press).
15. Mizock BA. "Lactic Acidosis." *Dis Mon* 1989;35:323.
16. Veech, RL. "The metabolism of lactate." *NMR Biomed* 1991;4:53.
17. Rooth G, Sjostedt S, Caligara F. "Bloodless determination of arterial oxygen tension by polarography." *Science Tools* 1957;*LKW Instru J* 4:37.
18. Cone JB. "Cellular oxygen utilization." *In Oxygen Transport in the Critically Ill.* Chicago: Year Book Medical Pubs, 1987, 164.
19. Brown M, Vender JS. "Noninvasive oxygen monitoring." *Crit Care Clin* 1988;4:493.
20. Tremper KK, Shoemaker WC. "Transcutaneous oxygen monitoring of critically ill adults, with and without low flow shock." *Crit Care Med* 1981;9:706.
21. Kram HB. "Noninvasive tissue oxygen monitoring in surgical and critical care medicine." *Surg Clin North Am* 1985;65:1005.
22. Nolan LS, Shoemaker WC. "Transcutaneous O_2 and CO_2 monitoring of high risk surgical patients during the perioperative period." *Crit Care Med* 1982;10:762.
23. Abraham E, Smith M, Silver L. "Conjunctival and transcutaneous oxygen monitoring during cardiac arrest and cardiopulmonary resuscitation." *Crit Care Med* 1984;12:410.
24. Gutierrez G, Palizas F, Doglio G, et al. (Division of Pulmonary and Critical Care Medicine, University of Texas Health Science Center, Houston 77030.) "Gastric intramucosal pH as a therapeutic index of tissue oxygenation in critically ill patients." *Lancet* 1992;Vol.339, 8787:195, U9211 4561.
25. Partain CL, Price RR, Patton JA, et al. "Nuclear magnetic resonance imaging." *Radiographics* 1984; 4:5.
26. Ter Pogossian MM, Raichle ME, Sobel BE. "Positron emission tomography." *Sci Am* 1980;243:171.

10
$S\bar{v}_{O_2}$ Monitoring

$S\bar{v}_{O_2}$ (mixed-venous hemoglobin saturation of oxygen) monitoring has been noted for several decades to potentially be of clinical value in the assessment of oxygenation.[1] Clinical uses of $S\bar{v}_{O_2}$ monitoring did not occur commonly, however, until the 1970s. $S\bar{v}_{O_2}$ monitoring from a continuous point of view became available (in adults) in 1981 with the development and integration of plastic fiberoptics and pulmonary-artery catheters.[2] This development allowed for continuous $S\bar{v}_{O_2}$ monitoring in the tracking of clinical events. The potential value for $S\bar{v}_{O_2}$ monitoring and the interest in its use stem from its ability (1) to correlate oxygen consumption (V_{O_2}) and oxygen delivery (D_{O_2}), and (2) to correlate these parameters more rapidly than other measures. $S\bar{v}_{O_2}$ monitoring usually gives an integrated view of all components of oxygen transport and consumption, and thereby offers the potential to be more valuable than any individual aspects of D_{O_2} and V_{O_2}.

$S\bar{v}_{O_2}$ monitoring, however, is not consistently used in the clinical setting, due to potential problems and an incomplete application of $S\bar{v}_{O_2}$ data. $S\bar{v}_{O_2}$ monitoring has potential limitations that are related to $S\bar{v}_{O_2}$ theory, the cellular use of oxygen, and the potential misapplication of $S\bar{v}_{O_2}$ monitoring. In order to understand $S\bar{v}_{O_2}$ monitoring and to use it correctly, $S\bar{v}_{O_2}$ principles must be understood regarding the relationship of oxygen transport, O_2 consumption, and cellular utilization of oxygen.

Presently, $S\bar{v}_{O_2}$ monitoring has inconsistent use in critical care settings for reasons related to the above limitations. These reasons can be classified in seven categories:

1. difficulty in identifying when a change in $S\bar{v}_{O_2}$ becomes clinically significant;
2. use of the $S\bar{v}_{O_2}$ to predict individual organ oxygenation;
3. use of $S\bar{v}_{O_2}$ as data points as opposed to trend analysis;
4. use of $S\bar{v}_{O_2}$ when cellular dysoxia results from local blood flow abnormalities;
5. technical difficulties associated with $S\bar{v}_{O_2}$ monitoring;
6. use of $S\bar{v}_{O_2}$ when the oxyhemoglobin-dissociation curve is abnormal;
7. economic issues associated with $S\bar{v}_{O_2}$ use.

Each of the potential problems of $S\bar{v}_{O_2}$ monitoring can be addressed, however, allowing appropriate use of $S\bar{v}_{O_2}$ monitoring in the clinical setting. In addition, $S\bar{v}_{O_2}$ monitoring can provide several valuable clinical concepts, including:

1. analysis of the balance between D_{O_2} and V_{O_2};
2. assessing a critical D_{O_2} point (when V_{O_2} becomes dependent on D_{O_2});

3. assessing when changes in Pa_{O_2} values are due to changes in $S\bar{v}_{O_2}$, not Qs/Qt (Chapter 3);
4. calculation of parameters requiring venous oxygen content ($C\bar{v}_{O_2}$) data:
   a. cardiac outputs;
   b. V_{O_2} [Chapter 8]; via Fick equation
   c. Qs/Qt [Chapter 3];
   d. caloric requirements [Chapter 8];
5. use of $S\bar{v}_{O_2}$ as an end point in establishing the effectiveness of treatment.

It is the clinician, however, that must make the proper application of these potential uses of $S\bar{v}_{O_2}$ information, or its value will be limited. $S\bar{v}_{O_2}$ monitoring has been referred to as a technology in search of a problem.[3] This statement does not give credit to the specific and appropriate use of $S\bar{v}_{O_2}$ monitoring. $S\bar{v}_{O_2}$ monitoring has clear potential value if the clinician understands both the indications and limitations of its use. Research reports criticizing $S\bar{v}_{O_2}$ monitoring have too frequently focused on correlating $S\bar{v}_{O_2}$ with specific components of oxygen transport, a concept which does not lend it-self to the theory of $S\bar{v}_{O_2}$ use.[4] This chapter reviews the theoretical principles of $S\bar{v}_{O_2}$ monitoring, clinical examples of $S\bar{v}_{O_2}$ use, as well as each of the seven potential clinical problems. During this presentation, the clinician will see that $S\bar{v}_{O_2}$ monitoring, if used appropriately, has clear potential to be a major aid in the assessment of overall oxygenation.

PRINCIPLES OF Sv̄O₂ MONITORING

$S\bar{v}_{O_2}$ monitoring is based on the basic premise that hemoglobin releases oxygen to the cells in a manner dependent on the cellular need for oxygen and the amount of oxygen being delivered. Under normal circumstances, hemoglobin is nearly completely saturated with oxygen upon arrival to the cells (Figure 10.1). Upon arrival to the cells, hemoglobin can unload oxygen and allow the cells to extract oxygen from the blood, dependent upon cellular oxygen demand and partial pressures of oxygen. As the cells unload oxygen, hemoglobin desaturates according to cellular oxygen requirements (Figure 10.2). The desaturation of

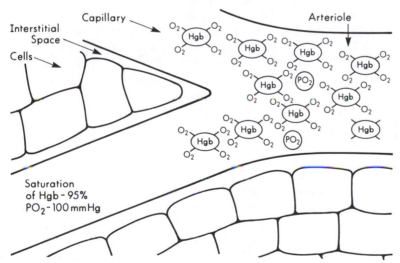

FIGURE 10.1. Saturation of hemoglobin on arrival to the cells. Upon arrival to the cells, most hemoblobin is fully loaded (saturated) with oxygen. Some dysfunctional hemoglobin is present (carboxyhemoglobin) or not all the binding sites are occupied by oxygen. However, most of the hemoglobin is carrying oxygen. Some oxygen is carried by the dissolved P_{O_2}.

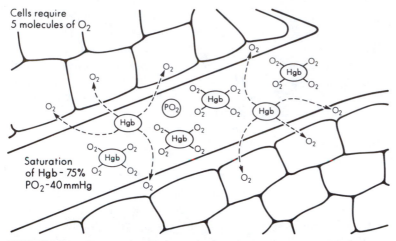

FIGURE 10.2. Desaturation of hemoglobin at the cellular level. As hemoglobin reaches the cells, oxygen is released according to the cellular need. Many factors influence the release of hemoglobin, including the difference between arterial and cellular-oxygen tension. Despite releasing oxygen for cellular use, the hemoglobin retains most of its oxygen.

hemoglobin is never complete; that is, hemoglobin never releases all of its oxygen.[5] Under normal circumstances, hemoglobin releases approximately one fourth of the oxygen attached to hemoglobin, releasing enough for the cellular need and resulting in a normal venous oxygen saturation of approximately 75%. If oxygen transport is inadequate or cellular demand increases, hemoglobin carries a reserve of oxygen in the sense that approximately 40–50% more oxygen can be extracted off hemoglobin.[6] Generally hemoglobin can never release all of the oxygen attached to hemoglobin molecules, but can release levels of up to nearly 70–80%.[7] This equates to a mixed-venous saturation of about 20–30%. The only oxygen reserve that truly is present in the body is hemoglobin's ability to release more oxygen than the 25% that is released during a normal oxygen pass by the tissues. If the cells require more oxygen, hemoglobin can release more, which would result in a lower venous oxygen saturation (Figure 10.3).

The clinical value of $S\bar{v}_{O_2}$ monitoring centers on its relationship with oxygen transport and O_2 consumption, and the reflection of potential cellular imbalance of these two components. If oxygen transport is inadequate, theoretically the cells will extract the same level of oxygen, resulting in a lower $S\bar{v}_{O_2}$ (Figure 10.4).[8] If oxygen consumption increases without a compensating increase in oxygen transport, $S\bar{v}_{O_2}$ levels will fall (Figure 10.5). Based on this logic, if $S\bar{v}_{O_2}$ levels decrease, the clinician realizes that one of two major problems could exist: either a decrease in oxygen transport or an increase in oxygen consumption. Should a $S\bar{v}_{O_2}$ level decrease, each of the four components of oxygen transport—cardiac output, hemoglobin, hemoglobin saturation (Sa_{O_2}), or Pa_{O_2}—would need to be assessed to determine if any of these levels had changed. If, on the other hand, oxygen transport remains constant, any change in the $S\bar{v}_{O_2}$ level is due to a change in oxygen consumption. If O_2 consumption levels increase, treatment should be focused on finding the cause of the increased O_2 consumption and treating this cause.

The value of $S\bar{v}_{O_2}$ monitoring also stems from its ability to serve as an early warning of problems in oxygenation. In theory, as soon as oxygen transport or O_2 consumption changes to the point where clinically

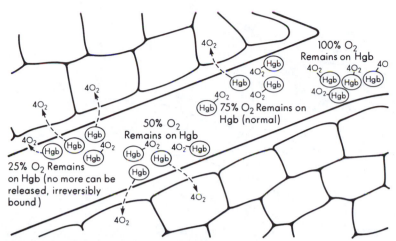

FIGURE 10.3. Hemoglobin changes the amount of oxygen released depending on changing supply and demand. Hemoglobin can release anywhere between 25 and 75% of the oxygen attached, depending on cellular requirements. Hemoglobin cannot release all oxygen, being irreversibly bound at levels near 25% saturation.

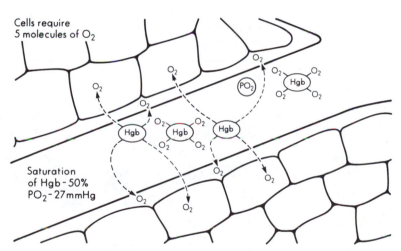

FIGURE 10.4. Decreased oxygen transport offset by increased extraction of oxygen from hemoglobin. If oxygen transport decreases, because of either a reduction in cardiac output or loss of hemoglobin, more oxygen can be removed from hemoglobin. Instead of losing 25% of the oxygen attached (S$_{O_2}$ of 75%), the hemoglobin can release more (S$_{O_2}$ of 50% in this illustration). The ability of hemoglobin to release more oxygen is the only real reserve of oxygen in the body.

more oxygen would be extracted from hemoglobin, the S$\overline{v}_{O_2}$ reflects the change (Figure 10.6).

S$\overline{v}_{O_2}$ monitoring will theoretically detect clinically significant problems in overall oxygenation, not changes in any one aspect of oxygenation. In other words, if one component of oxygenation changes, such as hemoglobin saturation (Sa$_{O_2}$), and another component, such as cardiac output, increases to offset the loss in saturation, S$\overline{v}_{O_2}$ levels may not change (Figure 10.7). If the S$\overline{v}_{O_2}$ level is

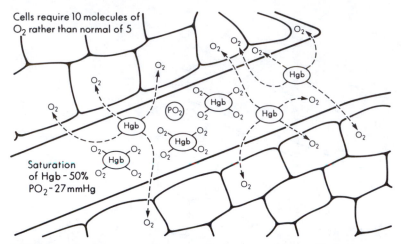

FIGURE 10.5. Increased oxygen consumption can be offset by increasing oxygen extraction from hemoglobin. If oxygen consumption increases without a rise in oxygen transport, cellular metabolism can be protected by extracting more oxygen from hemoglobin. The result is a lower venous hemoglobin saturation (Sv_{O_2}).

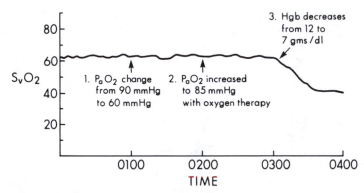

FIGURE 10.6. Sv_{O_2} can reflect clinically significant events. (1) No change in Sv_{O_2}. The decrease in Pa_{O_2} did not affect overall oxygenation. (2) No change in Sv_{O_2}. The increase in Pa_{O_2} did not affect overall oxygenation. (3) Decrease in hemoglobin affected the balance between oxygen transport and demand.

normal or unchanged, this indicates that any individual oxygenation change, such as Sa_{O_2}, has not caused a problem in cellular oxygenation. This means $S\bar{v}_{O_2}$ values should not be used to replace monitoring Sa_{O_2} levels or any other individual aspect of oxygenation. Rather, $S\bar{v}_{O_2}$ should be used as an indicator of when the change in one parameter starts to affect overall oxygenation.

$S\bar{v}_{O_2}$ monitoring is the assessment of overall balance between oxygen transport and consumption components, not individual components. The Sa_{O_2} level in the above example still needs to be assessed from the point of view that a drop in Sa_{O_2} (and also Pa_{O_2} levels) can, by itself, potentially cause clinical problems such as an increased work of breathing or pulmonary hypertension. $S\bar{v}_{O_2}$ monitoring is not intended as a replacement for other components of oxygenation but should be used to reflect overall clinical interactions. Multiple studies

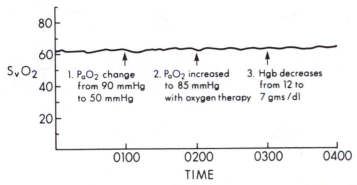

FIGURE 10.7. Compensation mechanisms may limit changes in Sv_{O_2}. (1) No change in Sv_{O_2}. Cardiac output increases slightly. (2) No change in Sv_{O_2}. Cardiac output returns to normal. (3) Decrease in hemoglobin is offset by an increase in the cardiac output.

have demonstrated the inconsistent correlation between S$\bar{v}_{O_2}$ and individual aspects of D$_{O_2}$.[9-12] These studies reinforce the importance of avoiding S$\bar{v}_{O_2}$ monitoring in isolation.

S$\bar{v}_{O_2}$ monitoring has been shown to be a relatively reliable indicator of overall balance of oxygenation, but it has not been demonstrated through research studies to be a parameter that should be used in isolation.[13-15] S$\bar{v}_{O_2}$ monitoring is best applied when used simultaneously with other components of oxygenation, including each of the four aspects of oxygen transport, the component of oxygen consumption, and assessment of cellular oxygenation utilization, such as serum-lactate levels.

INTEGRATION OF Sv_{O_2} AND Sa$_{O_2}$ FOR ASSESSMENT OF CARDIAC OUTPUT, OXYGEN CONSUMPTION (V$_{O_2}$), AND INTRAPULMONARY SHUNTING (Qs/Qt)

Both continuous and intermittent S$\bar{v}_{O_2}$ and Sa$_{O_2}$ values can be combined, either manually or with a computer program, to assess cardiac output, intrapulmonary shunting, or oxygen consumption. Cardiac output and V$_{O_2}$ are based on the Fick equation. Qs/Qt is measured from the classic shunt equation. Both the Fick and classic shunt equations are listed in Table 10.1.

TABLE 10.1.   Fick and Classic Shunt Equations

Fick Equation

$$CO = \frac{V_{O_2}}{Ca_{O_2} - Cv_{O_2}} \times 10$$

Classic Shunt Equation

$$Qs/Qt = \frac{Cc_{O_2} - Ca_{O_2}}{Cc_{O_2} - Cv_{O_2}}$$

Where

CO	= cardiac output
V$_{O_2}$	= oxygen consumption
C$\bar{v}_{O_2}$	= mixed-venous oxygen content
Ca$_{O_2}$	= arterial-oxygen content
Cc$_{O_2}$	= capillary-oxygen content

CARDIAC OUTPUT MEASUREMENT

In the Fick equation, S$\bar{v}_{O_2}$ and Sa$_{O_2}$ combine with hemoglobin to give the denominator. If oxygen consumption is measured or assumed, cardiac output can be obtained. A few key assumptions may be necessary for this measurement to be useful:

1. If pulse oximetry is employed, remember that a Sp$_{O_2}$ gives only an approximate Sa$_{O_2}$.
2. If oxygen consumption is not measured, estimation of V$_{O_2}$ must occur. An assumed V$_{O_2}$ at rest is about 3.5 cc/kg/min.[16]

3. Hemoglobin should be relatively constant if it is not measured.
4. The influence of Pa_{O_2} and $P\bar{v}_{O_2}$ on oxygen content may be eliminated without substantially affecting the computations.

Based on these assumptions, cardiac output can be measured or trended with $S\bar{v}_{O_2}$ and Sa_{O_2} data. The following example will give an analysis of cardiac output over time, without actually performing the cardiac-output measurement.

Example 1

Assume you have the following oxygenation information for a patient. At 1300, no cardiac output was obtained despite starting Lasix (20 mg orally), as well as initiating dobutamine at 3 mcg/kg/min. You would like to know if the cardiac output changed substantially from 1300 to 1400. Can you find out the cardiac output at 1300 from the given information?

	Time	
	1300	1400
Sa_{O_2}	.97	.94
$S\bar{v}_{O_2}$	.59	.64
Hgb	12	12
Weight	60 kg	

Using the information provided, the cardiac output can be computed for 1300, even if it was not actually measured at this time.

	Time	
	1300	1400
Measured Ca_{O_2}	15.6	15.1
Measured Cv_{O_2}	9.49	10.3
Measured Ca_{O_2} – Cv_{O_2}	6.11	4.8
Estimated V_{O_2}	60 × 3.5 cc/kg = 210 cc/min	
Estimated CO	$\frac{210}{6.11} \times 10 = 3.44$ l/min	
		$\frac{210}{4.8} \times 10 = 4.38$ l/min

The cardiac output is substantially higher at 1400 than at 1300, indicating a successful response to the initiation of the two drugs.

MEASUREMENT OF OXYGEN CONSUMPTION

The measurement of V_{O_2} is similar to the measurement of CO since the Fick equation is again used. When measuring V_{O_2}, the following data are necessary.

Sa_{O_2}
Hgb
$S\bar{v}_{O_2}$
Cardiac output

The Fick equation is adjusted to measure V_{O_2} in the following manner:

$$V_{O_2} = CO \times (Ca_{O_2} - Cv_{O_2}) \times 10$$

An example of measuring V_{O_2} is given below.

A 32-year-old man is in the unit with the diagnosis of acute respiratory failure following a bone-marrow transplant. He has a pulmonary-artery catheter in place to help monitor hemodynamics. Based on the information, what is the oxygen consumption? Completing the necessary computations generates the following information:

Sa_{O_2} .97
$S\bar{v}_{O_2}$ .56
Hgb   11 gm/dl
CO   7.2 LPM

Ca_{O_2} = 1.34 × 11 × .97 = 14.3
Cv_{O_2} = 1.34 × 11 × .56 = 8.3
Ca_{O_2} – Cv_{O_2} = 6.0
V_{O_2} = 7.2 × 6 × 10 = 432 cc/min

Measuring V_{O_2} is useful for several reasons, including both oxygenation and nutritional assessments. Understanding how to obtain V_{O_2} measurements is important since many ICUs do not routinely measure V_{O_2} (see Chapter 8).

DETERMINING INTRAPULMONARY SHUNT (Qs/Qt)

With both $S\bar{v}_{O_2}$ and Sa_{O_2} information, Qs/Qt can be measured via the classic-shunt equation.[17] Qs/Qt provides an estimate of the degree of lung dysfunction and is a useful clinical tool (Chapter 3). The classic-shunt equation is given below:

$$Qs/Qt = \frac{Cc_{O_2} - Ca_{O_2}}{Cc_{O_2} - Cv_{O_2}}$$

Measurement of the intrapulmonary shunt requires the following data:

Pa_{O_2}
Pa_{CO_2}
Sa_{O_2}
$P\bar{v}_{O_2}$
$S\bar{v}_{O_2}$
Hemoglobin
F_{IO_2}

From this data, pulmonary-capillary, arterial, and venous oxygen content can be computed. These computations are simplified if a computer software program containing these computations is employed. If no program is available, these computations can be performed by a calculator. The clinician will need to compute the alveolar-air equation to accurately account for P_{O_2} values (Chapter 3). While the alveolar-air equation was not as important in the measurement of CO and V_{O_2}, it is more important when measuring Qs/Qt because of the increased influence exerted by a high pulmonary-capillary oxygen pressure on the pulmonary oxygen content. The following clinical situation illustrates how to calculate the Qs/Qt.

A 71-year-old woman is in the unit for aspiration pneumonia. She has been in the unit for three days. Her current chest x-ray has evidence of consolidation in the right upper lobe. Given the following information, what is the degree of intrapulmonary shunting from the consolidation?

Pa_{O_2}	73 mm Hg
Sa_{O_2}	.92
Pa_{CO_2}	40 mm Hg
$P\bar{v}_{O_2}$	35 mm Hg
$S\bar{v}_{O_2}$	.61
Hemoglobin	10 gm/dl
F_{IO_2}	.50

PA_{O_2} (alveolar oxygen) = .50 (760 − 47) − 40/.8 = 306 mm Hg

Cc_{O_2} = 1.34 × 10 × 1.00 + (.003 × 306) = 14.3 gm/dl
Ca_{O_2} = 1.34 × 10 × .92 + (.003 × 73) = 12.6 gm/dl
Cv_{O_2} = 1.34 × 10 × .61 + (.003 × 35) = 8.3 gm/dl

$$Qs/Qt = \frac{14.3 - 12.6}{14.3 - 8.3} = .28$$

The Qs/Qt of .28 indicates a major disruption in the matching of ventilation to perfusion. This patient will have an increased work of breathing and cannot be removed from oxygen therapy.

For all of these calculated values—CO, V_{O_2}, and Qs/Qt—continuous measurement of both $S\bar{v}_{O_2}$ and Sa_{O_2} allows for computer-generated continuous readings. While many units do not currently have the computer capability to perform these computations, most units can have this capability in the near future.

$S\bar{v}_{O_2}$ AND THE V_{O_2}/D_{O_2} RELATIONSHIP

A key application of $S\bar{v}_{O_2}$ monitoring is the theoretical relationship between oxygen transport and oxygen consumption. Several investigations have demonstrated that a potential exists for oxygen consumption to be directly related to oxygen transport in various diseases states, including ARDS, sepsis, and congestive heart failure. The use of $S\bar{v}_{O_2}$ monitoring when oxygen transport may control changes in oxygen consumption limits the primary theoretical relationship of $S\bar{v}_{O_2}$ monitoring. Oxygen transport and O_2 consumption must be independent for $S\bar{v}_{O_2}$ values to give objective and reliable information regarding cellular oxygenation. When $S\bar{v}_{O_2}$ monitoring is used in clinical conditions where oxygen transport may determine oxygen consumption, the clinician must be aware that oxygen transport and oxygen consumption will not behave in the manner traditionally accepted for $S\bar{v}_{O_2}$ monitoring.

For $S\bar{v}_{O_2}$ monitoring to be used when oxygen consumption is dependent on oxygen transport, new guidelines must be established for $S\bar{v}_{O_2}$ monitoring. The oxygen transport/oxygen consumption relationship may exist at both high and low oxygen transport consumption.[18-19] Due to these extreme ranges, $S\bar{v}_{O_2}$ monitoring may not give an overt assessment of the relationship between transport and consumption. However, $S\bar{v}_{O_2}$ values may reach a plateau phase if transport and consumption are linearly related. Therefore $S\bar{v}_{O_2}$ may reflect the two situations where V_{O_2} has been indicated as being dependent on D_{O_2}, that is, low and high D_{O_2} states. For example, when D_{O_2} falls to a critically low point, V_{O_2} may become dependent on further reduction in D_{O_2}. At this point, $S\bar{v}_{O_2}$ will not markedly change, reflecting an apparent stable V_{O_2}/D_{O_2} relationship. Unfortunately, D_{O_2} may be decreasing with the V_{O_2} keeping pace.

Cellular hypoxia will develop in this case. The $S\bar{v}_{O_2}$, however, may not indicate any further worsening, since the balance between V_{O_2} and D_{O_2} may not be changing.

The same analysis applies to high D_{O_2} states; with high D_{O_2} levels, V_{O_2} may also be elevated. The high D_{O_2} levels usually produce elevated $S\bar{v}_{O_2}$, since the increased V_{O_2} is not high enough to reduce $S\bar{v}_{O_2}$ levels through an increase in oxygen extraction from hemoglobin. In addition, disruptions in cellular oxygen utilization may be present.

The $S\bar{v}_{O_2}$ catheter allows the clinician to establish whether a theoretical relationship exists between D_{O_2} and O_2 consumption by the following mechanism. If the $S\bar{v}_{O_2}$ level remains constant or elevated while either oxygen transport or O_2 consumption change, the assumption can be made that O_2 consumption is dependent on oxygen transport (Figure 10.8). $S\bar{v}_{O_2}$ monitoring would indicate that the O_2 consumption is dependent on oxygen transport, and might indicate that the patient requires improved D_{O_2}, V_{O_2}, or cellular utilization of oxygen. The primary advantage of $S\bar{v}_{O_2}$ monitoring if O_2 consumption is dependent on O_2 transport is the identification of when such a situation exists. When a situation exists in which O_2 consumption is dependent on O_2 transport, the clinician should be aware that cellular hypoxia may

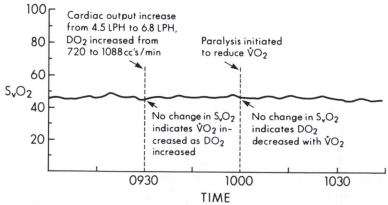

FIGURE 10.8. Stable Sv_{O_2} may occur when oxygen consumption (V_{O_2}) becomes dependent on oxygen delivery (D_{O_2}).

be present despite unchanging or elevated S$\bar{v}_{O_2}$ values. Immediate measures should be taken to try and improve oxygen transport, O_2 consumption, or cellular utilization of oxygen.

POTENTIAL PROBLEMS IN S$\bar{v}_{O_2}$ ANALYSIS
Importance of Specific S$\bar{v}_{O_2}$ Values

S$\bar{v}_{O_2}$ monitoring can be used in many clinical situations. In order to do this, however, specific changes in S$\bar{v}_{O_2}$ need to be quantified for their potential value. For example, normal S$\bar{v}_{O_2}$ levels are generally near 75%; however, levels as low as 60% have been stated as being clinically acceptable normals.[20-21] At what point below 60% S$\bar{v}_{O_2}$ signals cellular hypoxia has not been demonstrated.[22,23] As S$\bar{v}_{O_2}$ decreases, the clinician is alerted to begin an investigation of potential clinical problems rather than looking for a single S$\bar{v}_{O_2}$ value that may indicate cellular hypoxia. For example, the patient with an S$\bar{v}_{O_2}$ level that has decreased from 62% at 2200 to 54% at 0200 should cause the clinician to look at the decrease in S$\bar{v}_{O_2}$ as a potential problem with one of the aspects of oxygen transport or consumption, rather than to try to estimate how much of a change in oxygenation has occurred.

The point where the nurse should notify the physician of potential problems is also unclear. Since S$\bar{v}_{O_2}$ changes have not been able to be quantified specifically as to when cellular hypoxia may exist, it is best to collaborate with the physician beforehand in determining what level of change is to be viewed as clinically significant.

As the S$\bar{v}_{O_2}$ level decreases below 60%, the lower the value falls, the more potential problems exist in oxygenation. However, cellular hypoxia is difficult to quantify simply on S$\bar{v}_{O_2}$ levels. Clearly S$\bar{v}_{O_2}$ levels that fall below 50% have a higher risk of problems than values above 50%, but neither the absolute S$\bar{v}_{O_2}$ level nor a downward trend should be viewed in isolation.[24] Many patients have tolerated low values of S$\bar{v}_{O_2}$ (<40%) longer than would be expected.[25] Exceptions such as these preclude absolute guidelines for S$\bar{v}_{O_2}$ use.

Individual Organ Analysis

The S$\bar{v}_{O_2}$ catheter measures the mixed-venous blood from all organs. This invalidates its use as a measure of any individual organ. Each organ has a tendency to extract oxygen from hemoglobin at different levels. Organs that extract large amounts of oxygen from hemoglobin include the heart and brain (S$_{O_2}$ levels near 33%).[26] The kidneys and skeletal muscle (at rest) tend to extract less oxygen (S$_{O_2}$ levels > 75%).[27] Due to this variation in organ extraction of oxygen, the S$\bar{v}_{O_2}$ reflects the combination of all organs and cannot reflect an individual system (Figure 10.9).

Since the S$\bar{v}_{O_2}$ reflects all organs, a worsening or improvement in one system may not be reflected in overall S$\bar{v}_{O_2}$ values. For example, in cardiac failure the skeletal mus-

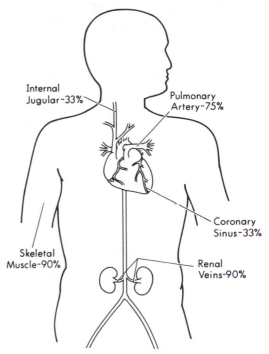

FIGURE 10.9. Venous hemoglobin saturation varies in each organ.

cle may have a decreased flow, decreased V_{O_2}, and higher $S\bar{v}_{O_2}$, whereas the heart may have a slight reduction in $S\bar{v}_{O_2}$. The higher S_{O_2} from the skeletal muscle may negate the slight decrease in cardiac S_{O_2}.

The use of $S\bar{v}_{O_2}$ has a practical limitation in the assessment of organ oxygenation. Some research studies have measured the S_{O_2} from individual organs, but this is not as yet a practical clinical alternative.

Trend Analysis in $S\bar{v}_{O_2}$ Monitoring

One of the most useful values of $S\bar{v}_{O_2}$ is trend analysis as opposed to individual-point analysis. As the $S\bar{v}_{O_2}$ level changes, either down or up, assessments of overall aspects of oxygenation are being reflected. A downward trend in $S\bar{v}_{O_2}$ levels is more likely to indicate a problem than is a single $S\bar{v}_{O_2}$ value obtained in isolation that may be lower than 60%. $S\bar{v}_{O_2}$ values that trend upward may be viewed as a potential improvement in oxygenation (in the absence of sepsis). $S\bar{v}_{O_2}$ levels have been shown to change frequently for short periods of time.[28] The trend analysis helps avoid sampling a single $S\bar{v}_{O_2}$ value in one of the tran-

sient, clinically insignificant periods (Figure 10.10). Sampling $S\bar{v}_{O_2}$ intermittently, rather than through continuous use, runs the risk of missing sudden changes in oxygenation that could occur with sampling in a non-representative time period. For $S\bar{v}_{O_2}$ to achieve optimal effect, particularly considering its rapid reflection of oxygenation changes, continuous use is preferable.

$S\bar{v}_{O_2}$ MONITORING AND CELLULAR DYSOXIA

$S\bar{v}_{O_2}$ monitoring has been restricted in assessment of cellular oxygenation in certain clinical conditions. In conditions where the cells do not properly use oxygen, or where blood does not perfuse tissues or unload oxygen normally, $S\bar{v}_{O_2}$ values will be artificially elevated relative to cellular oxygenation status. A review of the conditions that may cause inaccurate $S\bar{v}_{O_2}$ reflections of cellular oxygenation will help illustrate how to apply $S\bar{v}_{O_2}$ data appropriately. This category has similarities with the section on D_{O_2}/V_{O_2} relationships. It actually may be a subsection of the D_{O_2}/V_{O_2} relationship.

Cells may not utilize oxygen properly if a

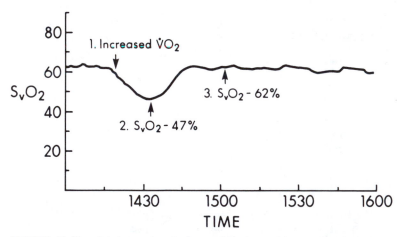

FIGURE 10.10. Continuous monitoring avoids errors that may result from intermittent sampling. (1) IM injection given which temporarily increases oxygen consumption. (2) Intermittent Sv_{O_2} sample obtained. Patient shows no overt evidence of an increased V_{O_2}. (3) Sv_{O_2} returns to normal after 20 minutes. If the Sv_{O_2} is obtained during the time of increased oxygen consumption, an assessment of overall oxygenation problems may be made, when actually the only problem is a transient oxygenation disturbance.

component of the energy-generation system in inhibited. For example, if cytochrome a3 is inhibited (as in cyanide poisoning), oxygen cannot be utilized. The lack of oxygen utilization may cause an increased S$\bar{v}_{O_2}$ value when the cells are in a state of hypoxia.

Lack of perfusion to an area can be the result of many factors, including pericapillary shunting, decreased capillary density, and microembolization (Figures 10.11 & 10.12).[29–32] In all of these conditions, oxygen will not be extracted as would be expected from the reduced blood flow into the tissue area. The S$\bar{v}_{O_2}$ value cannot reflect tissue oxygenation that does not have perfusion. The result is similar to that of arterial blood mixing with venous blood, elevating the S$\bar{v}_{O_2}$. In this situation, as with decreased oxygen utilization, the S$\bar{v}_{O_2}$ value will be artificially elevated relative to the cellular oxygenation status.

Conditions associated with the decreased flow into the area primarily involve loss of local vasoregulation, such as sepsis. Release of microemboli have also been proposed as a possible mechanism of cellular hypoxia in some shock states. Microembolization may be the result of local coagulation disturbances, such as thromboxane A2, precipitated by eicosanoid release. With conditions in which local vasoregulation is impaired, multiple factors are present that may cause the impairment of vascular tone. Alterations in local pH, electrolytes, osmolality, and prostaglandin levels all can mediate the loss of vasomotor regulation (see Chapter 1). As factors such as these decrease flow into a tissue bed, less blood is exposed to tissue for oxygen release. Overall blood return to the heart will not reflect tissue beds that have lost perfusion so the S$\bar{v}_{O_2}$ will not accurately reflect tissue oxygenation.

Technical Issues Associated with S$\bar{v}_{O_2}$ Monitoring

The technology for intermittently measuring mixed-venous samples of blood has existed since the early part of this century. Continuous pulmonary-artery measurement has been reported since 1961.[33] The primary concept of continuous S$\bar{v}_{O_2}$ monitoring centers around reflectance spectrophotometry. Reflectance spectrophotometry

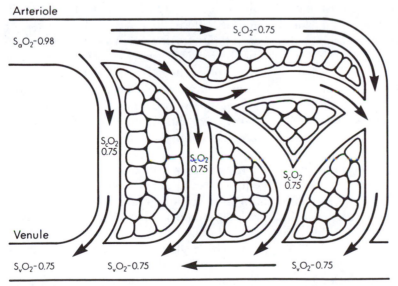

FIGURE 10.11. Normal capillary blood flow. Normal blood flow through the capillaries allows increasing amounts of oxygen to be extracted from hemoglobin. Normal levels of extraction are about 25%, yielding Sv$_{O_2}$ values of about 75%.

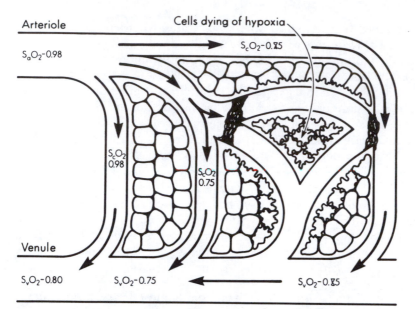

FIGURE 10.12. Pericapillary shunting owing to microemoboli phenomenon. In situations where pericapillary shunting develops, for example, sepsis, some arterial blood fails to come into contact with tissues. The result is an inability to provide oxygen to these cells, resulting in tissue hypoxia. Since the blood being shunted past the tissues now has abundant oxygen, the result is an increase in the Sv_{O_2} level and a decreased overall hemoglobin extraction.

is the measurement of the oxyhemoglobin saturation of blood. Different mechanisms of reflectance spectrophotometry have been developed to accurately measure oxygen saturation of the venous system. All of these mechanisms work approximately on the following principles.

TECHNICAL PRINCIPLES OF $S\bar{v}_{O_2}$ MONITORING

$S\bar{v}_{O_2}$ monitoring operates on concepts that have been developed and modified since the 1930s.[34] The primary concept in $S\bar{v}_{O_2}$ monitoring, that is, reflectance spectrophotometry, is slightly different from the absorptive (or transmission) spectrophotometry involved in pulse oximetry. Reflective spectrophotometry operates basically on the following principles:

All elements absorb light at a given wavelength. This absorption gives color to the object.[35] For example, oxyhemoglobin absorbs light in the 660-nm range (red), in contrast to reduced hemoglobin, which absorbs light in the 940-nm range (infrared).[36] The

different absorption characteristics give the hemoglobin different colors, oxyhemoglobin a red color and reduced hemoglobin a blue color (Figure 10.13). In addition to generating color, the wavelengths specific to each type of hemoglobin allow for measurement of each hemoglobin. Since multiple types of hemoglobin exist, a multi-wavelength system would need to be employed to measure all the hemoglobin types.[37] Unfortunately, the increased number of wavelengths required to measure the multiple types of hemoglobin adds to the complexity of the oximetry. Since the primary hemoglobin of interest is oxyhemoglobin, manufacturers have forgone measurement of all types of hemoglobin and have focused only on oxyhemoglobin.

Oxyhemoglobin is measured by emitting light at 660 nm, then quickly turning off the 660-nm light and switching to an 805-nm light. (A typical oximeter may perform this light pulsation over 200 times per second).[38] The 805-nm wavelength is equally absorbed by both oxyhemoglobin and deoxyhemo-

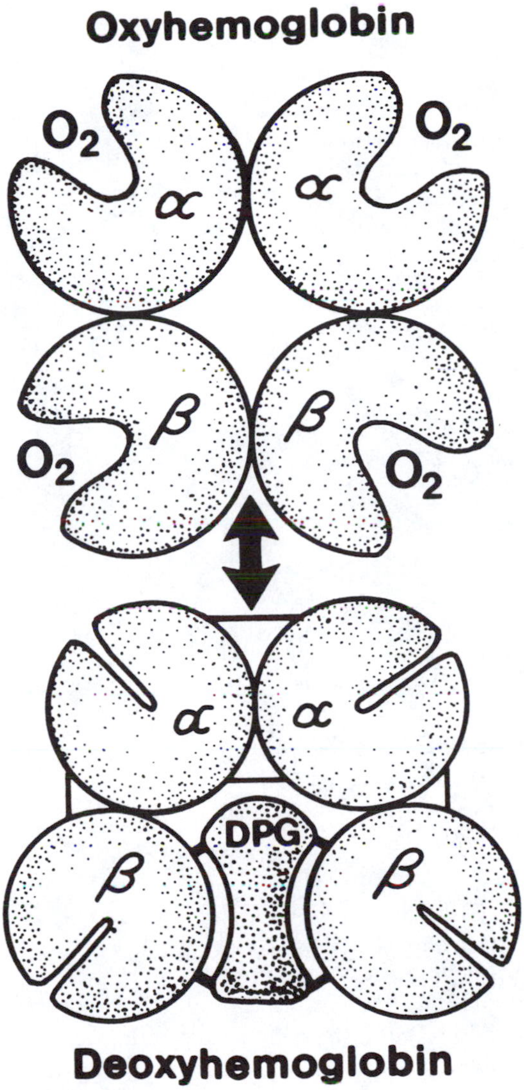

Oxyhemoglobin

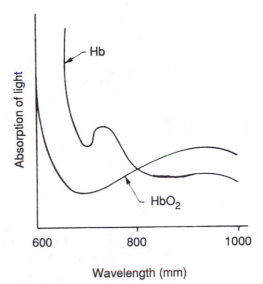

FIGURE 10.14. Oxyhemoglobin and deoxyhemoglobin absorb light in equal amounts at the isobestic point. Adapted from Fahey PJ. *Continuous measurement of blood oxygen saturation in the high risk patient.* Mountian View CA: Abbott Laboratories, 1987, p. 61.

Deoxyhemoglobin

FIGURE 10.13. Hemoglobin color characteristics are different because of different light-absorption characteristics. Adapted from Hillman RS, Finch CA. *Red Cell Manual,* 5th ed. Philadelphia: F.A. Davis, 1985.

globin (referred to as the isobestic point) (Figure 10.14). The two-wavelength-emitting system forms the basis for in vivo (inside the blood vessel) oximetry measurement.

The fiberoptics in the S$\overline{v}_{O_2}$ pulmonary-artery catheter are designed to both send and receive light (Figure 10.15). As light is pulsed at 660 nm, light is reflected from oxyhemoglobin back to the receiving optical fibers. In contrast, as the light is pulsed at the

805-nm wavelength, light from both oxy- and deoxyhemoglobin is reflected back to the receiving optical bundle (fibers). The comparison between the amount of light reflected between the two pulses allows for determination of the oxyhemoglobin concentration (Figure 10.16).

The components of the S$\overline{v}_{O_2}$ catheters include a light-emitting source, a receiving source, a photodetector for the increasing light, and a microprocessor for the analysis of the amount of light reflected from each pulse. The microprocessor determines the actual oxyhemoglobin saturation level (Figure 10.17).

One key limitation to the two-wavelength system is the potential to have elements in the blood other than oxyhemoglobin and reduced hemoglobin reflect light. While emitting specific wavelengths reduces most of these problems, it does not eliminate them. For example, variations in total hemoglobin, hematocrit, and blood flow and the presence of excess lipids (such as in TPN solution) or dye (radiology tests) can alter the S$\overline{v}_{O_2}$ signal. One manufacturer

FIBEROPTIC CATHETER

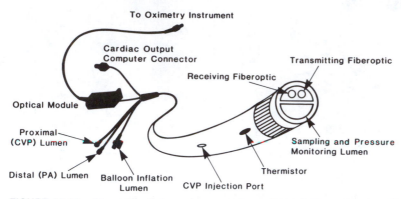

FIGURE 10.15. Fiberoptics in the pulmonary-artery catheter both send and receive light impulses. Adapted from Fahey PJ. *Continuous measurement of blood oxygen saturation in the high risk patient.* Mountian View CA: Abbott Laboratories, 1987, p. 71.

PRINCIPLES OF REFLECTION
SPECTROPHOTOMETRY

Fiberoptic catheter oximetry (*in vivo*)

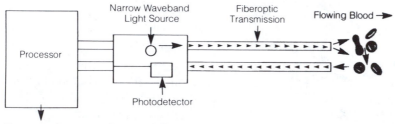

Output: Oxyhemoglobin Saturation (SO₂)

FIGURE 10.16. The processor analyzes the reflection of light to obtain an oxyhemoglobin value. Adapted from Fahey PJ. *Continuous measurement of blood oxygen saturation in the high risk patient.* Mountian View CA: Abbott Laboratories, 1987, p. 61.

developed and released a system in 1981 that incorporates a third wavelength to control some of the artifact induced by changing hematocrit levels.[39] Studies seem to support the improved accuracy of the three-wavelength systems.[40-41]

The nurse should check the accuracy of the $S\bar{v}_{O_2}$ catheter in order to correct for drifts in the $S\bar{v}_{O_2}$ values that may impair its ability to accurately reflect trends in oxygenation. This check should be performed at least once a day depending on the type of catheter and manufacturer recommendation. Two-wavelength systems may require more frequent analysis than three-wavelength systems. However, the technology in this area is frequently improving and one

needs to refer to the manufacturer guidelines to get specific information in regard to how frequently the oximeter should be calibrated.

NURSING AND TECHNICAL ISSUES

Care of the continuous $S\bar{v}_{O_2}$ catheter is not different from the normal pulmonary-artery catheter, with a few exceptions. One major difference is due to the presence of fiberoptic bundles in the catheter, care should be taken not to bend the catheter. The clinician must be aware that the $S\bar{v}_{O_2}$ catheter can be inaccurate if substances other than oxyhemoglobin and reduced hemoglobin are being reflected. Also, the $S\bar{v}_{O_2}$ will not correlate exactly with a mixed-

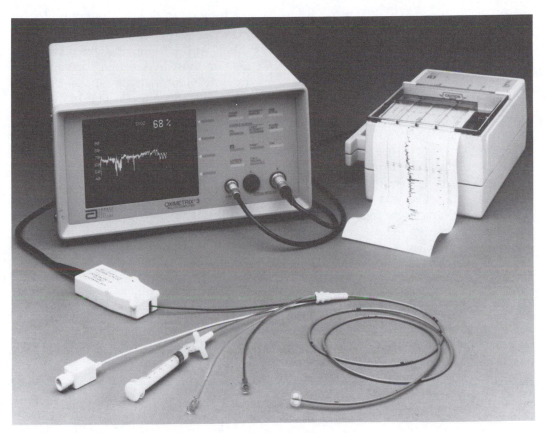

FIGURE 10.17. Equipment employed in the measurement of continuous mixed-venous hemoglobin saturation. Photo supplied by Abbott Laboratories (1991). Reproduced with permission. Abbott Critical Care, 1992.

venous blood sample analyzed by the laboratory. This is because the $S\bar{v}_{O_2}$ catheter does not measure all types of hemoglobins. The $S\bar{v}_{O_2}$ value will always read higher than the laboratory measure of $S\bar{v}_{O_2}$. In order to correct for the other types of hemoglobin and allow for comparison of $S\bar{v}_{O_2}$ from the laboratory catheter, use the following equation:

$$S\bar{v}_{O_2} \text{ (from catheter)} = \frac{S\bar{v}_{O_2} \text{ (from lab)}}{1 - (\text{carboxyhemoglobin (\%)} + \text{methemoglobin (\%)})}$$

For example, assume that the $S\bar{v}_{O_2}$ reading from the catheter is .66. A blood sample drawn at the same time of the catheter reading indicates the following:

$S\bar{v}_{O_2}$	.66
COHgb (carboxyhemoglobin)	.02
MetHgb (methemoglobin)	.01

Comparison of the $S\bar{v}_{O_2}$ from the catheter and the laboratory can take place after entering the lab data into the above equation:

$$S\bar{v}_{O_2} \text{ (from catheter)} = \frac{.66}{1 - (.02 + .01)} = \frac{.66}{.97} = .68$$

Based on the equation, the laboratory and catheter readings are within 2% of each other, indicating an accurate $S\bar{v}_{O_2}$ catheter reading.

Manufacturers provide specific information regarding requirements for obtaining accurate values and troubleshooting problems with $S\bar{v}_{O_2}$ catheters, but a few principles should be followed to obtain accurate readings:

1. If the $S\bar{v}_{O_2}$ value reads higher than 70–80%, the catheter may be reflecting capillary wall as opposed to blood (Figure 10.18). The catheter will usually warn of a problem with high light-intensity alarms. Flushing or repositioning the catheter may help eliminate this problem.

2. Check the $S\bar{v}_{O_2}$ value against the cooximeter value from the lab (an in vivo calibration) at least daily. Update the $S\bar{v}_{O_2}$ value when necessary. (When drawing blood from the distal port of the pulmonary-artery catheter to perform an in vivo calibration, draw the blood slowly in order to avoid pulling pulmonary-capillary blood into the sample.[42])

Changes in the Oxyhemoglobin-Dissociation Curve

Shifts in the oxyhemoglobin-dissociation curve can cause $S\bar{v}_{O_2}$ readings to have implications different than may appear simply by the absolute $S\bar{v}_{O_2}$ level. The oxyhemoglobin-dissociation curve illustrates the hemoglobin's affinity for oxygen (Figure 10.19). Changes in blood chemistries can cause the oxyhemoglobin curve to change from the normal hemoglobin oxygen affinity relationship. Conditions that can increase hemoglobin's affinity for oxygen include an alkalosis, low carbon-dioxide levels, insufficient levels of 2,3 diphosphoglycerate (2,3 DPG), and decreased body temperature.[43] The increased affinity of hemoglobin for oxygen will cause a higher hemoglobin saturation and lower partial pressures of oxygen (Figure 10.20). With these circumstances, hemoglobin has less ability to release oxygen and tends to hold on to oxygen longer. On

Normal

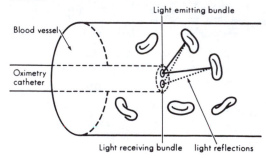

Catheter Reflecting Vessel Wall

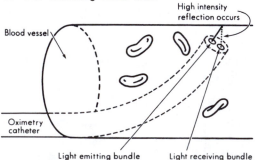

FIGURE 10.18. Oximetry catheter reading with a falsely elevated Sv_{O_2} owing to blood-vessel-wall reflection.

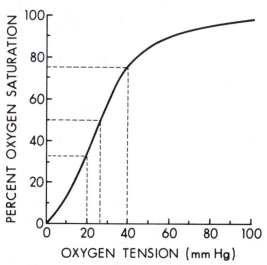

FIGURE 10.19. The oxyhemoglobin-dissociation curve at venous levels. Note that hemoglobin does not have a strong affinity for oxygen as the P_{O_2} decreases. At a normal venous P_{O_2} of about 40 mm Hg, the saturation of hemoglobin is 75%. If the P_{O_2} decreases by only 13 mm Hg, hemoglobin loses another 25% of the oxygen (S_{O_2} of 50%). This loss of affinity for oxygen is important in that it allows oxygen to leave hemoglobin and enter the cells without reattaching to hemoglobin.

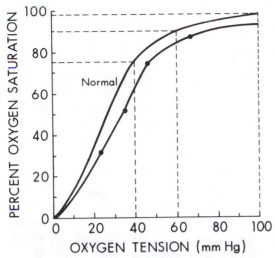

FIGURE 10.20. Left shift in the oxyhemoglobin-dissociation curve. Several conditions cause hemoglobin to bind tighter to oxygen, a situation referred to as a left shift in the oxyhemoglobin-dissociation curve. When conditions such as an alkalosis, hypocarbia, decreased, 2, 3, DPG levels, and hypothermia exist, higher hemoglobin saturations are present than normally anticipated relative to the P_{O_2} value.

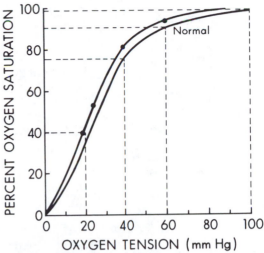

FIGURE 10.21. Right shift in the oxyhemoglobin dissociation curve. Several conditions cause hemoglobin to bind more loosely with oxygen, a stituation referred to as a right shift in the oxyhemoglobin-dissociation curve. When conditions such as an acidosis, hypercarbia, increased, 2, 3, DPG levels, and hyperthermia exist, lower hemoglobin saturations are present than normally anticipated relative to the P_{O_2} value.

the other hand, the right-sided shift in the oxyhemoglobin dissociation curve, which is precipitated by such things as acidosis, chronic carbon-dioxide levels, excess quantities of 2,3 DPG, or an increased temperature, tend to reduce hemoglobin's affinity for oxygen (Figure 10.21).[43] The right shift causes S$\bar{v}_{O_2}$ levels to be associated with higher than expected P_{O_2} levels at a given S$\bar{v}_{O_2}$. An example of the normal left- and right-sided P_{O_2} and S$\bar{v}_{O_2}$ levels are given in Table 10.2. One major reason for correlating S$\bar{v}_{O_2}$ and P$\bar{v}_{O_2}$ levels is the potential value of P$\bar{v}_{O_2}$ levels in the assessment of tissue oxygenation.

P$\bar{v}_{O_2}$ AND CELLULAR OXYGENATION

P$\bar{v}_{O_2}$ levels are thought to be near tissue-capillary oxygen levels.[44–45] Tissue-capillary levels of oxygen are a primary factor in driving oxygen into cells, that is, generating the pressure necessary to facilitate oxygen movement out of the vascular space and into the tissue level (Figure 10.22). The nor-

mal P$\bar{v}_{O_2}$ of 40 mm Hg is adequate to drive oxygen into the cell.[46] As the P$\bar{v}_{O_2}$ level decreases and driving pressure falls, oxygen diffusion into the cells may be inhibited.[47]

The point where a decrease in the P$\bar{v}_{O_2}$ level inhibits oxygen diffusion into the cell is unclear. Mitochondrial oxygen tensions have been documented to be less than 2 mm Hg.[48] Due to the low mitochondrial pressure, the pressure gradient from the vascular space to the cells is likely to be maintained, even at low vascular-oxygen

TABLE 10.2. Effect on the P_{O_2}/Sa$_{O_2}$ Relationship with Shifts in the Oxyhemoglobin-Dissociation Curve

Sa$_{O_2}$	P_{O_2} (Sample Values)		
	Expected	Left Shift	Right Shift
33%	20	15	25
50%	27	20	33
75%	40	34	46
90%	60	50	70
95%	85	76	92

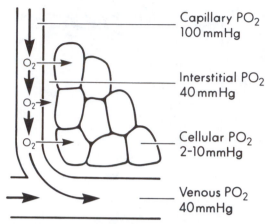

Capillary PO2
100 mmHg

Interstitial PO2
40 mmHg

Cellular PO2
2–10 mmHg

Venous PO2
40 mmHg

FIGURE 10.22. Capillary pressure of oxygen as a driving force pushing oxygen into the cells. Note that venous-oxygen tensions approximate capillary-oxygen tensions.

pressure levels. Clinical observations coupled with available research, however, indicate that vascular-oxygen pressures should be no lower than about 20 mm Hg in order to maintain adequate driving pressures.[49–50]

According to the oxyhemoglobin-dissociation curve, $P\bar{v}_{O_2}$ values of 27 mm Hg correlate with $S\bar{v}_{O_2}$ values of 50%. Hemoglobin can dissociate from oxygen only to levels of about 33%, at which time the $P\bar{v}_{O_2}$ is about 20 mm Hg. As a rule of thumb, when the $S\bar{v}_{O_2}$ is below 0.75, every $S\bar{v}_{O_2}$ decrease of 2% changes the $P\bar{v}_{O_2}$ by about 1 mm Hg. While the change in $S\bar{v}_{O_2}$ and $P\bar{v}_{O_2}$ is not a linear relationship, use of this guideline allows the approximation of the $P\bar{v}_{O_2}$ from the $S\bar{v}_{O_2}$ (assuming a normal oxyhemoglobin-dissociation curve).

The use of $P\bar{v}_{O_2}$ values in clinical practice is similar to $S\bar{v}_{O_2}$ application: the use of $P\bar{v}_{O_2}$ trends is more valuable than a single $P\bar{v}_{O_2}$ value. While evidence exists that $P\bar{v}_{O_2}$ levels less than 27 mm Hg may indicate cellular hypoxia, there is no specific $P\bar{v}_{O_2}$ value that correlates with cellular anoxia.[51] The clinician can use the $P\bar{v}_{O_2}$ as a guideline, however, for estimating overall oxygenation. For example, as the $P\bar{v}_{O_2}$ falls below 27 mm Hg, difficulties in oxygen diffusion into the cells may be developing. At $P\bar{v}_{O_2}$ levels less than 20 mm Hg, cellular hypoxia

is likely. Aggressive support of oxygen transport and consumption should be given if the $P\bar{v}_{O_2}$ falls to levels less than 27 mm Hg.

Shifts in the oxyhemoglobin curve can be somewhat misleading regarding $P\bar{v}_{O_2}$ levels. As the oxyhemoglobin curve shifts to the left, higher hemoglobin saturation is evident, which may give a false indication of adequate oxygenation. However, these higher $S\bar{v}_{O_2}$ levels are associated with lower $P\bar{v}_{O_2}$ levels. When the oxyhemoglobin curve is shifted to the left, the higher $S\bar{v}_{O_2}$ can mislead the clinician into thinking that the oxygenation is adequate when the $P\bar{v}_{O_2}$ may indicate that the patient has some degree of potential for hypoxia.

On the other hand, right-sided shifts of the oxyhemoglobin dissociation curve can cause the clinician to be misled in believing the person may be worse than anticipated. The low $S\bar{v}_{O_2}$ levels are associated with a higher $P\bar{v}_{O_2}$ level and may give an indication of hypoxia when tissue or $P\bar{v}_{O_2}$ levels are adequate. In order to assess the patient's oxyhemoglobin-dissociation curve and its relationship to $S\bar{v}_{O_2}$ and $P\bar{v}_{O_2}$ levels, the clinician should draw a blood sample for $S\bar{v}_{O_2}$ and $P\bar{v}_{O_2}$ values. From this sample, the clinical should note whether the $P\bar{v}_{O_2}$ and $S\bar{v}_{O_2}$ information can identify where the oxyhemoglobin-dissociation curve is located regarding a left- or right-sided shift. Unfortunately, the oxyhemoglobin-dissociation curve is dynamic and not fixed for long periods of time; the oxyhemoglobin curve could shift its position very rapidly. It is important however, to try and get an idea of current $S\bar{v}_{O_2}$ values relative to $P\bar{v}_{O_2}$ value.

Economic Issues of the $S\bar{v}_{O_2}$ Catheter

Controversial issues regarding $S\bar{v}_{O_2}$ monitoring include whether the $S\bar{v}_{O_2}$ catheter should be utilized instead of a normal pulmonary catheter,[52–53] and whether continuous versus intermittent $S\bar{v}_{O_2}$ analysis should be used. The most obvious limitation of the fiberoptic pulmonary-artery catheter capable of continuously measuring $S\bar{v}_{O_2}$ levels is the price. These catheters generally cost substantially more than the simple pulmonary catheter (approximately $100 more). Research has not been able to demonstrate cost effectiveness of many types of technological advances in equipment, including pulmonary-artery and S$\bar{v}_{O_2}$ catheters.

The value in S$\bar{v}_{O_2}$ monitoring clearly will come from its appropriate utilization by clinicians. The use of S$\bar{v}_{O_2}$ monitoring to assess the D$_{O_2}$/V$_{O_2}$ balance, as an end point in determining the effectiveness of treatments, identifying a critical D$_{O_2}$ point and use of C$\bar{v}_{O_2}$ calculations (cardiac output, V$_{O_2}$, caloric determination and Qs/Qt measurement) is required to truly assess the value of S$\bar{v}_{O_2}$ monitoring. If the clinician is able to use the S$\bar{v}_{O_2}$ catheter for all these purposes, cost-effective use is possible. If the S$\bar{v}_{O_2}$ catheter is not actively utilized in the treatment and assessment of the patient, then it is unlikely that S$\bar{v}_{O_2}$ monitoring will achieve economic (or clinical) effectiveness. The general effectiveness of the S$\bar{v}_{O_2}$ catheter seems obvious, but it is important to remember that it is only as useful as the clinician responsible for applying its values.

The question of whether the S$\bar{v}_{O_2}$ catheter has been demonstrated to be cost effective is not easy to answer. However, with the use of the S$\bar{v}_{O_2}$ to guide clinical decisions regarding the end point of treatment, one would expect the S$\bar{v}_{O_2}$ value to be of enough clinical use to potentially reduce the overall number of therapeutic interventions and reduce the length of stay in the ICU. These two objectives, reducing the overall interventions and length of stay, remain to be demonstrated in a research study. However, clinicians can get an approximation of how valuable the S$\bar{v}_{O_2}$ catheter is to their particular institution by asking these questions: (1) Does the S$\bar{v}_{O_2}$ information help direct practice and avoid or reduce the number of interventions? and (2) Does the S$\bar{v}_{O_2}$ catheter perhaps increase the number of interventions, yet help the patient to leave the unit in a shorter period

of time? The S$\bar{v}_{O_2}$ catheter, like many other pieces of technology, undoubtedly is more effective in the hands of a good clinician. The question of whether the S$\bar{v}_{O_2}$ catheters are cost effective is at this point in time likely related to individual clinician use and application.

Intermittent sampling of mixed venous blood gases as opposed to use of a continuous S$\bar{v}_{O_2}$ catheter has several practical limitations. Blood-gas samples require extra nursing or technician time and are costly. More importantly, for S$\bar{v}_{O_2}$ monitoring to achieve a clinical benefit and therefore a cost benefit, early changes in oxygenation must be detected. Intermittent sampling is likely to miss these early changes.[46] The continuous use of S$\bar{v}_{O_2}$ monitoring is the most likely method of achieving a clinical and economic impact.

SUMMARY

S$\bar{v}_{O_2}$ monitoring has been suggested by several literature sources to be potentially useful for its ability to serve as an end point in assessing overall oxygenation or the monitoring of individual parameters. For S$\bar{v}_{O_2}$ monitoring to be used correctly, it should not be used to monitor a single parameter of either D$_{O_2}$ or V$_{O_2}$. S$\bar{v}_{O_2}$ monitoring can, however, be utilized in assessing overall oxygenation as individual components of D$_{O_2}$ or V$_{O_2}$ change. For example, the use of S$\bar{v}_{O_2}$ to identify changes in the specific parameters, such as arterial P$_{O_2}$ levels, hemoglobin saturation, hemoglobin, or cardiac output, has found limited accuracy. This is expected, however, due to the relationship that exists between each of the oxygenation components, and to the dynamic interaction as one component can compensate for changes in another without substantially changing S$\bar{v}_{O_2}$ levels. In addition, local blood flow changes prevent S$\bar{v}_{O_2}$ levels from changing as one would expect. The use of S$\bar{v}_{O_2}$ monitoring as an end point in treatment is primarily designed to determine the effectiveness or the impact of a particular component on overall oxygenation and not to replace the measurement of those concepts. For example, if reducing the FI_{O_2} on a patient, the $S\bar{v}_{O_2}$ can aid in assessing the overall impact on oxygenation but should not be used to replace measurements of Sa_{O_2} or Pa_{O_2}. The fact that changes in individual components, such as Pa_{O_2}, give us important information by themselves is another reason why $S\bar{v}_{O_2}$ measurements should not replace individual parameters. If the Pa_{O_2}, for example, decreases below a level of approximately 60 mm Hg, three primary conditions can occur, decreasing affinity of hemoglobin for oxygen, increasing work of breathing through stimulation of carotid and aortic bodies, and decreasing pulmonary-vasomotor tone causing an increase in pulmonary-vascular resistance. While a decrease in Pa_{O_2} below 60 may not affect overall oxygenation as reflected by the $S\bar{v}_{O_2}$, the clinician would want to know the change in the Pa_{O_2} in order to avoid these potential deleterious effects of changes in the Pa_{O_2}. $S\bar{v}_{O_2}$ data obtained from continuous monitoring is designed to reflect the overall oxygenation changes, not to replace an individual component of oxygenation. Use of $S\bar{v}_{O_2}$ data offers the clinician an important tool in the assessment of oxygenation; but it needs to be applied with the knowledge of both theoretical formulation of oxygenation and the potential problem of $S\bar{v}_{O_2}$ use. Only with the appropriate application of $S\bar{v}_{O_2}$ data will the clinician be better able to assess overall oxygenation.

REFERENCES

1. Gamble WJ, Hugenholtz PG, Monroe RG, Polanyi M, Nadas AS. "The use of fiberoptics in clinical cardiac catheterization." *Circulation* 1965;31:328.
2. Waller JL, Kaplan JA, Bauman DI, et al. "Clinical evaluation of new fiberoptic catheter oximeter during cardiac surgery." *Anesth Analg* 1982;61:676.
3. McPherson RW. *Yearbook of Critical Care Medicine 1987*. Chicago: Year Book Medical Pubs, 1987, 432.
4. Ahrens T. "$S\bar{v}_{O_2}$ monitoring: is it being used appropriately?" *Crit Care Nurse* 1990;10:70.
5. Bunn HF. *Hemoglobin: Molecular, Genetic and Clinical Aspects*. Philadelphia: WB Saunders, 1986, 94.
6. White KM. "Completing the hemodynamic picture: $S\bar{v}_{O_2}$." *Heart & Lung* 1985;14:272.
7. Dickerson RE. *Hemoglobin: Structure, Function, Evolution and Pathology*. Menlo Park: Benjamin/Cummings Pub, 1983, 3:42.
8. Dudell G, Cornish JD, Bartlett RH. "What constitutes adequate oxygenation?" *Pediatrics* 1990; 85:39.
9. Carlile PV, Barry AG. "Effect of opposite changes in cardiac output and arterial P_{O_2} on the relationship between mixed venous P_{O_2} and oxygen transport." *Am Rev Respir Dis* 1989;140:891.
10. Vaughn S, Puri VK. "Cardiac output changes and continuous mixed venous oxygen saturation measurements in the critically ill." *Crit Care Med* 1988;16:495.
11. Hassan E, Gree JA, Nara AR, Jarvis RC, Kasmer RJ, Pospisil R. "Continuous monitoring of mixed venous oxygen saturation as an indicator of pharmacologic intervention." *Chest* 1989;95:406.
12. Magilligan DJ, Teasdall R, Eisinminger R, Peterson E. "Mixed venous oxygen saturation as a predictor of cardiac output in the postoperative cardiac surgical patient." *Annals of Thoracic Surgery* 1987;44:260.
13. Chodosowska E, Skwarski K, Zielinski J. "Mixed venous blood oxygen tension is not a good predictor of survival in patients with chronic obstructive lung disease." *European Journal of Respiratory Diseases* 1987;71:233.
14. Shenaq SA, Casar G, Chelly JE, Ott H, Crawford ES. "Continuous monitoring of mixed venous oxygen saturation during aortic surgery." *Chest* 1987;92:796.
15. Nelson L. "Continuous venous oximetry in critically ill surgical patients." *Annals of Surgery* 1986;203:329.
16. Shapiro BA, Harrison QA, Kacmarck RN, Cane RD. *Clinical Application of Respiratory Care*. Chicago: Year Book Medical Pubs, 1979, 423.
17. Rasanen J, Downs JB, Malec DJ, DeHaven B, Seidman P. "Estimation of oxygen utilization by dual oximetry." *Annals of Surgery* 1987;206:621.
18. Mohsenifar A, Goldbach P, Tashkin DP, et al. "Relationship between O_2 delivery and O_2 consumption in the adult respiratory distress syndrome." *Chest* 1983;84:267.
19. Shibutani K, Komatsu T, Kubal K, et al. "Critical level of oxygen delivery in anesthetized man." *Crit Care Med* 1983;11:640.
20. Kersten LD. *Comprehensive Respiratory Nursing*. Philadelphia: WB Saunders, 1989, 46.
21. Gore JM, Sloan K. "Use of continuous monitoring of mixed venous saturation in the coronary care unit." *Chest* 1984;86:757.
22. Mims BC. "Physiologic rationale of $S\bar{v}_{O_2}$ monitoring." *Crit Care Nurs Clin of North Amer* 1989;1:619.
23. Bryan-Brown CW. "Gas transport and delivery." *In* Shoemaker WC, Thompson WL, Holbrook RR (eds). *Textbook of Critical Care*. Philadelphia: WB Saunders, 1984, 212.
24. McArthur KT, Clark LC, Lyons C, Edwards S.

"Continuous recording of blood oxygen saturation in open-heart operations." *Surgery* 1962;51:121.

25. Schlichtig R, Cowden WL, Chaitman BR. "Mixed venous oxygen saturation in chronic low cardiac output." *Am J Med* 1986;80:813.

26. Bruns FJ, Fraley DS, Haigh J, Marquez JM, et al. "Control of organ blood flow." *In* Snyder JV, Pinsky MR (eds). *Oxygen Transport in the Critically Ill* Chicago: Year Book Medical Pubs, 1987, 94.

27. Forster RE, DuBois AB, Briscoe WA, Fisher AB. *The Lung: Physiologic Basis of Pulmonary Function Tests.* Chicago: Year Book Medical Pubs, 1986, 234.

28. Heiselman D, Jones J, Cannon L. "Continuous monitoring of mixed venous oxygen saturation in septic shock." *Journal of Clinical Monitoring* 1986;2:237.

29. Astiz ME, Rackow EC, Kaufman B, Falk JL, Weil MH. "Relationship of oxygen delivery and mixed venous oxygenation to lactic acidosis in patients with sepsis and acute myocardial infarction." *Crit Care Med* 1988;16:655.

30. Dahn MS, Lange MP, Jacobs LA. "Central mixed and splanchnic venous oxygen saturation monitoring." *Intensive Care Medicine* 1988;14:373.

31. Cain SM. "Assessment of tissue oxygenation." *Crit Care Clin* 1986;2:537.

32. Rackow EC, Astiz ME, Weil MH. "Cellular oxygen metabolism during sepsis and shock. The relationship of oxygen consumption to delivery." *JAMA* 1989;259:1989.

33. Enson Y, Briscoe WA, Polanyi ML, Cournand A. "In vivo studies with an intravascular and intracardiac reflection oximeter." *J Appl Physiol* 1962;17:552.

34. Millikan GA. "A simple photoelectric colorimeter." *J Physiol* 1933;79:152.

35. Severinghaus JW, Astrup PB. "History of blood gas analysis. VI Oximetry." *J Clin Monit* 1986;2:270.

36. Tremper KT, Barker SJ. "Pulse Oximetry." *Anesthesiology* 1989;70:98.

37. Barker SJ, Tremper KK, Hyatt J. "Effects of methemoglobinemia on pulse oximetry and mixed venous oximetry." *Anesthesiology* 1989;70:112.

38. Schweiss JF. "Mixed venous hemoglobin saturation: Theory and application." *International Anesthesiology Clinics* 1987;25:113.

39. Baele PL, McMichan JC, Marsh HM, et al. "Continuous monitoring of mixed venous oxygen saturation in critically ill patients." *Anesth Analg* 1982;61:513.

40. Gettinger A, DeTraglia MC, Glass DD. "In vivo comparison of two mixed venous saturation catheters." *Anesthesiology* 1987;66:373.

41. Palmer J, Neblett J, Chulay M. "Clinical evaluation of continuous S$\bar{\text{v}}_{O_2}$ systems in cardiac surgical patients." *Heart & Lung* 1988;17:311.

42. Suter PM, Lindauer JM, Fairly HB, et al. "Errors in data derived from pulmonary artery blood gas values." *Crit Care Med* 1975;3:175.

43. Shapiro BA, Harrison RA, Cane R, Templin R. *Clinical Application of Blood Gases.* Chicago: Year Book Medical Pubs, 1989, 159.

44. Tenney SM. "A theoretical analysis of the relationship between venous blood and mean tissue oxygen pressures." *Respir Physiol* 1974;20:283.

45. Kirby RR, Taylor RW. *Respiratory Failure.* Chicago: Year Book Medical Pubs, 1986, 574.

46. Snyder JV, Carroll GC. "Tissue oxygenation: A physiologic approach to a clinical problem." *Curr Probl Surg* 1982;19:11.

47. McConachie IW, Edwards JD, Nightingale P, Mortimer AJ. "Relationship of oxygen delivery and mixed venous oxygenation to lactic acidosis in patients with sepsis and myocardial infarction (letter)." *Crit Care Med* 1989;17:844.

48. Denison DM. "Oxygen supply and uses in tissue." *In* Reihart K, Eyrich K (eds). *Clinical Aspects of O_2 Transport and Tissue Oxygenation.* Berlin: Springer-Verlag, 1989, 77.

49. Miller MJ. "Tissue oxygenation in clinical medicine: A historical review." *Anesth Analg* 1982; 61:527.

50. Kasnitz P, Druger GL, Yorra F, Simmons DH. "Mixed venous oxygen tension and hyperlactemia." *JAMA* 1976;236:570.

51. Dantzker DR. "Physiological and biochemical indicators of impaired tissue oxygenation." *In* Reihart K, Eyrich K (eds). *Clinical Aspects of O_2 Transport and Tissue Oxygenation.* Berlin: Springer-Verlag, 1989, 187.

52. Jastremski MS, Chelluri L, Beney KM, Bailly RT. "Analysis of the effects of continuous on-line monitoring of mixed venous oxygen saturation on patient outcome and cost effectiveness." *Crit Care Med* 1989;17:148.

53. Boutros AR, Lee C. "Value of continuous monitoring of mixed venous blood oxygen saturation in the management of critically ill patients." *Crit Care Med* 1986;14:132.

11
Physical Assessment of Oxygenation

Physical assessment is one area in which nursing places much emphasis in establishing initial assessments. Reliance by nursing on physical assessments stems partially from two reasons: (1) nurses usually cannot order laboratory tests to aid in making assessments, and (2) nurses spend large amounts of time in physical contact with the patient. The assessment of oxygenation has traditionally involved physical assessment to varying degrees. This assessment, however, is without a lot of basis in scientific evidence. A common phrase when referring to a problem with a patient is that "something is wrong" or "I feel something is wrong, but can't explain what it is that is wrong." This makes it very difficult to communicate to another health professional, such as physician or another nurse, what problem exists or requires treatment. Problems in oxygenation are commonly described this way. The focus of this chapter will be to review problems of oxygenation that are detectable by physical assessment and to review the limitations of physical assessments in oxygenation assessment. Physical assessment can be a useful tool for the nurse in the assessment of disturbances in oxygenation, although one has to be aware of which signs are reliable and which signs are ambiguous or unclear.

PHYSICAL ASSESSMENT OF P_{O_2}

Physical assessment of changes in the Pa_{O_2} (arterial oxygen pressure) level has little basis in the area of obvious physical changes. The P_{O_2} by itself is difficult to detect owing to the properties of oxygen. Oxygen is an odorless, colorless, tasteless gas that cannot be detected by any physical sense.[1] The P_{O_2} can change markedly, for example, from 80 mm Hg to 50 mm Hg, and not cause any detectable changes. However, one can estimate the Pa_{O_2} from changes in the oxyhemoglobin value.

OXYHEMOGLOBIN (Sa_{O_2}) ASSESSMENT

Oxyhemoglobin values can give some physical indication of change. The ability for oxyhemoglobin values to reflect in physical signs is tied into the properties that are present in hemoglobin as it changes its oxygen-carrying ability. Based on the oxyhemoglobin-dissociation curve, hemoglobin changes in its affinity for oxygen depending on the level of P_{O_2}. It is the relationship with P_{O_2} and oxyhemoglobin that allows one to infer changes in the P_{O_2} as changes in the oxyhemoglobin level occur.

Hemoglobin, when well saturated with oxygen (generally in values in excess of 90%), absorbs more red light and gives the blood a color of a reddish tint. In areas of the body that are peripherally well perfused, this gives the mucous membrane a reddish tint.[2] The coloration due to oxyhemoglobin levels is best noted on mucous membrane, such as the lips, inside the mouth, and beneath the eyelids (Figure 11.1). Subsequently, whenever the oxyhemoglobin level

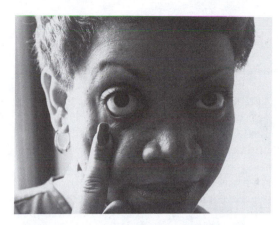

FIGURE 11.1.   Checking for central cyanosis under the eyelid.

is greater than approximately 90%, the mucous membranes or the nailbeds of the fingers and toes will typically take on a reddish appearance. As the oxyhemoglobin level falls below 90% into the 80% level, the larger quantity of deoxyhemoglobin starts to exert more of an influence. Deoxyhemoglobin tends to absorb light in the blue region of the light spectrum, giving the color of blood a more bluish tint. The bluish tint is frequently described by the term cyanosis. Cyanosis, derived from the color cyan (a light bluish color), is one of the most common descriptions of arterial hypoxemia. Cyanosis will not become evident until greater than 5 gms. of reduced hemoglobin are present. Therefore, cyanosis will not be common in any patient with a reduced total hemoglobin.

If the oxyhemoglobin value is in excess of 90%, the P_{O_2} is generally higher than 60 mm Hg. Therefore, in the absence of cyanosis, Pa_{O_2} levels higher than 60 may be present. When cyanosis is present, Pa_{O_2} may be less than 60. From skin and mucous membranes coloration, rough estimates of both Pa_{O_2} and Sa_{O_2} are possible (Table 11.1).

How well cyanosis can reflect changes in the oxyhemoglobin level is not well substantiated in scientific literature. In the early part of the century, clinicians first noted that cyanosis and physical changes were inconsistent in reflecting changes in P_{O_2} and hemoglobin saturation.[3] In addition, other studies have indicated that physical assessment does not readily indicate changes in blood oxygen levels.[4-6]

Two types of cyanosis exist, compounding the problem with the use of cyanosis as an indicator of oxygenation. The two types of cyanosis are peripheral cyanosis and central cyanosis.[7] Central cyanosis, which is the more important clinical concept in terms of overall oxygenation, is the result of having low arterial-oxygen-saturation values. Peripheral cyanosis is more the result of having low capillary-oxygen levels. Low capillary-oxygen levels manifest themselves in superficial parts of the body (i.e., near the skin) and reflect low blood flow to an area as opposed to low arterial oxygen levels. Some examples will help illustrate these two types of cyanosis.

A person with peripheral vascular disease may have peripheral cyanosis due to poor blood supply in a region.[8] Lower extremities in these individuals frequently have a bluish tint, or are cyanotic. Yet if arterial blood gases are obtained, one would find normal Pa_{O_2} and Sa_{O_2} values. The low peripheral capillary-oxygen tensions are due to diminished blood flow in the region. A practical example of this can be seen in a normal per-

TABLE 11.1. Pa_{O_2} and Sa_{O_2} Values Associated with Cyanosis

When	then the	Pa_{O_2} is	Sa_{O_2} is
Cyanosis is present		<60 mm Hg	<90%
Cyanosis is absent		>60 mm Hg	>90%

*NOTE: Cyanosis is unlikely to be present unless at least 5 gms of reduced hemoglobin is present in the peripheral circulation. The above Pa_{O_2} and Sa_{O_2} values are simple guidelines but do not take into account the crucial rule of peripheral (near capillary) level of reduced hemoglobin.

son. If a normal person is out in the cold with skin exposed, it is common to note the skin or mucous membrane of the lip turning a bluish color. Another example would be in the summer after swimming. When one steps out of the pool and is met with a sudden cool breeze, the coolness may cause a temporary bluish discoloration of the mucous membranes. These forms of peripheral cyanosis do not indicate a problem with oxygenation of the blood. The problem is in a reduction of blood flow to the area. The reduction of blood flow to the area is treated by improving blood flow rather than by trying to improve arterial oxygenation. People that have peripheral oxygenation problems and manifest peripheral cyanosis do not have a response to increasing the Fi_{O_2} (fraction of inspired oxygen) since the Pa_{O_2} and Sa_{O_2} are already normal.

Central cyanosis, on the other hand, is primarily due to pulmonary dysfunction, such as an increase in intrapulmonary shunt, that decreases the Pa_{O_2} and Sa_{O_2} levels. The reduction in the arterial saturation levels causes an overall cyanosis that is treatable by oxygen therapy. In theory, as long as the Pa_{O_2} and Sa_{O_2} are kept above normal levels, Pa_{O_2} of 60 and Sa_{O_2} of 90%, cyanosis will not exist.

Differentiating the peripheral cyanosis from central cyanosis is sometimes clinically difficult. One recommendation is to avoid using areas of the body that can also show peripheral cyanosis, such as the hands and the feet. Unfortunately, most clinicians have been taught that cyanosis of the hands or the fingertips, and clubbing of the fingers, is an excellent indicator of arterial hypoxemia. This may not always be the case. A better place to observe for cyanosis may be the lips, inside the mouth, or under the eyelids. Inside the mouth would be an ideal location except that it is difficult to identify color changes by visualization. Under the eyelids is a potentially good location since this area of the eyes is fed with the blood supply from the internal carotid arteries and is unlikely to be affected by factors that nor-

mally affect peripheral cyanosis. Pulling the eyelids down and looking under them to see if cyanosis is present may be a method of assessing oxygenation problems, specifically the hemoglobin saturation level. This location may be superior to looking at peripheral body parts, such as the hands and feet. Little research has been done in this area and certainly more is required to determine the adequacy of eyelid examination as a useful assessment tool. Unfortunately, most research done for the past several decades has indicated that cyanosis is not a reliable indicator of hemoglobin saturation levels.[9-10] In addition, factors other than body parts, such as fluorescent lighting, can limit the usefulness of detecting cyanosis.[11]

Practically, cyanosis can be used in a very simple manner. When noting the presence of cyanosis, the nurse is faced with the possibility that one of two causes exist: (1) peripheral cyanosis is present and a decreased blood flow to that area is possible; or (2) central cyanosis exists and the person has a low arterial oxygen saturation. The clinician should try to determine which of these types of saturation and cyanosis are present. Leading causes of central cyanosis include pulmonary disturbances, such as pneumonia, chronic lung disease, atelectasis, pulmonary edema, and other conditions that would cause intrapulmonary shunts. Conditions that cause peripheral cyanosis are mainly conditions that cause, for one reason or another, decreased blood supply to the area, for example, peripheral vascular disease or vasoconstricting drugs. Central cyanosis can be distinguished from peripheral cyanosis if the person responds well to oxygen therapy. The key point to remember is if cyanosis is observed, the clinician must suspect that the arterial oxygen saturation is threatened.

Lower arterial oxygen saturations, by themselves, do not necessarily indicate a problem with oxygenation. However, if cyanosis is present, the clinician must check to make sure the other aspects of oxygen transport are adequate. For example, if cyanosis is present, it now becomes more important that an adequate hemoglobin level exists and an adequate cardiac output is present. Low oxygen-saturation levels which produce cyanosis by themselves will not indicate a problem with low oxygen-transport levels but do threaten the patient with low oxygen content (e.g., from low hemoglobin values) or diminished cardiac output values. When cyanosis is present, the cyanosis serves simply as a clue to assess reasons for the cyanosis and to assess all aspects of oxygen transport.

AUSCULTATION OF THE LUNGS

Auscultation of the lungs is a common physical assessment parameter in the assessment of oxygenation. Information primarily revealed in the auscultation of the lungs is in regard to the Pa_{O_2}, Sa_{O_2}, and Pa_{CO_2} levels. The most important concept to keep in mind with auscultation of the lungs is the physiological impact on oxygenation with changes in lung sounds. The physiological changes can be categorized as one of two effects: (1) a change in intrapulmonary shunting (Qs/Qt), or (2) an increase in dead space (V_D/V_T). Only a change in intrapulmonary shunting will be reviewed owing to the common conditions that present with Qs/Qt changes.

Intrapulmonary shunting results from situations in which pulmonary perfusion exceeds ventilation (Chapter 3). Clinical conditions causing an increase in intrapulmonary shunting include atelectasis, pulmonary edema, pneumonia, asthma, chronic bronchitis, and ARDS. These conditions can present during auscultation in several ways, possibly in opposite manners. For example, if consolidation of lung tissue is present (pneumonia), the sound transmission to the stethoscope may be improved.[12] The improved sound transmission makes the lung sound increase in area. On the other hand, if ventilation is markedly reduced in an area without consolidation (atelectasis), the lung sound in the area will decrease.[13] In both situations, the end result is to increase the intrapulmonary shunt.

Perhaps the most common abnormal lung sound is the sound referred to as crackles. Crackles can occur when airway walls are weak or have excessive extra-airway pressures (Figure 11.2).[14-16] Crackles are likely to develop in conditions of weak airways, for example, chronic bronchitis, or of increased extra-airway pressures, such as ARDS and both early and late development of left-ventricular failure. Crackles are potentially significant because they can indicate the presence of a low ventilation/perfusion ratio (an increased Qs/Qt).

The increased intrapulmonary shunt produced by the above conditions has one primary problem: the production of reduced Pa_{O_2} and Sa_{O_2}. For any of the above clinical conditions to cause a problem with oxygenation, it must cause an increased Qs/Qt and produce a decrease in the Pa_{O_2}/Sa_{O_2} values. For the physical assessment via auscultation to be of value, it must be combined with an assessment of the Pa_{O_2}/Sa_{O_2} values. For example, if crackles are present, the potential for an increase in Qs/Qt is present. However, unless the Pa_{O_2} or Sa_{O_2} are abnormal, no active threat to oxygenation is present. The clinician must attempt to improve the condition causing the crackles, but must also be aware that the clinical importance of crackles is as a warning of the production of an increased intrapulmonary shunt. The danger of an increased intrapulmonary shunt is a reduction in the Pa_{O_2} and Sa_{O_2}. If the Pa_{O_2} and Sa_{O_2} are normal in the presence of crackles or other abnormal lung sounds, no major active threat to oxygenation exists.

ASSESSMENT OF HEMOGLOBIN

Physical assessment of hemoglobin is also difficult. Hemoglobin typically will give color to mucous membranes based on the oxyhemoglobin-saturation percent. For example, if a normal oxyhemoglobin level is present, a reddish color is given to hemoglo-

A) Air bubbling through secretions

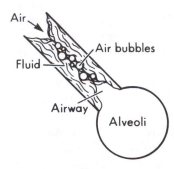

B) Equilibration of unequal pressures

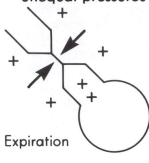

Expiration

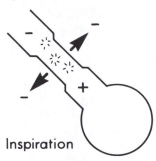

Inspiration

FIGURE 11.2.   Potential origins of crackles. (A) Air bubbling through secretions in the airways is a potential source of auscultated crackles. (B) Equilibration of unequal presures following reopening of closed airways represents another potential cause of crackles. Closure of the airway may be due to weakness of the airway structure (lung disease) or excessive extra-airway pressures (commonly seen in left-ventricular failure).

bin. The level of hemoglobin determines how bright this color will be (Table 11.2). If the person has a normal saturation and a normal hemoglobin, the color of the mucous membrane will be a pinkish-red. If the person has a normal oxyhemoglobin level and a low hemoglobin saturation, this color is diminished, and the mucous membranes appear pink or pale. The opposite occurs when oxyhemoglobin levels diminish and give more of a bluish color. When the oxyhemoglobin level is low and the hemoglobin level is normal, a mild bluish tint is given to mucous membranes. If the oxyhemoglobin level is low and hemoglobin is low, the oxyhemogoblin low value will manifest in a light blue. If the hemoglobin level is elevated, a bright blue or red appearance will occur, depending on the Sa_{O_2} level.

A common example of color change is the patient who has chronic bronchitis. A chronic-bronchitic patient, also called the "blue bloater," is identified as a blue bloater because of the chronically low Pa_{O_2} levels that may be present, causing low hemoglo-

TABLE 11.2.   Hemoglobin and Sa_{O_2} Influence on Mucous Membrane Coloration

Hgb Level	Sa_{O_2} Level	Mucous Membrane Color
Normal	Normal	Red
Low	Normal	Light red (pale)
High	Normal	Bright red
Normal	Low	Blue
Low	Low	Light Blue
High	Low	Bright Blue

bin saturation. The low Pa_{O_2} and Sa_{O_2} are compensated with an increased hemoglobin level. An increased hemoglobin level coupled with a decreased oxyhemoglobin level cause a brighter bluish tint to be given to mucous membranes. This brighter bluish tint gives the person an appearance of being blue. The "bloating" term comes from the right-sided heart failure that occurs from the chronically elevated pulmonary-artery pressures and systemic engorgement secondary to the right-ventricular failure. The mucous membranes, primarily the hands, lips, and underneath the eye, are again used to assess the hemoglobin level. Physical assessment of hemoglobin has very little scientific support in the literature. When noting a patient's physical appearance, changes in appearance will be one of the more inconsistent indicators of changes in hemoglobin, e.g., a patient who is bleeding. Generally, changes in hemoglobin will not markedly change a patient's coloration, at least not perceptibly to the human eye. As such, the physical assessment of hemoglobin is generally an unreliable indicator of oxygenation disturbances.

PHYSICAL ASSESSMENT OF THE CARDIAC OUTPUT

The assessment of cardiac output is based on the concept that the output is regulated by two factors, stroke volume and heart rate. Heart rate is the easiest mechanism to use for physical assessment of oxygenation. Stroke volume is not as easy to assess, which is unfortunate since if the clinician had some indicators of stroke volume, assessment of cardiac output would be relatively straightforward.

Heart Rate

Heart rate is the most obvious change that usually occurs with the change in oxygen transport. The reason for this is that cardiac output (CO) is the primary mechanism by which oxygen transport is regulated, and a heart-rate increase (tachycardia) is the first response necessary to increase

the CO. Reductions in oxygen content, for example, can be compensated through increases in cardiac output. Unfortunately, it is difficult sometimes to identify why a heart-rate change may occur. From an oxygenation point of view, a heart-rate change is likely to occur for two reasons: (1) to increase and offset a loss of stroke volume and maintain cardiac output; or (2) to increase overall cardiac output to meet an increase in oxygen demand.

Decreases in heart rate are potentially important as they can act as an indication of low cardiac-output states. Changes in oxygenation can occur with both a bradycardia and a tachycardia. Due to the more likely clinical occurrence of a tachycardia, the following section will focus on an increase in heart rate as the mechanism by which cardiac output attempts to adjust changes in oxygenation. Brachycardias, however, are important and should always be viewed as a possible threat to cardiac output and oxygenation.

The heart rate will increase for one of two oxygenation reasons, either to compensate for low stroke volume or to increase the total oxygen transport. A patient developing a heart rate greater than 100 beats per minute requires an assessment of potential reasons for the increase. Separate clinical indicators that favor overall low oxygen transport, such as reduced hemoglobin, indicate that the heart rate increased in an attempt to offset loss of another component of oxygenation. For example, if the person who suffers a MI has congestive heart failure or is hypovolemic, the heart-rate increase may be an indication of an attempt to compensate for lost stroke volume. If the person has a low hemoglobin level or low hemoglobin saturation and an increase in heart rate, an attempt by the heart to compensate for a loss of oxygen content (Ca_{O_2}) is indicated.

If the person has an increased metabolic rate, as is clinically common in presence of temperature elevation, the heart rate can respond by increasing in a somewhat predictable manner. One guideline given for assessing changes in the heart rate caused by increased metabolic rate is for every one degree increase in temperature Celsius, the heart rate will increase by fifteen beats.[17] If the resting heart rate is known, the increase in heart rate secondary to an increase in temperature can be assessed. If the heart rate starts at a resting level, for example 70 beats per minute, and a person has a temperature elevation of 39°C then a 2° elevation over the normal body temperature of 37°C exists. A 2° temperature elevation provides, according to this guideline, an increase in heart rate of 30 beats per minute. The heart rate would be 100 beats per minutes with a temperature of 39° in this patient with a resting heart rate of 70 beats per minute. The use of changes in the heart rate to assess changes in the cardiac output is limited primarily by one feature, the inability to understand what the stroke volume is.

Stroke Volume

Increases in heart rate due to decreases in stroke volume are difficult to assess clinically because no clear physical sign exists that can measure stroke volume. The clinician is limited to identifying when a tachycardia is caused by decreased stroke volume due to the lack of physical measures reflecting stroke volume. Since stroke volume is one of the three components that determines systolic blood pressure, systolic blood pressure can be used as an estimate of stroke volume. Systolic blood pressure is comprised of stroke volume, aortic distensibility, and left-ventricular ejection rate.[18] If aortic distensibility and left-ventricular ejection rate are constant, stroke volume will be the primary determinant to systolic blood pressure. Unfortunately, in clinical settings aortic distensibility and left-ventricular ejection capabilities are not constant. They are fluctuating components and depend to a large extent on medications being given and on the patient's ventricular compliance.

In a patient who has constant aortic distensibility and left-ventricular ejection consistency, stroke volume may be a reliable indicator within a fairly narrow blood-pressure range. The correlation of blood pressure and stroke volume can be approximated if one understands that stroke volumes in clinical settings usually are limited. Changes in blood pressure due simply to stroke volume are primarily at a lower level of blood pressure. For example, if the blood pressure increases to levels over 120 mm Hg, the change usually is not caused by changes in stroke volume. Blood-pressure increases over 120 mm Hg are more likely caused by changes in aortic distensibility. Subsequently, the upper limit of approximately 120 mm Hg can be used as a guideline when applying stroke volume to systolic blood-pressure estimates. Table 11.3 has an example of pairing stroke volume to approximate levels of systolic blood pressure. The guideline generally followed when estimating systolic blood pressure by stroke volume is that stroke volume starts in a clinical level between 50 and 100 cc per beat. Ranges in excess of 70 cc per beat are less common except in the septic patient. As stroke volume drops below 70, the blood-pressure fall reflects these decreases in stroke volume: as blood pressure decreases, stroke volume may be decreasing. The primary relationship between stroke volume and systolic blood pressure has never been clearly established, although the concept that as blood pressure changes, stroke volume most likely changes in the same direction, is one that

TABLE 11.3. Estimating Stroke Volume from Systolic Blood Pressure (In the Absence of Sepsis as Low Systemic Vascular Resistance)

Approximate Stroke Volume (ccs)	Systolic Blood Pressure (mm Hg)
70	120
60	110
50	100
40	90
30	80

has some degree of clinical value. If the patient has a decrease in systolic blood pressure, stroke volume may be falling as well. In this setting, a falling blood pressure is a major indicator of loss of oxygenation through the loss of cardiac output. An increase in heart rate may offset this loss of stroke volume, and cardiac output may be maintained. From a clinical point of view, however, and from a physical assessment point of view, this answer cannot be known for certain. A drop in blood pressure, even with the presence of a tachycardia, has to be considered a possible threat to overall oxygenation.

INTEGRATING PHYSICAL ASSESSMENT SIGNS

From a practical point of view, the use of physical assessment parameters can be summarized in the following guidelines. If cyanosis exists in a patient, a low oxyhemoglobin is probably present. If this cyanosis is a central cyanosis, then the person probably would benefit from oxygen therapy. Though hemoglobin levels are difficult to assess, if a person has a pale color to mucous membrane, then low hemoglobin levels may be present. The cardiac output assessment is probably the most important parameter, as noted in the following principles. If the person exhibits a tachycardia, for whatever reason, he or she must be assessed as having a potential threat to oxygenation.[19] When a sinus tachycardia exists, the clinician must assess the possibility that overall oxygen transport is being threatened and that the increase in heart rate is a compensation response to this threat. For example, if the heart rate changes from 100 to 120 beats per minute, then the clinician should check for indications that may be accompanying a worsening O_2 transport, that is, low stroke volume, loss of hemoglobin, or loss of hemoglobin saturation. If the person has a low blood pressure or if the blood pressure is falling from 120 mm Hg to lower values, the clinician should be aware that there may be a loss of stroke volume. Loss of stroke volume may reflect a loss of oxygenation through the loss of cardiac output. All these measures of oxygen transport in physical assessment are highly subjective and may be difficult to quantify. However, if one is trying to communicate the possibility of a problem with oxygenation, then the use of these simple guidelines at least gives some scientific credence to an assessment that something "may be wrong with the patient." Identifying these types of symptoms tells the clinician that a disturbance in oxygen transport may exist.

OXYGEN CONSUMPTION ASSESSMENT

The measurement of oxygen consumption from physical assessment is based on the relationship between oxygen consumption and carbon-dioxide production. In order for changes in oxygen consumption to be assessed physically, one must understand the basis for how oxygen consumption is reflected through breathing patterns.

Oxygen is brought into the oxygenation cycle through the respiratory system. Changes in breathing are the primary mechanisms for physical assessment of disturbances in oxygen consumption. In order to understand how breathing changes can affect the physical presentation of oxygen consumption, one must understand the relationships between carbon-dioxide (CO_2) and oxygen consumption and between carbon-dioxide production (V_{CO_2}) and the control of breathing.

Control of Breathing

Respiration is controlled primarily through the influence of carbon-dioxide on hydrogen-ion concentration in the ventral lateral surface of the medulla. CO_2 production indirectly is a primary determinant of breathing patterns. The reason that CO_2 production is a determinant to breathing patterns can be seen through the following concepts.

Arterial CO_2 (Pa_{CO_2}) levels bathe the central nervous system at the medullary region. Pa_{CO_2} levels influence the pH or hydrogen-ion concentration of the cerebral spinal fluid, as demonstrated by the Henderson–Hasselbach equation:

$$CO_2 + H_2O \leftrightarrow H_2CO_3 \leftrightarrow HCO_3^- + H^+$$

The relationship between hydrogen and Pa_{CO_2} is evident in the Henderson–Hasselbach equation: carbon dioxide, in the presence of water and through the enzyme carbonic anhydrase (CA), is converted to carbonic acid (H_2CO_3) which again, in the presence of carbonic anhydrase, will be dissociated into hydrogen and bicarbonate (HCO_3^-). Current theories of breathing are that the hydrogen-ion concentration acts as a primary determinant to breathing.[20-22] If too much hydrogen ion is present in the cerebral spinal fluid, breathing increases. If too little hydrogen ion is present, breathing decreases. As the carbon-dioxide levels increase, they will decrease the cerebral spinal fluid pH, making the cerebral spinal fluid more acidic. This acidic pH will then cause an increase in breathing. If too little carbon dioxide is present, this will create an alkalosis in the cerebral spinal fluid pH and cause breathing to slow down. Therefore, carbon-dioxide levels can have a strong influence on breathing through their indirect effect on cerebral spinal fluid pH. As a rule of thumb, if the Pa_{CO_2} level rises, breathing is stimulated. If the Pa_{CO_2} level falls, breathing is inhibited.

Examples of the Pa_{CO_2} influence on breathing are readily apparent in everyday examples. If we go to sleep where it is cold, we can warm ourselves fairly quickly by pulling the blankets over our heads. When these blankets are pulled overhead, it only takes a matter of minutes before we feel warm and have a need to take breaths of fresh air. Why do we need to take the blankets off of our heads after a few minutes? Because we are rebreathing carbon dioxide, which elevates the Pa_{CO_2} levels until a stim-

ulus is created to take a breath of fresh air. To illustrate the opposite example, where the carbon-dioxide level is low, consider what happens if we try to hold our breath for a long period of time. One way of increasing our breathholding abilities is to breathe excessively just before attempting to hold our breath. If we hyperventilate and lower the Pa_{CO_2} breathing will be inhibited. The inhibition to breathing produced by the low Pa_{CO_2} increases our ability to hold our breath for a longer period of time.

The illustration of Pa_{CO_2} influence on breathing is one of the key aspects of understanding how oxygen consumption is related to breathing. Another key aspect is in understanding how CO_2 production relates to breathing patterns. If one breathes excessively, alveolar ventilation (V_A) is increased and the Pa_{CO_2} level decreases. As the Pa_{CO_2} decreases, breathing will be inhibited and one will return to a slower form of breathing. If alveolar ventilation is decreased, then the person's breathing pattern will be stimulated as the Pa_{CO_2} levels increase.

Alveolar ventilation is a product of minute ventilation minus dead space (Table 11.4). Minute ventilation (V_E) is the amount of air that is inspired in a minute's period of time. V_E comprises respiratory rate and tidal volume. Respiratory rate and tidal volume are two key physical parameters in the assessment of oxygen consumption. Tidal volume is the volume of air inspired with every breath, and respiratory rate is how many breaths are taken per minute. Respiratory rate multiplied by tidal volume equals minute ventilation. Minute ventilation does

TABLE 11.4. Determination of Alveolar Ventilation (V_A)

$$V_A = V_E - V_D$$

V_A = alveolar ventilation (air reaching alveoli in one minute)

V_E = minute ventilation (air inspired in one minute)

V_D = dead space (inspired air not reaching alveoli)

not directly equal alveolar ventilation but can be used to approximate alveolar ventilation by subtracting the amount of air that does not participate in gas exchange, that is, the dead space. Minute ventilation minus dead space equals alveolar ventilation. The amount of air that is inspired in one minute is measurable from the physical point of view by measuring respiratory rate and tidal volume, and can give an approximation of alveolar ventilation (provided dead space remains at least stable). For example, if a person's respiratory rate increases and tidal volume remains constant, the following will occur: (1) overall minute ventilation will increase, (2) if dead space is normal, alveolar ventilation will increase, and (3) if alveolar ventilation increases, the net result will be a drop in Pa_{CO_2} values. The primary exceptions to an increased V_E, which do not produce a decrease in Pa_{CO_2} levels, are: (1) an increase in dead space, and (2) an elevation of carbon-dioxide production, as in exercise or temperature elevation. More on the respiratory rate and tidal volume will be presented shortly.

The last important concept in understanding the relationship between carbon-dioxide production and oxygen consumption is that carbon-dioxide production is the primary component of Pa_{CO_2} levels. Carbon-dioxide production, under normal circumstances, provides the carbon dioxide returning to the lung. If the lung can clear the normal metabolic production of carbon dioxide, Pa_{CO_2} levels will remain within normal levels. If the body is unable to clear the normal metabolically produced carbon dioxide, Pa_{CO_2} levels will rise and the person's breathing pattern will be stimulated. If the person breathes in excess of the amount of carbon dioxide produced, the Pa_{CO_2} will drop and inhibition of breathing patterns will be inhibited. The value of understanding carbon-dioxide production is in understanding that it has a very close relationship with oxygen consumption.[23] Normally, carbon-dioxide production is slightly less than oxygen consumption.[24] The direct relationship between carbon-dioxide production and oxygen consumption is dependent upon the substrate (food) being utilized for energy. For example, fats tend to produce less carbon dioxide in relationship to oxygen consumed than do carbohydrates, which tend to produce equal amounts of carbon dioxide and oxygen consumption.[25] As a rule, carbon-dioxide production is slightly less than oxygen consumption, but they are fairly close to being linearly related. To tie these terms together, remember that as carbon dioxide levels change, oxygen consumption levels are probably changing in the same direction (proportionately and linearly).

O_2 Consumption Relationship to Breathing Patterns

Oxygen consumption can be tied to breathing patterns by noting the following principles: (1) An increase in minute ventilation is likely to be a result of an increase in carbon-dioxide production and, therefore, oxygen consumption (provided dead space does not increase). When noting breathing patterns, it is important to note increases in respiratory rate and tidal volume, since they may reflect an increase in oxygen consumption. If O_2 consumption increases, oxygen transport should increase. (2) If O_2 consumption decreases, one may experience an overall decrease in minute ventilation.

The difficulty associated with measuring or assessing oxygen consumption through minute ventilation is a fairly obvious one: several features, which are assumed to be constant, such as dead space and tidal volume, may not actually be constant. For example, if a person has an elevated respiratory rate, an increased O_2 consumption may be present unless two key exceptions exist—a change in dead space or a reduction of tidal volume.

An increase in respiratory rate may be secondary to an enlarging dead space (the part of the lung that does not participate in gas exchange). This would be seen commonly in forms of COPD and pulmonary embolism. (Figure 11.3.) As the dead space enlarges, the overall minute ventilation must increase to provide the same level of alveolar ventilation. Clinically, one can identify this change in dead space by noting an increase in minute ventilation. An increase in V_E under normal circumstances will drop the person's Pa_{CO_2} level. If the person's Pa_{CO_2} level stays within normal levels in the presence of an increased minute ventilation, it is likely that the dead space level has increased. The second example of difficulty in assessing V_{O_2} through breathing patterns is a respiratory rate that increases while the tidal volume falls. The decrease in tidal volume is a common compensation mechanism to maintain minute ventilation and reduce work of breathing.[26] The increased respiratory rate would not be caused by an increase in oxygen consumption but by an effort to compensate for a loss in tidal volume.

A clinician who is trying to make an assessment of oxygen consumption through physical assessment must remember that an increase in minute ventilation, which can be assessed through an increased respiratory rate or tidal volume, may be an indicator of an increased O_2 consumption. The opposite is also true: a decreased respiratory rate and a decreased tidal volume may indicate a decrease in O_2 consumption. These physical signs are obscured by many other factors that may also cause the respiratory rate to change and the minute ventilation to increase without having a direct relationship with oxygen consumption.

A simple practical guideline is useful when caring for a patient with an increased respiratory rate. If the respiratory rate is increased, the nurse should make sure that the respiratory-rate increase is not due to voluntary mechanisms such an anxiety, pain, or fear. If a person exhibits an increased respiratory rate, the clinician should make sure that oxygen transport variables are optimized as much as possible in order to prevent a problem with oxygen balance. If the respiratory rate is increased and overall minute ventilation may be increased, note the Pa_{CO_2} level. If the Pa_{CO_2} level is within normal range, the person may have an increased dead space. This increased dead space does not rule out the possibility of an increased O_2 consumption, but it decreases the likelihood. Simply noting an in-

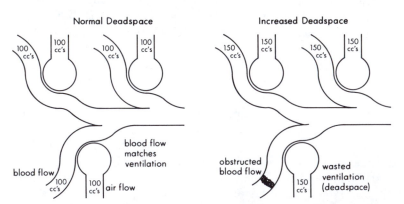

FIGURE 11.3. Increased dead space. Increased dead space occurs when the functioning alveolar unit serviced by the obstructed blood vessel still receives ventilation. The net result is increased ventilation. Blood flow is diverted around the obstructed blood vessel to other pulmonary capillaries. The blood flow increases in the other capillaries to maintain adequate pulmonary blood flow. Alveolar ventilation also increases to keep pace with the increased pulmonary blood flow in the nonobstructed capillaries.

creased respiratory rate or increased ventilation should signal the clinician that an increased O_2 consumption may exist.

SUMMARY

Of the physical assessment signs employed in estimating oxygen consumption and oxygen transport, it is important to remember that some of the changes occurring in physical presentation can signal a problem in oxygenation. Unfortunately, many of these parameters are ambiguous, are not consistent, or are not related solely to changes in oxygenation. This inconsistency makes it difficult to establish any one of these parameters as a primary assessment tool in oxygenation. Physical assessment of oxygenation, unfortunately, is a late and not completely reliable method by which oxygenation should be assessed. Oxygenation assessments can use changes in physical patterns as aids to the identification of an impending problem. The clinician must be aware, however, that the lack of consistently reliable physical indicators makes the use of physical assessments of oxygenation an inconsistent value.

Many physical assessment parameters in use to assess oxygenation are without direct relationships to oxygenation specifically. For example, if one listens to lung sounds and hears crackles, this by itself does not indicate a problem with oxygenation. For a problem with oxygenation to exist that is clinically related to crackles in the lungs, there must be a change in one of the components of oxygen transport. As a rule, crackles in the lungs have the direct potential to decrease hemoglobin saturation and Pa_{O_2} levels. If hemoglobin saturation and P_{O_2} levels are adequate and crackles in the lungs exist, then the crackles are not clinically significant as a threat to oxygenation. It may be a warning sign or an indicator that the crackles should be treated to help the patient maintain oxygenation, but by itself this does not indicate a problem with oxygenation. On the other hand, crackles in the lungs may indicate that the person has decreased cardiac output, which may be a threat to oxygenation. If the crackles are caused by a reduced cardiac output, however, it should manifest itself through either a direct measurement of cardiac output, a tachycardia, or a low-normal blood pressure. Any physical signs not mentioned as having an impact on oxygenation must affect one of the four parameters of oxygen transport or affect O_2 consumption. If, for example, the person has decreased breath sounds but maintains normal oxygen-saturation levels, then there is no immediate threat from that decreased lung sound to oxygenation. This does not mean that the decreased lung sound should not be investigated, only that it presents no apparent impediment to oxygenation.

CLINICAL EXAMPLES OF A PHYSICAL ASSESSMENT OF OXYGENATION

Example 1

A 62-year-old man is admitted into the intensive care unit with a chief complaint of shortness of breath and marked dyspnea on exertion. He has a history of chronic lung disease and has a 35-pack per year history of smoking. On initial examination, you note that his blood pressure is 138/88, pulse 112, respiration 32, and temperature 37.8°C. He has inspiratory crackles throughout his lungs, heard most prominently in the posterior lobes. Breath sounds are equal bilaterally and no cyanosis exists. A finger-oximeter reading indicates that he has a Sp_{O_2} value of 0.89. Blood gases are drawn and indicate a pH of 7.34, Pa_{CO_2} of 79, and Pa_{O_2} of 58, with a bicarbonate level of 37. Hemoglobin level is 14.5.

Based on this information, what do you estimate his overall oxygenation status to be?

ANSWER

The patient has the presence of arterial hypoxemia as evidenced by a Pa_{O_2} level in the 50s and hemoglobin saturation levels less than 90%. His oxygen content is actually normal, however, as obtained by the O_2 content formula (1.3 × 14.5 × .87). The O_2 content in this patient is about 16.9, which is within the normal limits of O_2 content. The normal blood pressure, even in the presence of a tachycardia, indicates that cardiac output is probably not low. If a relatively normal cardiac output exists in the presence of a normal O_2 content, overall oxygen transport is adequate. The respiratory rate of 32 may indicate an increased minute ventilation. Tidal volume must be measured to actually compute the minute ventilation. If the minute ventilation is adequate, then the O_2 transport is likely sufficient for adequate oxygenation. If the minute ventilation is elevated, then oxygen transport may not be sufficient for his O_2 consumption. More sophisticated information is necessary to make a better assessment of overall oxygenation.

ally not a wise idea. The inconsistency or unreliability of physical assessment makes the reliance on these symptoms a decision that could result with incorrect assessment parameters. Subsequently, the physical assessment of oxygenation primarily directs the nurse or clinician to note that when a physical change occurs more information is necessary in the form of laboratory tests or, perhaps, insertion of invasive hemodynamic monitoring.

Example 2

A 37-year-old woman is admitted to the unit following a gunshot wound to the left upper thigh. She returns from the OR after evacuation of the wound and internal fixation of a fractured femur. Blood loss has been estimated at 900 cc. The hemoglobin level on return to the unit is 8 gm/dl. Blood gases reveal a P_{O_2} of 119, Sa_{O_2} of 99%, Pa_{CO_2} of 29, and a pH of 7.46. Blood pressure shows a value of 102/56 and a heart rate of 116 beats per minute. Her respiratory rate is 28 breaths per minute. Mucous membranes beneath the eyes are pink.

Based on this information, what do you estimate her overall oxygenation to be?

ANSWER

In this patient, the low hemoglobin coupled with the low normal blood pressure and tachycardia are obvious threats of oxygen transport. The low hemoglobin, if it presents physically, may be reflected by a change in mucous membrane coloration, yet the change may be subtle and not evident. With the availability of hemoglobin levels, the physical assessment of changes in hemoglobin becomes less necessary. This person has the potential risk for overall oxygenation problems primarily because of low O_2 content, which in her case is about 10.6. A low normal blood pressure and tachycardia indicates a potential low cardiac output. The exact cardiac output, however, is unknown and may be high enough to compensate for low hemoglobin levels. However, more information will be needed to sufficiently assess this patient's oxygenation status.

ECONOMIC CONSIDERATIONS

From an economic point of view, the substitution of physical assessment for laboratory data or invasive monitoring is gener-

REFERENCES

1. Gilbert DL. *Oxygen and Living Processes: An Interdisciplinary Approach.* New York: Springer-Verlag, 1981.
2. Lundsgaard C, Val Slykk DD. "Cyanosis." *Medicine* 1923;2:1.
3. Stadie WC. "The oxygen of the arterial and venous blood in pneumonia and its relation to cyanosis." *J Exp Med* 1919;30:215.
4. Comroe JH, Botelho S. "The unreliability of cyanosis in the recognition of arterial anoxemia." *Am J Med Sci* 1947;214:1.
5. Carroll PL. "Cyanosis: The sign you can't count on." *Nursing* 1988;18:50.
6. Nitchey RV. "Cyanosis." *In* Horwitz LD, Groves BM (eds). *Signs and Symptoms in Cardiology.* Philadelphia: JB Lippincott, 1985, 118.
7. Lundsgaard C. "Studies in cyanosis: Secondary causes of cyanosis." *J Exp Med* 1919;30:271.
8. Martin L, Khalil H. "How much reduced hemoglobin is necessary to generate central cyanosis." *Chest* 1990;97:182.
9. Morgan-Hughes JO. "Lighting and cyanosis." *Br J Anaesth* 1968;40:503.
10. Medd WE, French EB, Wyllie VMcA. "Cyanosis as a guide to arterial oxygen desaturation." *Thorax* 1959;14:247.
11. Kelman GR, Nunn JF. "Clinical recognition of hypoxemia under fluorescent lamps." *Lancet* 1966;6:125.
12. Bates B. *A Guide to Physical Examination and History Taking.* 4th ed. Philadelphia: JB Lippincott, 1987, 251.
13. Swartz MH. *Textbook of Physical Diagnosis.* Philadelphia: WB Saunders, 1989, 236.
14. Forgacs P. "The functional basis of pulmonary sounds." *Chest* 1978;73:399.
15. Murphy RLH, Holford SK. "Lung sounds." *Basics of RD* 1980;8:1.
16. Loudon R, Murphy RLH. "Lung sounds." *Am Rev Resp Dis* 1984;130:663.
17. Cunha BA, Digamom-Beltran M, Gobbo PN. "Implications of fever in the critical care setting." *Heart & Lung* 1984;13:460.
18. Caris TN. *Hypertension.* Littleton: PS 6 Pub Co, 1985;14.

19. Ahrens TS. "Concepts in the assessment of oxygenation." *Focus Crit Care* 1987;14:36.
20. Loeschcke HH. "Central chemosensitivity and the reaction theory." *Journal of Physiology* 1982;332:1.
21. Millhorn DE, Eldridge FL. "Role of ventrolateral medulla in regulation of respiratory and cardiovascular systems." *J Appl Physiol* 1986;60:1249.
22. Pallet DJ. *Control of Breathing.* New York: Oxford University Press, 1983, 41.
23. Hagan RD, Smith MG. "Pulmonary ventilation in relation to oxygen uptake and V_{CO_2} during incremental load work." *Inter J Sports Med* 1984;5:193.
24. Benotti PN, Bistrian BR. "Practical aspects and complications of total parenteral nutrition." *Crit Care Clin* 1987;3:115.
25. Abbott WC, Brakauskas AM, Bistrian BR, et al. "Metabolic and respiratory effects of continuous and discontinuous lipid infusion." *Archives of Surgery* 1984;119:1367.
26. Milic-Emili G, Petit JM. "Mechanical efficiency of breathing." *J Appl Phys* 1960;15:359.

12
Treatments for Pa_{O_2} and Sa_{O_2}

Pamela Becker Weilitz, MSN(R), RN

Treatments for Pa_{O_2} and Sa_{O_2} disturbances are treatments for hypoxemia. Hypoxemia is defined as an inadequate amount of oxygen in the blood, a Pa_{O_2} less than 60–65 mm Hg.[1] Hypoxia can be the result of ventilation-perfusion changes, a true shunt, or changes in venous admixture. Patients can have oxygenation disturbances independent of problems with ventilation. Oxygenation is assessed by the Pa_{O_2} and the Sa_{O_2}, as well as by the a/A ratio, ventilation-perfusion ratios, Pv_{O_2} and the arteriovenous oxygen content difference. Ventilation is assessed by the Pa_{CO_2} and the pH.

Hypoxia is defined as an inadequate amount of oxygen available at the tissue level for cellular respiration. Hypoxia can occur as the result of a decreased ability to carry oxygen, an alteration in the cardiac output, changes in the tissues abilities to use oxygen, or decreases in oxygen diffusion across the alveolar capillary membranes. Table 12.1 defines hypoxia by ranges of the Pa_{O_2}.[1]

Examples of hypoxemia that result in hypoxia include a low inspired F_{IO_2}, ventilation-perfusion inequalities, increased true shunt, cardiac anomalies, and diffusion defects.[1]

WHEN TO INITIATE TREATMENT

When ventilation-perfusion (V/Q) ratios are not markedly decreased, or shunt (Qs/Qt) ratios are less than 25%, arterial hypoxemia usually can be corrected by simple oxygen therapy. Hypoxemia caused by a physiologic shunt or a very low V/Q ratio is generally less responsive to supplemental oxygen therapy.[2] Moderate-to-high concentrations of oxygen therapy are effective in maintaining a Pa_{O_2} at 60 mm Hg or greater when the shunt fraction is less than 25% with normal or near-normal cardiovascular function.[2] As the shunt fraction increases beyond 25%, supplemental oxygen therapy may not be able to correct the hypoxemia. In these instances, the addition of continuous positive airway pressure (CPAP), positive end-expiratory pressure (PEEP), and mechanical ventilation may be required.[2]

METHODS TO INCREASE Pa_{O_2} AND Sa_{O_2}

Oxygen Therapy

Supplemental oxygen therapy is used alone to treat mild to moderate hypoxemia. A Pa_{O_2} less that 60 mm Hg and a Sa_{O_2} less

TABLE 12.1. Degrees of Hypoxemia

Degree	Pa_{O_2}
Normal	80–100 mm Hg
Elderly (> 60 years)	Decrease by 1 mm Hg per year over 60
Mild	60–79 mm Hg
Moderate	40–59 mm Hg
Severe	< 40 mm Hg

Adapted from Kacmarek. *Essentials of Respiratory Therapy.* 2nd ed. Chicago: Year Book Medical Pubs, 1985, 371.

than 0.90 are indications for initiation of oxygen therapy. With a resting Pa_{O_2} and Sa_{O_2} within the acceptable range, it may be necessary to exercise the patient to determine oxygen needs. Two types of oxygen therapy are available, high-flow and low-flow systems. Table 12.2 lists the supplemental oxygen devices by high- and low-flow systems. Understanding each type of system is essential for appropriate clinical application. High flow does not mean high F_{IO_2}. The flow refers to the liters per minute of oxygen delivered to the patient.

Low-Flow Oxygen-Delivery Systems

Low-flow oxygen-delivery systems are used in more clinically stable patients. Low-flow systems provide oxygen flows from 0 to 15 liters per minute. The average inspiratory-flow rate in a patient with a normal minute ventilation is greater than 15 liters per minute.[2] To calculate a patient's inspiratory-flow needs, the clinician multiplies the patient's tidal volume by the inspiratory time divided into 60 seconds. For example, a patient with an inspiratory time of 1 sec and a tidal volume of 500 ml requires 30 l/min. V_T 500 ml $\times$ 60 sec = 30,000 ml/min, or 30 l/min inspiratory flow.

Entrainment of ambient air by the patient during inspiration dilutes the 100% oxygen delivered from the gas source. The amount of dilution is directly proportional to the amount of ambient air entrained. Delivery of a precise F_{IO_2} cannot be accomplished with a low-flow system because of the uncontrolled air entrainment. It is possible to deliver a high F_{IO_2} with a low-flow system; however, the actual amount of oxygen delivered may vary breath to breath. A low-flow oxygen-delivery system will provide relatively stable F_{IO_2} levels if the patient's ventilatory pattern is regular, the tidal volume is between 300 and 700 cc, and the respiratory rate is less that 25 breaths per minute.[1]

Examples of low-flow delivery systems include nasal cannulas, nasal catheters, simple face masks, partial rebreathing masks, and nonrebreathing masks (Figures 12.1–12.4). A nasal cannula at 1 l/min provides approximately 0.24 F_{IO_2} in a patient with a normal tidal volume and inspiratory-flow rate. Table 12.3 lists the approximate F_{IO_2} for nasal cannulas and simple face masks.[1] The rule of thumb is that each 1-l/min increase in the flow will result in a 3–4% increase in the F_{IO_2}, provided the V_T is 500 ml.

The major advantages of a low-flow delivery system are the ease of use and patient comfort. One of the disadvantages is the fit of the equipment on the patient's face and nose. To maximize oxygen delivery, masks and cannulas must fit properly.

Nasal cannulas are used for patients with COPD, mild hypoxemia, and Pa_{CO_2} retainers. In patients with COPD, 1- to 4-l/min flow rates are recommended. Higher liter flows may result in a depressed respiratory drive. The primary drive to breathe is the stimulation of the central chemoreceptors, which react to changes in the Pa_{CO_2}. Patients with chronic hypercarbia rely on the secondary stimuli to breath, stimulation of

TABLE 12.2. Low- and High-Flow Oxygen-Delivery Systems

Low-Flow	High-Flow
Nasal cannula	Venturi system
Simple face mask	T-piece with a Venturi
Face tent	adaptor
Partial rebreathing	Mechanical ventilation
mask	
Nonrebreathing mask	
T-piece	
Trach collar	

TABLE 12.3. Approximate Delivery of F_{IO_2} with a Nasal Cannula and Face Mask

	Liter Flow (l/min)	Approximate F_{IO_2} (%)
Nasal Cannula	1	24
	2	28
	3	32
	4	36
	5	40
	6	44
Mask	5–6	40
	6–7	50
	7–8	60

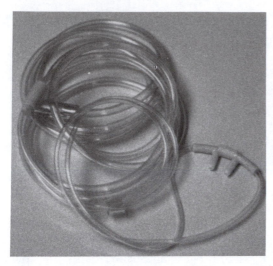

FIGURE 12.1. Sample low-flow oxygen therapy with nasal cannula.

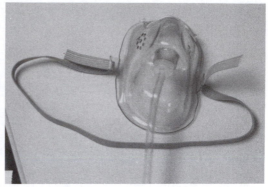

FIGURE 12.2. Sample low-flow oxygen therapy with simple face mask.

the peripheral chemoreceptors in the carotid and aortic bodies, which respond to changes in Pa_{O_2}.[3] When high F_{IO_2} levels are delivered, the hypoxic drive to breathe may be depressed and overall breathing reduced. Oxygen administration should be guided by the Pa_{O_2} and Pa_{CO_2}/pH in combination.

Example 1

A patient presents with the following ABGs: pH 7.46, Pa_{CO_2} 32 mm Hg, Pa_{O_2} 55 mm Hg. Can this patient receive oxygen therapy safely?

ANSWER

Yes, she is breathing from her Pa_{CO_2} drive, as indicated by a low Pa_{CO_2}.

Face masks are indicated in moderate hypoxemia for short-term administration of F_{IO_2} at 0.40 or greater. The major disadvantage is the interference with communication and eating. Simple face masks are not recommended for patients with COPD and CO_2 retainers because of possible respiratory depression caused by uncontrolled F_{IO_2}.

Partial rebreathing masks are indicated in moderate to severe hypoxemia. A flow rate of 6 l/min provides approximately 0.60

F_{IO_2}. Each 1-liter increase in the flow rate increases the F_{IO_2} approximately 10%. It is important to observe the reservoir bag during inspiration. The bag should not completely collapse. If it does collapse, the patient's peak inspiratory-flow requirement is greater than that delivered. It will be necessary to increase the flow rate to meet the patient's inspiratory demands.

The nonrebreathing mask is used for severe hypoxemia and provides a F_{IO_2} between 0.60 and 0.90. The reservoir bag should be observed to determine whether the patient's inspiratory-flow needs are met, as in the partial rebreathing mask. The mask has small flaps on either side that should be observed for sticking. If the humidification causes the flaps to stick, inhalation and

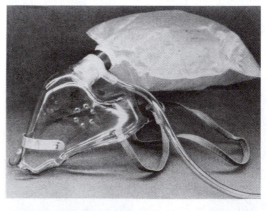

FIGURE 12.3. Sample low-flow oxygen therapy with partial rebreathing face mask. From McPherson SP, Spearman CB. *Respiratory Therapy Equipment*, 4th ed. St. Louis: CV Mosby, 1990.

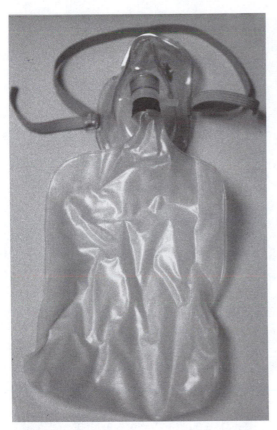

FIGURE 12.4. Sample low-flow oxygen therapy with nonrebreathing face mask.

exhalation can be obstructed. The non-rebreathing mask is contraindicated in patients with CO_2 retention due to the high oxygen concentration and possible respiratory depression.

HIGH-FLOW OXYGEN THERAPY

High-flow oxygen-delivery systems are indicated in patients with a variable respiratory rate and pattern. High-flow systems provide F_{IO_2} at flow rates that meet or exceed the patient's peak inspiratory demands. The high flow prevents entrainment of ambient air and dilution of the delivered F_{IO_2}. High-flow systems should provide flows of at least 50–60 liters per minute.[2] Although peak inspiratory flows are difficult to measure, they can be approximated at four times the patient's measured minute ventilation (V_E).[1] Some patients may re-quire flow rates that approach 100 liters per minute.[2]

High-flow delivery systems are either air-entrainment devices or blending systems (Figure 12.5). Entrainment devices, such as the Venturi mask, entrain ambient air at a fixed ratio to oxygen. Blending systems premix high-pressure oxygen and air sources to achieve the desired F_{IO_2}.

Nurses generally do not set up high-flow oxygen systems except in an emergency. Understanding how to set up the system is helpful. Do not attempt to set up a high-flow system that requires a bleed in. The clinician can easily set up oxygen systems that deliver 0.60 F_{IO_2} or less; adjust the F_{IO_2} on the nebulizer to any F_{IO_2} less than 0.60 and turn the flow meter to 15 l/min. At a F_{IO_2} of 0.60, air is entrained with the oxygen delivery at a 1:1 ratio. Table 12.4 lists the air-entrainment ratios for various values of F_{IO_2}. At 15 l/min, 15 liters of room air will be entrained to give a total flow of 30 l/min.

Actually, a F_{IO_2} of less than 60% can be achieved by setting the flow meter to 15 l/min. The resultant total flow is very high. For example, a F_{IO_2} of 0.28 could be achieved with 15 l/min and an air entrainment ratio of 1:10, yielding a total flow of 165 l/min.

A F_{IO_2} greater than 0.60 has an entrainment ratio less than 1:1 and requires a second flow meter. The clinician should allow a respiratory therapist or clinician skilled in oxygen delivery to assemble the system.

Air-entrainment systems include the Venturi mask system and the mechanical aerosol. Venturi masks are recommended in alert patients without upper-airway blockage or alterations. Nebulizer systems are used in patients who do not have normal mechanisms for humidifying the inspired air. Air entrainment systems are used to provide moderate levels of oxygen therapy between 0.21 and 0.50 F_{IO_2}.[3–4]

The Venturi mask system works by controlling the ratio of entrained ambient air in proportion to the amount of oxygen. The oxygen is delivered at high velocities

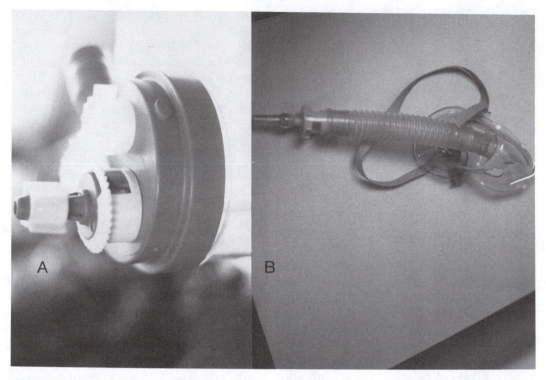

FIGURE 12.5.   Sample high-flow oxygen therapy with entrainment devices.

through the jet adaptor. Each adaptor has a different size entrainment port and jet orifice. Specific liter flows are required to produce the desired F_{IO_2}. The required liter flows and delivered F_{IO_2} for the Venturi mask system are summarized in Table 12.5.

An important consideration in delivery of oxygen with the Venturi system is humidification of the airway. The high flows of oxygen are very drying to the nasal and oral mucosa and to the upper airway. The use of an air-powered jet or ultrasonic nebulizer

TABLE 12.5.   Venturi Mask System

Desired F_{IO_2} (%)	Required Liter Flow	Entrainment Ratio	Delivered Liter Flow
0.24	4	1:25	104
0.28	4	1:10	44
0.31	6	1:7	48
0.35	8	1:5	48
0.40	8	1:3	32
0.50	12	1:1.7	32

Adapted from Shapiro et al. *Clinical Application of Blood Gases.* 3rd ed. Chicago: Year Book Medical Pubs, 1985.

TABLE 12.4.   Air Entrainment Ratios

Desired F_{IO_2} (%)	Entrainment Ratio
0.24	1:25
0.28	1:10
0.31	1:7
0.35	1:5
0.40	1:3
0.50	1:1.7
0.60	1:1

with a standard 22-mm collar may be necessary to provide humidification.[2]

The mechanical aerosol or gas-powered nebulizer has a fixed orifice for oxygen and a variable orifice for ambient-air entrainment. Oxygen concentrations range from 0.40 to 1.0 F_{IO_2}. To achieve 0.60 to 0.70 F_{IO_2} with a mechanical aerosol, 12 liters of oxygen are required to deliver 24 to 19 l/min to the patient, respectively.

Example 2

A patient complains of chest pain and shortness of breath. The physician orders 100% oxygen. How can this be accomplished?

ANSWER

Simply turning the dial on the nebulizer to 100% will not provide the patient with the desired oxygen concentration. A second flow meter will need to be added to the system and both flow meters must be turned to 15 l/min.

Oxygen blenders use a 50-psi source of oxygen and compressed air. The gases are mixed in the blender and delivered to the patient at the prescribed F_{IO_2}. Oxygen blenders can deliver 0.21 to 1.0 F_{IO_2} at flow rates of 2 to 100 l/min. As with all high-flow systems, humidification of the airway is recommended.

OXYGEN TOXICITY

Oxygen therapy is not without complications and risks. Levels of oxygen at 0.40 F_{IO_2} or less are considered to be safe.[1,3,5] An F_{IO_2} of greater than 0.50 for greater than 24 to 48 hours has been associated with oxygen toxicity.

Oxygen toxicity is manifested by destruction of the alveolar Type II cells, alveolar edema and hemorrhage, interstitial edema, and capillary endothelial cell damage. The acute phase is characterized by perivascular, interstitial, and intra-alveolar edema with destruction and necrosis of the endothelial cells.[1] After 6 hours of oxygen therapy at 1.0 F_{IO_2}, there is decreased trachael mucus flow, decreased macrophage function, and tracheobronchitis.[3] By 30 hours, impaired gas exchange across the alveolar capillary membrane can be seen. Increasing atelectasis is the result of the loss of surfactant, inactivation of plasma complements, and loss of alveolar Type II cell function.[3] Oxygen-free radicals increase with the increasing alveolar partial pressure (PA_{O_2}). The effects of these radicals include inhibition of glycolysis, interference with surfactant production and DNA and RNA synthesis, and mitochondria damage.[2]

The early clinical picture of oxygen toxicity, if one exists, includes chest pain and lower-lobe diffuse patchy infiltrates by chest x-ray. The clinical picture looks much like a diffuse bacterial pneumonia.[2] Signs and symptoms include tracheobronchitis, cough, refractory hypoxemia, and decreased lung compliance. Altered assessment parameters include Pa_{O_2} and Sa_{O_2}, decreased a/A ratio, increased dead space (VD/VT), increased work of breathing,[5] decreasing vital capacity, increased peak inspiratory pressure, and decreased diffusion capacity.[3]

END POINTS OF OXYGEN THERAPY

The best or safest levels of oxygen therapy continue to be researched.[1–2] It is generally accepted that F_{IO_2} at levels of less than 0.40 to maintain a Pa_{O_2} greater than 60 mm Hg or an Sa_{O_2} greater than 0.90 are safest. It is always wise to use the least amount of oxygen needed. When oxygen alone cannot provide the desired Pa_{O_2} and Sa_{O_2}, other techniques can be added to aid in oxygenation.

PEEP/CPAP

Positive end-expiratory pressure (PEEP) is defined as the establishment and maintenance of a preset airway pressure greater than ambient air at end exhalation.[1,3–4] Continuous positive airway pressure (CPAP) is PEEP applied to the spontaneously breathing patient when inspiratory and expiratory airway pressures are maintained above atmosphere.[1,3–4] Positive pressure airway techniques, specifically PEEP and CPAP, are used in patients with refractory hypoxemia and when oxygen toxicity is possible from high F_{IO_2} levels.[6–7] (Figure 12.6).

During airway closure, low V/Q ratios are created.[7] By increasing airway pressure at end exhalation, functional residual capacity is increased and alveoli are stabilized above

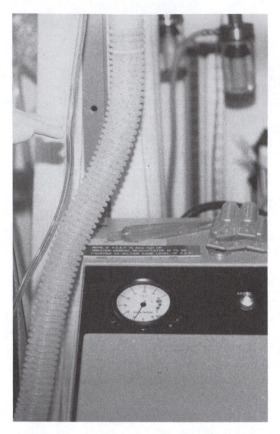

FIGURE 12.6. Positive end expiratory pressures. Note that the airway-pressure manometer does not return to zero, but remains supra-atmospheric (positive).

their closing volumes.[5] Recruitment of collapsed alveoli, expansion of open alveoli, and redistribution of pulmonary perfusion improve lung compliance.[3] Reduced intrapulmonary shunting and increased alveolar patency improve the Pa_{O_2}.[5]

The addition of PEEP to the patient on mechanical ventilation or CPAP to the spontaneously breathing patient is used to improve oxygenation or reduce existing F_{IO_2}. Usually PEEP is started at 5–10 cm H_2O in the adult.[8] The amount of PEEP used is adjusted to deliver the best oxygenation at the lowest F_{IO_2} with the least cardiovascular compromise. Best PEEP may be the level at which intrapulmonary shunt (Qs/Qt) is the lowest without a detrimental drop in the cardiac output.[4]

PEEP has been associated with decreased cardiac output.[1,9] This results from increased intrathoracic pressure, decreased venous return, increased right-ventricular afterload, and decreased left-ventricular distensibility.[8] A decrease in left-ventricular function has been shown, particularly with levels of PEEP at 15 cm H_2O or greater.[9]

High levels of PEEP, greater that 10 cm H_2O, have been associated with a significant incidence of barotrauma.[4] Barotrauma occurs when alveoli rupture from the positive airway pressure. Gas can then move into the tissue, mediastinum, and pleura, producing pneumomediastinum, subcutaneous emphysema, and pneumothorax. Patients with COPD or bullous lung disease are at increased risk of developing barotrauma when PEEP is added. However, there is no good statistical correlation between PEEP levels, mortality, and incidence of pneumothorax.[1]

The clinician should monitor the patient's response to the addition of PEEP. Assessment parameters include arterial blood gases, blood pressure, cardiac output, and lung compliance.[10] The key parameter to measure is the loss of stroke volume.[7] Monitor for decreased systolic blood pressure and increased heart rate to approximate the stroke volume changes in patients without a pulmonary artery (PA) catheter.

Example 3

A 40-year-old woman was admitted to the ICU following a motor-vehicle accident. She was intubated and placed on mechanical ventilation, and two chest tubes were inserted in the right thorax for a hemo/pneumothorax. Suddenly the patient was observed to be restless, diaphoretic, tachycardic, and tachypenic. Arterial blood gases revealed a Pa_{O_2} of 38 on 0.40 F_{IO_2}. Increasing the F_{IO_2} to 0.60 did not improve the Pa_{O_2} or Sa_{O_2}. PEEP was added at varying levels to improve oxygenation and decrease the delivered F_{IO_2}. Table 12.6 lists assessment findings at various levels of PEEP.

ANSWER

A PEEP of 6 cm H_2O at a F_{IO_2} of 0.60 provided the best oxygen transport of 958 cc. A PEEP of 9 cm H_2O at a F_{IO_2} of 0.40 provided the best Pa_{O_2} (70 mm Hg) and Sa_{O_2} (.91) at a lower F_{IO_2} (0.50). The small drop in cardiac output and oxygen transport are insignificant to the reduction in F_{IO_2}. A PEEP of 12 cm H_2O and a F_{IO_2} of 0.40 resulted in a significant fall in the cardiac output and the oxygen transport. In this example, the PEEP of 6 or 9 cm H_2O at a F_{IO_2} of 0.50 would be the intervention of choice. When a F_{IO_2} can be reduced to 0.50 or lower without significantly reducing oxygen transport, PEEP therapy is considered successful.[7]

INVERSE RATIO VENTILATION

Inverse ratio ventilation (IRV) is a method of mechanical ventilation used to improve oxygenation. IRV is an increased inspiratory-to-expiratory ratio of 1.1:1 or greater. Normal inspiratory-to-expiratory ratios are 1:2 to 1:4. The ratio is determined by the amount of time spent in each phase of respiration. For example, an inspiratory time of 2 seconds to an expiratory time of 6 seconds translates to a 1:3 I-E ratio.

Inverse-ratio ventilation has been reported to achieve higher levels of oxygenation at lower peak airway pressures.[11-13] Oxygenation is thought to improve by some of the same mechanisms as in PEEP. Prolonging the time the airways are exposed to higher airway pressure increases recruitment of closed alveoli.[7] The increased inspiratory time and increased mean airway pressure probably allows for stabilization of alveoli and redistribution and diffusion of gases.[11,14] The shortened expiratory phase

TABLE 12.6. Assessment Findings at Various Levels of PEEP

Parameters	Levels of PEEP (cm H_2O)				
	Baseline	3	6	9	12
F_{IO_2}	.60	.60	.50	.50	.50
Pa_{O_2}	44	50	58	70	89
Sa_{O_2}	.78	.80	.86	.91	.97
Cardiac Output (l/min)	6.5	6.6	6.5	6.2	5.5
Oxygen Transport (cc)	860	882	958	954	900

Adapted from Rutherford KA. "Advances in the treatment of oxygenation disturbances." *Crit Care Nurs Clin NA* 1989; 1:665.

allows an adequate tidal volume to escape without allowing alveoli to fall below their closing volume.[11] The improved ventilation elevates the V/Q ratio and improves the Pa_{O_2} and Sa_{O_2}.[4] The use of inverse ratio ventilation may be preferable to the use of PEEP because CO_2 elimination is more efficient and peak pressure is less, thus diminishing the risk of barotrauma.[15]

Inverse-ratio ventilation is useful in patients with diffuse lung disease and oxygenation failure who do not respond to high levels of PEEP.[11,14,16] It has been used with success in patients with adult respiratory distress syndrome (ARDS).

Patients who require inverse-ratio ventilation need continuous monitoring of their hemodynamic status.[12] Like PEEP, IRV has been associated with decreases in venous return to the right side of the heart, increased pulmonary-artery pressure, and reduced cardiac output. Hypotension is the major side effect of inverse ratio ventilation. Tachycardias and arrhythmias should be anticipated.[17] Inverse ratio ventilation at ratios between 1.1:1 and 1.7:1 may produce better gas exchange and less detrimental effect to the cardiac output.[15]

Neuromuscular paralysis and sedation is recommended to reduce patient anxiety and feelings of discomfort, and to improve pulmonary compliance.[14,17] The improvement in oxygenation may be related to the decreased oxygen consumption from respiratory muscle paralysis and to the reduced work of breathing.[11]

Application of IRV is gradual, usually starting at 1.1:1 and progressing over time.[7] Continual assessment of cardiac output, heart rate, oxygen transport, Sa_{O_2}, and Pa_{O_2} should occur as the inverse ratio is increased. The optimal ratio allows for the lowest F_{IO_2} with a Pa_{O_2} greater than 60 mm Hg.[7]

AIRWAY PRESSURE-RELEASE VENTILATION

Airway pressure-release ventilation (APRV) provides continuous positive airway pressure (CPAP), so the patient can breathe spontaneously without airway pressure fluctuations.[18] The APRV delivers CPAP and augments ventilation as an adjunct.[19] APRV is considered a variation of IRV.[5] Cyclical release of the airway pressure allows for a rapid decrease in lung volumes and passive elimination of CO_2 from the lungs.[20] When the release valve closes, the airway pressure rapidly returns to the original CPAP level, thus increasing the lung volume.[18] Frequency, duration, CPAP, pressure-relief level, lung compliance, airway resistance, and the pressure-relief valve determine the level of ventilatory assistance.[17–18]

APRV augments spontaneous ventilation, providing improved oxygenation, probably because of the prolonged inspiratory time and increased functional residual capacity.[17,20] The maintenance of airway pressure at or below CPAP reduces the risk of barotrauma.[18,20] This is believed to provide improvement in oxygenation without the depressant effect on cardiac function.[18]

HYPERBARIC OXYGEN THERAPY

Hyperbaric oxygen therapy calls for the administration of 1.0 F_{IO_2} at an increased atmospheric pressure of 2 to 3 atmospheres.[3] Hyperbaric oxygen therapy can provide a 22-fold increase in the alveolar P_{O_2}.[3] The resulting increased Pa_{O_2} provides more oxygen at the tissue level. The improvement in tissue oxygenation theoretically promotes healing. Although not proven clinically, there are those that believe sleeping in a hyperbaric oxygen chamber will improve skin, reduce aging, and promote youthfulness. Hyperbaric oxygen therapy is used clinically for the treatment of diving accidents and development of air emboli at depth. It also has been useful in the treatment of severe carbon-monoxide poisoning.[3]

SUMMARY

There are many options available for treating Pa_{O_2} and Sa_{O_2} disturbances. These include high flow and low flow oxygen delivery systems, modes of ventilation such as IRV and APRV and adjuncts to oxygen therapy such as PEEP and CPAP. It is important for the clinician to carefully assess the patient and select the method that will provide the patient with the greatest improvement in oxygenation at the least cost to cardiovascular function.

REFERENCES

1. Kacmarek RM, Mack CW, Dimas S. *The Essentials of Respiratory Care*. 3rd ed. Chicago: Mosby-Yearbook, Inc., 1990.
2. Thalken FR. "Medical gas therapy." *In* Scanlan CL, Spearman CB, Sheldon RL. *Egan's Fundamentals of Respiratory Care*. 5th ed. St. Louis: CV Mosby, 1990.
3. Kersten LD. *Comprehensive Respiratory Nursing Care*. Philadelphia: WB Saunders Company, 1989.
4. Shapiro B. "General principles of airway pressure therapy." *In* Shoemaker WC, Ayres S, Grenvik A, Holbrook PR, Thompson WL (eds). *Textbook of Critical Care*. 2nd ed. Philadelphia: WB Saunders, 1989.
5. Harper RW. A *Guide to Respiratory Care Physiology and Clinical Applications*. Philadelphia: JB Lippincott, 1981.
6. Kirby R, Smith R, DeSautels D. *Mechanical Ventilation*. New York: Churchill Livingston, 1985.
7. Rutherford KA. "Advances in the treatment of oxygenation disturbances." *Crit Care Nurs Clin N Am* 1989;1:659–667.
8. Abels L. *Critical Care Nursing: A Physiologic Approach*. St. Louis: CV Mosby, 1986.
9. Pick R, Handler JB, Murata GH, Friedman AS. "The cardiovascular effects of positive end-expiratory pressure." *Chest* 1982;82:345–350.
10. Murray J, Nadel J. *Textbook of Respiratory Medicine*. Philadelphia: WB Saunders, 1988.
11. Gurevitch MJ, Van Dyke J, Young ES, Jackson K. "Improved oxygenation and lower peak airway pressure in severe adult respiratory distress syndrome treatment with inverse ratio ventilation." *Chest* 1986;89:211–213.
12. Tharratt RS, Allen RP, Albertson TE. "Pressure controlled inverse ratio ventilation in severe adult respiratory failure." *Chest* 1988;94:755–762.
13. Toben BP, Lewandowski V. "Nontraditional and new ventilatory techniques." *Crit Care Nurs Quarterly* 1988;11:12–28.
14. Schuster DP. "A physiologic approach to initiating, maintaining, and withdrawing mechanical ventilatory support during acute respiratory failure." *Am J Med* 1990;88:268–278.
15. Cole AGH, Weller SF, Sykes MK. "Inverse ratio ventilation compared with PEEP in adult respiratory failure." *Intensive Care Med* 1984;10:227–232.

16. MacIntyre NR. "New forms of mechanical ventilation in the adult." *Clinical Chest Medicine* 1988;9:47–54.

17. Weilitz PB. "New modes of mechanical ventilation." *Crit Care Nurs Clin N Am* 1989;1:689–695.

18. Downs JB, Stock MC. "Airway pressure release ventilation: A new concept in ventilatory support." *Crit Care Med* 1987;15:459–461.

19. Garner W, Downs JB, Stock MC, Rasanen J. "Airway pressure release ventilation (APRV): A human trial." *Chest* 1988;94:779–781.

20. Stock MC, Downs JB. "Airway pressure release ventilation: A new approach to ventilatory support during acute lung injury." *Respir Care* 1987; 32:517–524.

13
Treatment of Hemoglobin Deficits

Kim Rutherford MSN, RN, CCRN

Janice Zaiger MSN, RN

Hemoglobin (Hgb) is the main carrier of oxygen. Without hemoglobin, the body would have to rely on the oxygen dissolved in plasma to meet minimal oxygen-consumption requirements. The heart would need to generate a cardiac output of 66–67 l/min to meet this minimal oxygen requirement. Illustration of the contributory value of hemoglobin to oxygen transport has been presented in previous chapters. Loss of hemoglobin compromises oxygen transport via reduction of arterial oxygen content (Table 13.1). Low hemoglobin states may be caused by anemia, hypovolemia, and/or hemorrhagic shock. A brief review of causes of abnormally low Hgb will help introduce strategies for treatment.

ANEMIA

Anemia, a lack of red blood cells, may be caused by a rapid loss or retarded production of new cells. Hemoglobin concentrations as low as 3.8 gm/dl may be tolerated as long as compensatory mechanisms of the

TABLE 13.1. Varying Hemoglobin Level and Effect on Ca_{O_2}

Hemoglobin	Ca_{O_2}
15	15 × 1.34 × .96 = 19.30
12	12 × 1.34 × .96 = 15.44
10	10 × 1.34 × .96 = 12.86
8	8 × 1.34 × .96 = 10.29
5	5 × 1.34 × .96 = 6.43

circulatory system are intact.[1] For instance, cardiac output will increase as hemoglobin drops below 7 gm/dl. Vasodilatation of vital organs and the decreased viscosity of the blood help to improve flow to areas where oxygen is critical.[2-3] Oxygen extraction at the tissue level is promoted by an increased production of the enzyme 2,3 DPG, which in chronic anemia states may as much as double.[3,4] These compensatory mechanisms minimize the negative effects of anemia. Several types of anemia exist:

1. Aplastic anemia is characterized by a nonfunctioning bone marrow in which red blood cells are not produced. It is caused by drugs, infection, or radiation exposure.

2. A deficiency of vitamins, minerals, and/or other factors necessary for the maturation process of erythropoiesis may cause maturation failure anemia. Examples of this type include iron deficiency anemia or pernicious anemia, characterized by loss of an intrinsic factor from the mucosal lining of the stomach.[2] Malnutrition may promote anemia from a lack of protein.

3. Hemolytic anemias refer to a process of destruction of the red blood cell. The altered red blood cells are sequestrated as they pass through capillary beds commonly in the spleen, resulting in a shorter life span. Types of hemolytic anemias are listed in Table 13.2.[2,5]

TABLE 13.2.   Hemolytic Anemias

Type	Abnormality	Result
Hereditary spherocytosis	Small, spherical RBCs	Easily ruptured in capillaries
Sickle cell anemia	S-shaped Hgb	Sickling process causes hemolysis
Thalassemia (Cooley's anemia)	Abnormal globin formation	RBCs without Hgb easily ruptured

Treatment of anemia focuses on the degree and specific cause. Symptoms associated with anemia are uncommon when the hemoglobin is greater than 8 gm/dl. A lower exercise tolerance, fatigue, and palpitations may occur in patients with a hemoglobin of 5–8 gm/dl. More severe cardiac and neurologic deficits, such as lethargy, confusion, or obtundation, will be apparent with hemoglobin levels less than 5 gm/dl.[3] Patient education regarding early indicators of poor tissue oxygenation, such as tachycardia, tachypnea, dyspnea on exertion, shortness of breath, fatigue, vomiting, or nausea, must be emphasized.[5]

HYPOVOLEMIA

Low circulating volume may occur without bleeding owing to fluid volume deficits (loss of volume and electrolytes) or dehydration (low volume). Fluid volume deficits (FVD) occur with vomiting, excessive gastrointestinal suctioning, diarrhea, burns, low intake of water and electrolytes, and polyuria.[6] Clinical assessment of FVD will include the following: (1) dry mucous membranes, (2) poor skin turgor, (3) urine output < 30 cc/hr, (4) orthostatic hypotension (20 mm Hg decrease in systolic blood pressure and/or a 20-beat per minute increase in heart rate when the patient is sitting as compared to lying), (5) weight loss, and (6) low central venous pressure (< 2 mm Hg). Laboratory values consistent with FVD will include a rising blood-urea-nitrogen (BUN) and slightly elevated serum creatine (SCr). Even though both values rise, the rise in BUN will exceed the increase of SCr, making the BUN/SCr ratio greater than the normal 10–20/1. Hemoglobin and hematocrit values may be elevated due to hemoconcentration. Urine specific gravity and urine osmolality will be elevated.[6] Severe FVD causes symptoms similar to those of hemorrhagic shock.

Dehydration is caused by a low intake or excessive loss of fluid. Patients who cannot recognize a thirst response will be at risk for dehydration. For instance, patients with cerebral vascular accidents (CVA) commonly lose their sense of thirst.[7] Immobilized patients or infants who are unable to respond to thirst may be prone to dehydration.[7] Metabolic dysfunction such as diabetic ketoacidosis may cause polyuria, promoting an excessive loss of fluid. Clinical assessment and laboratory data in dehydration is similar to that with FVD except that the serum sodium (Na+) is elevated, indicating a greater loss of fluid alone versus fluid and electrolytes.

Treatment of FVD and/or dehydration requires prompt replacement of fluid, usually with a Lactated Ringers solution. Severe hypovolemia may lead to renal dysfunction (acute tubular necrosis). Prolonged hypovolemia will generate a shock response similar to that described under hemorrhagic shock. Attention must be given to the cause and prevention of fluid volume deficits/dehydration once the acute hypovolemia is corrected.

HEMORRHAGIC SHOCK

Blood-loss anemia may occur with acute or chronic bleeding. Mild blood loss (< 500 cc) may cause restlessness, anxiety, cool skin, pallor of the conjunctiva of the eye and nail beds, and loss of brisk capillary refill.[7] Profuse bleeding may lead to hemorrhagic shock. Initially, if plasma volume and red blood cells are lost, the concentration of hemoglobin may be normal. However, if bleeding continues, fluid will be shifted from intracellular to extracellular spaces, and hemoglobin concentration will fall.[1,4]

The low arterial oxygen content caused by loss of hemoglobin coupled with a low cardiac output markedly reduces oxygen transport. The low stroke volume stimulates baroreceptors in the aorta and carotid arteries, resulting in three important neuronal sympathetic responses[4]:

1. Vasoconstriction of the arterioles will increase blood pressure and systemic vascular resistance.
2. Capacitance vessels increase drainage, promoting a greater venous return.
3. Positive inotropic (strength of cardiac contraction) and chronotropic (heart rate) effects occur.

Greater blood loss (> 500 cc) may result in hypotension, tachycardia, and low urine output. Orthostatic changes may indicate strain on the sympathetic nervous system compensation.[7] Hormonal influences are activated to promote water retention. Hypoperfusion in the kidneys activates the renin-angiotension cycle which causes vasoconstriction, thus increasing the blood pressure. Increased water reabsorption from the distal tubules also occurs. Antidiuretic-hormone secretion further limits urine excretion and promotes reabsorption.[4] Other hormonal changes, such as the production of glucagon and increased resistance to insulin, elevate blood glucose which causes an osmotic pull of fluid from intracellular spaces to the circulating volume.[4]

If greater than 1000 cc of blood is lost, lethargy, confusion, a decreased level of consciousness, tachycardia, tachypnea, and further reduction in urine output may occur.[1,4,7] Autoregulatory changes in the microcirculation occur, causing changes in hydrostatic pressure that promote the movement of fluid from intracellular spaces to the capillaries.[4] This accounts for the hemodilutional effect of blood counts commonly seen 3–4 hours after bleeding.[1,4] Changes in the microcirculation redistribute blood flow to major organ systems. For instance, the heart may receive up to 25% of the cardiac output in hemorrhagic shock (normally the heart receives 5–8%).[8] The combined neuronal, hormonal, and autoregulatory mechanisms help compensate for the alterations of hemorrhagic shock. Though tissue perfusion may be inadequate in some capillary beds, resulting in anaerobic metabolism, the process remains reversible.[4] Prompt treatment, obviously centering on the source of bleeding and fluid replacement, will reverse the negative effects of hemorrhage.

If bleeding continues and blood loss approximates 3000 cc, severe hemorrhagic shock develops and death may be imminent if the process is not reversed. Further anaerobic metabolism leads to lactic acidosis, which negatively affects the cardiopulmonary system. Sludging of blood through capillary beds may cause microemboli, further insulting tissue perfusion.[4,7] A low pulse pressure, cold clammy skin, and oliguria characterize severe hemorrhagic shock. These symptoms of shock are similar to other shock states such as cardiogenic or late septic shock. Physical assessment parameters specific to hemorrhagic shock that may help to differentiate shock states are orthostatic changes (typically not seen in cardiogenic or septic shock) and the lack of crackles (commonly associated with cardiogenic shock).

TREATMENT OF HEMORRHAGIC SHOCK

Treatment priorities logically will center on the cause(s) of hemorrhage and volume replacement. Since subtle differences separate progressive hemorrhagic shock from irreversible shock, rapid replacement of blood cells and volume (crystalliods and colloidal agents) will be necessary.

Crystalloids Versus Colloids

Much controversy exists over whether crystalloids (IV salts) or colloids (plasma volume expanders) should primarily be used in addition to blood products for fluid replacement. In clinical studies comparing crystalloids versus colloids for fluid replacement, no significant differences were found when comparing outcome parameters such as pulmonary-function tests, intrapulmonary shunting, lung compliance, or extravascular lung water.[4] Crystalloid solutions such as Lactated Ringers or normal saline are most commonly used. Volume replacement can be achieved fairly rapidly; however, much of this fluid is excreted rapidly. Improvement in circulating volume may be challenging to maintain.[7] Colloidal agents such as albumin, plasma protein fraction (plasminate), Dextran, and hetastarch (Hespan) each contain proteins that increase the plasma colloidal osmotic pressure, enhancing fluid movement from the interstitium.[4,7] Despite which strategy is used for fluid replacement, careful attention must be given to avoid fluid overload, especially in patients with prior renal or cardiovascular dysfunction. Fluid resuscitation should continue until the patient has an adequate blood pressure, normal heart rate, urine output > .5 cc/kg, normal sensorium, and brisk capillary refill. If fluid therapy is based on blood pressure alone, volume replacement may be underestimated because of the body's vast compensatory efforts to maintain normal blood pressure in adverse conditions.[4]

Blood Transfusions

In hemorrhagic states in which the hemoglobin decreases below 10 gm/dl, the effect on oxygen transport should be assessed. Hypovolemia has a much more dramatic effect on oxygen transport than simply loss of hemoglobin from anemia. All of the compensatory efforts of the cardiovascular and circulatory systems are not possible with the loss of volume.[3] Hemorrhagic states are typically a more acute onset anemia. Treatment should focus on maintenance of mean arterial pressure, organ perfusion, and cause of hemorrhage. Blood transfusions should be considered if oxygen transport variables are compromised.

Though blood transfusions (Figure 13.1)

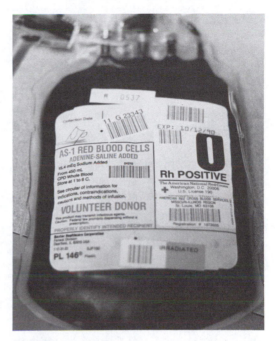

FIGURE 13.1.   Blood to be transfused.

are common in critical care settings, they are not without risk. Transfusion reactions may result in hemolysis, fever, chills, anaphylaxis, and death.[9–12] Fatal hemolytic reactions most commonly occur with transfusion of ABO-incompatible blood. A hemolytic reaction may occur with as little as 10–15 cc of an incompatible blood.[13–14] Symptoms associated with hemolytic reactions include: (1) fever, (2) chills, (3) nausea, (4) vomiting, (5) urticaria, (6) shortness of breath, (7) substernal and/or lumbar pain and (8) myalgias.[12,14] Over half of transfusion-related deaths are caused by hemolytic reactions, usually renal failure, refractory hypotension, and/or disseminated intravascular coagulation (DIC).[12–13] Judicial attention to blood-transfusion protocols may limit the occurrence of incompatible blood transfusion.

Febrile reactions may indicate the presence of leukoagglutins precipitating agranulocytosis. The incidence of these antileukocyte antibodies is directly proportional to the number of transfusions received. Symptoms usually begin 30–120 minutes after beginning the transfusion. Symptoms include fever, sensation of coldness, pallor, tachycardia, hypotension, tachypnea, and leukopenia. Use of leukocyte-poor blood (buffy coated blood) usually will prevent further such febrile reactions.[12] Currently used microaggregate filters also help to decrease the amount of white blood cells in transfused blood.

Other complications associated with massive blood transfusion (greater than 15 units and/or an amount greater than the patient's blood volume transfused within 24 hours) include circulatory overload, hypothermia, hyperkalemia, decreased 2,3 DPG, hypomagnesemia, citrate poisoning, decreased clotting factors, and dilutional thrombocytopenia.[2,4,9,13,15–17] Infections such as hepatitis, cytomegalovirus (CMV), and acquired immunodeficiency syndrome (AIDS) have been transmitted to patients via contaminated blood. Public awareness

of these serious complications of blood transfusions have resulted in many patients refusing to accept blood products.

Autologous blood transfusions decrease many of the aforementioned risks. Hemolytic reactions and transmission of infectious diseases are avoided. Patients who refuse blood products because of religious beliefs sometimes view autologous transfusions as an acceptable alternative.[18] Blood donation may begin 35 days prior to surgery. The blood is mixed with the preservative CPDA-1 (citrate-phosphate-dextrose-adenine). If the blood is stored as packed red cells, blood collection may begin 42 days prior to surgery. Maximal blood donation may be collected every 3 days up to 72 hours prior to surgery.[18] Retrieval of blood in a closed-chest tube system during an operative procedure or traumatic injury for reperfusion as whole blood or washed cells is another type of autologous blood transfusion (Figure 13.2).

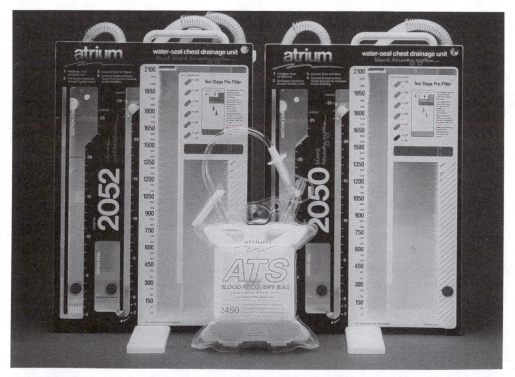

FIGURE 13.2. Single and dual collection auto transfusion systems. Adapted from Atrium Medical Corporation. Copyright © 1990 Atrium Medical Corporation, Hollis, NH. All rights reserved.

An anticoagulant is used (usually CPDA-1) to prevent clotting. Filtering of the blood both on collection and transfusion decreases the risk of microemboli from hemolytic-cell debris or platelet clumping, which can be potentially dangerous.

Blood Substitutes

Refusals of blood products in the clinical setting owing to personal and/or religious beliefs have prompted researchers to look for alternative oxygen-carrying compounds. Two such substances include stroma-free hemoglobins and perfluorocarbons. Clinical trials have been encouraging.

STROMA-FREE HEMOGLOBINS

Stroma-free hemoglobins are prepared from red blood cells that are membrane (stroma) free. Complications such as nephrotoxicity and/or coagulopathy have been associated with the stromal lipid component of hemoglobin. Stroma-free hemoglobins decrease the nephrotoxic/coagulopathy risks yet have desirable oxygen-carrying capacity.[19-21] Limitations such as a short half life (87 minutes) and decreased 2,3 DPG have limited clinical trials.[22-23] Mixture of stroma-free hemoglobins with glutaraldehyde produces polyhemoglobin, which increases life span up to three hours.[19,22-23] Other alterations elevate the P_{50} value, reversing the increased affinity-of-oxygen effect caused by low 2,3 DPG levels.[19,22] Clinical trials have compared stroma-free hemoglobins to autotransfusion or Lactated Ringers solution as resuscitative measures in dogs subjected to hemorrhagic shock. Marks et al. concluded that stroma-free hemoglobins may be a safe resuscitative fluid alternative, although it offers no advantage over Lactated Ringers. Side effects, including elevated liver enzymes, leukocytosis, and slightly elevated clotting times after transfusion, were noted in the dogs receiving stroma-free hemoglobins.[19]

Before practical consideration of stroma-free hemoglobins as a resuscitative alternative may occur, further research must focus on its efficacy as an oxygen-carrying component and address potentially negative immunotoxic and liver-dysfunction effects.[19]

PERFLUOROCARBONS

Perfluorocarbons (PFCs) have been investigated as another alternative for oxygen transport in plasma. Unlike hemoglobin, PFCs do not have a binding affinity for oxygen. Perfluorocarbons are hydrocarbons in which the hydrogen atoms have been substituted with fluorine. The end product has a high solubility coefficient for oxygen, which makes it a desirable oxygen-transport compound. Perfluorocarbons can dissolve over 40 cc/dl of oxygen. The average amount of oxygen dissolved in plasma is 2–3 cc/dl.[21,24] Perfluorochemicals must be combined with an emulsifying agent since PFCs are immiscible in water.[24-25]

Several key issues regarding PFC administration must be settled before vast clinical usage will occur. The ideal concentration, particle size, and viscosity of PFC in the emulsion has yet to be determined. Also, a high fraction of inspired oxygen (FI_{O_2}) must be used for the emulsifying fluid to dissolve oxygen. Oxygen toxicity may occur with high FI_{O_2}. Perfluorocarbons are eliminated at a rapid rate from circulating blood by the reticuloendothelial system, lung excretion, and through the skin, usually within 24 hours. Currently used dosages range between 20–40 cc/kg. A test dose of Fluosol-DA 20% (FDA-20%) is given before administration of the blood substitute. The test dose may produce a short-term decrease in neutrophils and platelets, which usually resolves spontaneously. Adverse effects such as hypotension, decreased leukocyte count, and abnormal hepatic and/or pulmonary function have limited widespread clinical use.[21,25-26]

The major PFC used to date is FDA-20%. Most clinical trials have involved severely anemic patients that refused blood products based on religious beliefs. Reports of the efficacy of PFCs as oxygen-carrying components have been inconsistent. Waxman reported a moderate increase of arterial oxygen content in six severely anemic patients who received FDA-20%, but also found higher oxygen consumption. Several of the aforementioned adverse effects were seen.[26] Gould et al. used FDA-20% in eight anemic surgical patients and found that it was unnecessary in moderate anemia and ineffective for severe anemia. No adverse reactions were noted.[27] Mitsuno and Ohyanagi reported the use of FDA-20% in 401 patients in Japan. They found a transient decrease in neutrophils and platelets. Although they reported a longer recovery to preoperative levels in patients receiving FDA-20% as compared to the control group, they reported FDA-20% as being an effective blood-gas carrier and plasma expander.[28] The inconsistent data on Fluosol-DA 20% as an oxygen-carrying agent has resulted in denial of Food and Drug Administration licensure for severe anemia.[3] Recently another PFC, perfluoroocytylbromide (PFOB) has been introduced. It has a greater ability than FDA-20% to dissolve oxygen and is not retained in organ systems as long.[29]

Clinical applications of PFC other than in anemia include cerebral ischemia, myocardial ischemia, cardiopulmonary bypass, and radiation therapy. The low viscosity of the PFC coupled with its small size allow it to penetrate ischemic areas that may not have been perfused by red blood cells.[24-25] Use of FDA-20% is being investigated with percutaneous transluminal coronary angioplasty (PCTA). Balloon inflation necessary to open partially occluded coronary vessels disrupts coronary blood flow, temporarily causing myocardial ischemia. The use of FDA-20% infused distal to the balloon maintains normal levels of oxygenation, even with balloon inflation. Normal or increased oxygenation provided by FDA-20% allows longer balloon inflation time, increasing success of PCTA.[24,29-30] Perfluorocarbons have been used in oncology in conjunction with radiation. The uptake of radiation in hypoxic tumor cells is limited. Perfluorocarbons enhance oxygenation of the tumor cells, therefore increasing the effectiveness of radiation and/or chemotherapy.[24,29]

Blood substitutes have promising potential as alternatives for blood products in the acutely ill. Current research must clarify their safety, effectiveness as an oxygen-transport medium, and the dosage requirements to minimize adverse effects.

CLINICAL EXAMPLES

Example 1

Mr. R was a 42-year-old man who experienced sudden vomiting of bright red blood while at home. His wife called 911 immediately and went to check on her husband. He had fallen to the floor and was having a seizure. Upon arrival of the emergency medical crew, Mr. R was lethargic, tachycardic, and hypotensive, with a weak thready pulse. He was rushed to the local emergency room. Admission vital signs were:

BP 80/50
HR 150
RR 30

He was pale, diaphoretic, and had cool clammy skin. Capillary refill of the nailbeds was sluggish, and the conjunctiva of his eyes were pale white. Estimated blood loss was 500–1000 cc. Intravenous fluids of Lactated Ringers solution were run at a wide-open rate through two 18-gauge IVs. A nasogastric tube was inserted so he could be ice lavaged. A foley catheter was placed so hourly urine output could be measured. He was typed and crossed for 8 units of blood. His hemoglobin was 7 gm/dl and hematocrit was 27 gm/dl. Electrolytes were within normal range. He was given 4 units of whole blood and 2 units of packed cells over the next 10 hours. His sensorium cleared and lethargy disappeared as the blood was transfused. Intravenous fluids were gradually slowed to 150 cc/hr. His BP stabilized at 110/65 and HR decreased to 85. His urine output gradually increased to 40 cc/hr. Once Mr. R was stabilized, the gastroenterologist was contacted for an endoscopy. A small lesion was found in the gastric mucosal lining. The location of the ulcer, however, was adjacent to an artery, thus the profound effects. He was medically managed for his ulcer.

Example 2

Mrs. S was recently diagnosed with ovarian cancer. She received chemotherapy and radiation. She contacted her physician complaining of diarrhea, nausea, and vomiting two days after the last dose of chemotherapy. She presented in the physician's office with weakness, dizziness, and weight loss of 5 pounds over two days. Her BP was 90/60 and HR 120. She was admitted to the MICU for hypovolemia. Clinical assessment revealed dry mucous membranes, poor skin turgor, and collapsed neck veins. Her BP was 100/60 and HR 125 when lying. Upon sitting, her BP fell to 78/50 and HR increased to 145. Laboratory data showed Na+ 150, K+ 3.0, Cl 115, glucose 90, SCr 1.8, BUN 55, bicarbonate 18, and Hgb 18 gm/dl. She admitted to her nurse that she had not had much food or fluids over the last couple of days due to her nausea.

What is your interpretation of these symptoms— FVD or hemorrhage?

ANSWER

The fluid volume deficit/dehydration was related to vomiting and diarrhea. Mrs. S was hypovolemic because of her vomiting and diarrhea. Her elevated Na+ demonstrated that she lost fluid in excess of her electrolyte loss. She admitted that she had not taken many fluids prior to admission. This contributed to her dehydration and hemoconcentration of 18 gm/dl.

She was treated with intravenous fluids, bedrest, and antiemetic drugs. A foley catheter was inserted to monitor urine output, and a stool culture was done to rule out infectious cause of diarrhea. Fluid resuscitation with Lactated Ringers solution stabilized her hemodynamic status.

Example 3

Mr. E was a 57-year-old man admitted to the SICU after an abdominal aortic aneurysm repair. Postoperatively, his vital signs were:

HR	120
BP	100/60
RR	30
Temperature	98°F
Hgb	9 gm/dl
Hct	28 gm/dl

Mr. E was arousable and could answer appropriate questions but would immediately fall back asleep. His urine output was 25 cc/hr. He complained of some abdominal discomfort so was given 75 mg Demerol intramuscularly. His surgeon decided to monitor his postoperative status and opted not to treat his slightly low Hgb/Hct because of Mr. E's religious beliefs as a Jehovah's Witness. Two hours later, Mr. E was barely arousable and complained of lower back pain and nausea. His HR was up to 140 and BP was 90/60. Physical assessment included dry skin turgor, pale mucous membranes, a urine output of 10 cc/hr, and an enlarged scrotum.

1. What is your interpretation of the above symptoms?

ANSWER

Mr. E is hemorrhaging, as evidenced by physical assessment, BP, and HR.

Mr. E's surgeon was contacted immediately. A blood count revealed Hgb 5 gm/dl and Hct 15 gm/dl. Mr. E was given Lactated Ringers solution at 400 cc/hour and told of his critical condition. He was asked if he would accept his own blood returned to him and he nodded approval. He was taken back to surgery in order to stop the bleeding. On return to the SICU, he was intubated on assist-control ventilation with 100% FI$_{O_2}$. His blood had been salvaged during surgery and he was currently being autotransfused. His Hgb was now 4 gm/dl and Hct 12 gm/dl. His BP was 90/60 with a HR of 135. He required norepinephrine and renal-dose dopamine to maintain his BP.

2. What are some treatment alternatives consistent with his religious beliefs?

ANSWER

Mr. E's hemodynamic status must be aggressively managed with fluids. Plasma volume expanders such as Hetastarch may be used to augment the circulating volume. Perfluorocarbons have been used also to enhance oxygen transport.

Mr. E was given 0.5 cc Fluosol-DA 20% test dose and a total infusion of 2800 cc (40 cc/kg). His BP decreased transiently to 80 systolic and normal saline was run at wide-open rate. Over the next several hours, his condition stabilized, and his BP was maintained at 100 systolic. His vasopressors were weaned.

3. What are the potential side effects of Fluosol-DA?

ANSWER

Adverse effects of Fluosol-DA 20% include hypotension, leukopenia, ARDS, decreased platelets, and abnormal liver function.

Mr. E's hemodynamic condition stabilized. His BP was 100 systolic and HR 120. Urine output was 20–25 cc/hr. Complications of his clinical course included adult respiratory distress syndrome (ARDS) and leukopenia. He was placed on prophylactic antibiotics and supported symptomatically. Twenty-one days later, he was discharged from the hospital.

ECONOMIC IMPLICATIONS

Optimal hemoglobin values for oxygen transport are difficult to identify. As hemoglobin deficits occur, optimal hemoglobin becomes even more obscure. Physiologic and economic risks and benefits must be evaluated prior to therapeutic interventions. For instance, consider the patient with chronic anemia. Chronic anemia over time may strain the cardiovascular compensatory mechanisms. If the ability of the heart to compensate is exceeded, higher ventricular-filling pressures are needed, which may lead to myocardial hypertrophy and/or cardiomegaly.[3] Blood transfusions given to these patients to improve their oxygen-carrying capacity may exceed the volume their heart can tolerate and exacerbate their congestive heart failure. Not only would this be a negative result physiologically, but also economically, as it would likely increase the length of hospitalization.

In hemorrhagic states, more emphasis should be placed on maintaining adequate mean arterial pressure and tissue perfusion versus an arbitrary hemoglobin value. Initial focus in acute hemorrhagic states will be to replace volume. Even though colloidal agents will increase circulating volume much more effectively than a similar amount of crystalloids, colloidal agents typically cost 4–5 times as much as crystalloids. Since studies have failed to show a significant advantage of colloidal agents over crystalloids, economic aspects should be considered when deciding treatment alternatives. When blood transfusions are necessary to improve oxygen transport, careful consideration of the potential risks of blood therapy should be evaluated. If a patient has a hemoglobin of 9 gm/dl, but cardiac output and oxygen transport are normal, blood transfusions should not be automatic. The physiologic and economic disadvantages may outweigh the assumed benefit. The escalating cost of overtreatment may be magnified if complications develop from unnecessary therapies.

SUMMARY

Hemoglobin deficits may negatively affect oxygen transport. However, an optimal hemoglobin is difficult to ascertain especially in conjunction with hemoglobin deficits. Compensatory mechanisms occur to negate the adverse effects of low hemoglobin levels. The ability or inability of these compensatory mechanisms to maintain adequate oxygen transport will determine the urgency of treating hemoglobin deficits. Current therapeutic options for hemoglobin deficits are somewhat limited. Blood transfusions, which are most commonly utilized for low hemoglobin states, have been associated with serious adverse effects and should not be given lightly. Artificial blood products seem promising, but as of yet are not practical alternatives since they are not currently available in the clinical practice. Therapeutic interventions for hemoglobin deficits must be evaluated on an individual basis with careful consideration of risk versus benefit.

REFERENCES

1. Ayres SM, Schlichtig R, Sterling M. *Circulatory Monitoring In Care of the Critically Ill.* Chicago: Year Book Medical Pubs, 1988, 43.
2. Guyton AC. "Red blood cells, anemia, and polycythemia." *Textbook of Medical Physiology.* Philadelphia: WB Saunders, 1981, 56.
3. Kruskall MS. "Clinical management of transfusions to patients with red cell antibodies." Nance SJ (ed). *Immune Destruction of Red Blood Cells.* Arlington, VA: American Association of Blood Banks, 1989, 263.
4. Snyder JV. "Oxygen transport: The model and reality." Snyder JV, Pinsky MR (ed). *Oxygen Transport in the Critically Ill.* Chicago: Year Book Medical Pubs, 1987, 3.

5. Langfitt DE. "Pathologic Hematologic Conditions." *Critical Care Certification Preparation and Review.* Bowie, MD: Brady Communications Co, 1984, 419.

6. Metheny NM. "Fluid Volume Imbalances." *Quick Reference to Fluid Balance.* Philadelphia: JP Lippincott, 1984, 81.

7. McAdams RC, McClure K. "Hypovolemia: When to suspect it." *RN,* Dec. 1986;34.

8. Peitzman A. "Principles of circulatory support and the treatment of hemorrhagic shock." Snyder JV, Pinsky MR (eds). *Oxygen Transport in the Critically Ill.* Chicago: Year Book Medical Pubs, 1987, 407.

9. Niinikoski J. "Tissue Oxygenation in Hypovolemic Shock." *Ann Clin Res* 1977;9:151.

10. Smith LG. "Reactions to blood transfusions." *Am J Nurs* 1984;84:1096.

11. Masoorli ST, Piercy S. "A step-by-step guide to trouble free transfusions." *RN,* May 1984;34.

12. Committee on Transfusion Practices. "The Latest Protocols for Blood Transfusions." *Nurs* 1986; 16:34.

13. Dutcher JP. *Modern Transfusion Therapy.* Boca Raton, FL: CRC Press, 1990, 58.

14. Walker RH. "Adverse effects of blood transfusion." *American Association of Blood Banks Technical Manual.* Arlington, VA: American Association of Blood Banks, 1990, 411.

15. Collins JA. "Problems associated with the massive transfusion of stored blood." *Surg* 1974;75:274.

16. McLellan BA, Reid SR, Lane PL. "Massive blood transfusion causing hypomagnesemia." *Crit Care Med* 1984;12:146.

17. Counts RB, Haisch C, Simon TL, et al. "Hemostasis in massively transfused trauma patients." *Ann Surg* 1979;190:91.

18. Butler S. "Current trends in autologous transfusion." *RN,* Nov. 1989;44.

19. Marks DH, Lynett JE, Letscher RM, et al. "Pyridoxalated polymerized stroma-free hemoglobin solution (SFHS-PP) as an oxygen-carrying fluid replacement for hemorrhagic shock in dogs." *Mil Med* 1987;152:265.

20. Messmer K. "Oxygen-carrying blood substitutes." *Int Anes Clin* 1983;21:137.

21. Rutherford KA. "Advances in the treatment of oxygenation disturbances." *Crit Care Nurs Clin* 1989;1:659.

22. Chang TMS, Farmer M, Geyer RP, et al. "Blood substitutes based on modified hemoglobin and fluorochemicals." *Trans Am Soc Artif Int Org* 1987;33:819.

23. Keipert P, Minkowitz J, Chang TM. "Cross-linked stroma-free polyhemoglobin as a potential blood substitute." *Int J Artif Organs* 1982;5:383.

24. Lowe KC. "Perfluorocarbons as oxygen-transport fluids." *Comp Biochem Physiol* 1987;87A:825.

25. Waxman K. "Perfluorocarbons as blood substitutes." *Ann Emer Med* 1986;15:1423.

26. Waxman K, Tremper KK, Cullen BF, et al. "Perfluorocarbon infusion in bleeding patients refusing blood transfusions." *Arch Surg* 1984;119:721.

27. Gould SA, Rosen AL, Sehgal LR, et al. "Fluosol-DA as a red cell substitute in acute anemia." *N Engl J Med* 1986;314:1653.

28. Mitsuno T, Ohyanagi H. "Present status of clinical studies of fluosol-DA (20%) in Japan." *Int Anesthesiol Clin* 1985;23:169.

29. Reiss JG. "Blood substitutes: Where do we stand with the fluorocarbon approach? *Curr Surg,* Sept–Oct 1988;365.

30. Cleman M, Jaffee CC, Wohlgelernter D. "Prevention of ischemia during percutaneous transluminal coronary angioplasty by transcatheter infusion of oxygenated fluosol-DA (20%)." *Circ* 1986;74:555.

Part IV
Treatment of Oxygenation Disturbances

14
Treatment of Low Cardiac Outputs

Treatment of cardiac output helps point out the close relationship between oxygenation and hemodynamics. As presented in the assessment of cardiac output (Chapter 6), the key role of cardiac output in overall oxygenation cannot be over estimated. If a patient can maintain an adequate cardiac output, the chance of maintaining normal oxygenation is greatly enhanced. The goal of this chapter is to review the primary treatment modalities available to improve cardiac output. Cardiac output can be improved by three primary mechanisms: alteration of preload, afterload, or contractility. Each of these potential modes will be addressed separately. A fourth mechanism is treatment of heart-rate disturbances. Treatment of heart rate is primarily treatment of dysrhythmias. Due to the extensive material already available in the literature, the treatment of dysrhythmias will be reviewed briefly.

TREATMENT OF PRELOAD

Treatment of preload classically addresses the concept of left-ventricular muscle stretch (muscle stretching). Right-ventricular (RV) assessment is also an important aspect of hemodynamic assessment. Parameters estimating RV preload include right-atrial and central venous pressures (CVP). For the purpose of assessing the role of cardiac output in oxygen transport, left-ventricular assessment and treatment will be the primary focus of this chapter. Despite the value of right-ventricular assessment, it is the left-ventricular output that plays the primary role in oxygen transport.

Adequate left-ventricular muscle stretching will equate to effective contractility (strength) status in the left ventricle. According to Starling's law, preload, which is measured by left-ventricular end diastolic volume, pressure, and compliance, is frequently estimated clinically through such factors as the pulmonary-capillary wedge (PCWP) or left-atrial pressures (Figure 14.1).[1-2] Both PCWP and LA pressures attempt to estimate left-ventricular pressure. Neither of these truly measure preload, but are employed clinically in an attempt to help estimate or approximate the preload of the left ventricle.[3] Since preload involves more components than pressure, that is, volume and muscle compliance, pressure estimates of preload are limited in accurately reflecting preload.[4] However, pressure measurements are readily available through pulmonary-artery catheters. Owing to the ease of obtaining PCWP values, the use of pressure to estimate preload is common practice. The clinician must be aware of the potential limitation of using pressure in isolation from other hemodynamics such as stroke volume, cardiac output and ejection fractions that are influenced by preload.

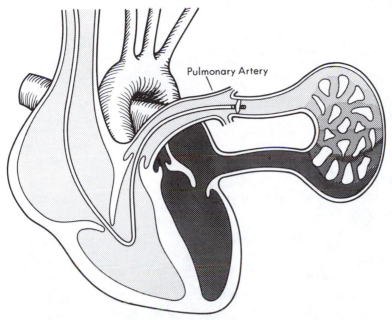

FIGURE 14.1. Why the wedge pressure (PCWP) reflects left-ventricular events. When the balloon of the pulmonary-artery catheter is inflated, a continuous uninterrupted pathway exists between the end of the catheter and the left atrium. In addition, when the mitral valve is open in diastole, the pathway extends to the left ventricle.

Use of the preload as an estimate of left-ventricular function can be grossly simplified by the following guidelines (see Table 14.1). (1) If the preload is decreased, inadequate fluid is returning to the heart. A low preload is reflected by PCWP less than 8 mm Hg and low stroke volumes (less than 50 cc or 25 cc/m[2]).[5] (2) If the preload is increased, the contractile strength of the heart is likely reduced. An elevated PCWP is usually present (over 18 mm Hg) with an increased preload. In both low and high preload, a decreased stroke volume will be present with clinically significant preload values.[6]

Treatment of Low Preload

If preload is low, as reflected clinically by low pulmonary-capillary wedge pressures and low stroke volumes, augmentation of preload could take place by one of two methods: the administration of (1) crystalloidal or (2) colloidal solutions.

Controversy exists over the use of crystalloidal solutions (such as Lactated Ringers and normal saline) and colloidal solutions (such as hetastarch (Hespan), albumin, or blood products) to treat low preloads. The use of colloidal solutions centers primarily around replacing acute volume loss such as may occur postoperatively, in trauma, or in acute GI bleeding. The purpose of colloidal solutions is to replace volume that would be lost primarily from the vascular space (Figure 14.2).[7-8] The major benefit of colloidal solutions is in replacement of vascular space

TABLE 14.1. Hemodynamic Pressure Guidelines

Preload Measure	Value (mm Hg)	Potential Condition
PCWP	< 8	Hypovolemia
CVP	< 5	Hypovolemia
PCWP	> 18	Left-ventricular failure
CVP	> 10	Right-ventricular failure
PCWP	12–18	No clear problem present,
CVP	5–10	adaptive responses likely occurring.

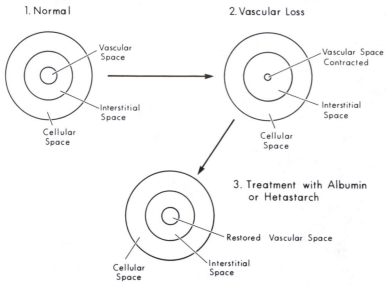

FIGURE 14.2. Loss of vascular volume may be best treated with colloidal solutions.

volume when major fluid loss from interstitial or intercellular compartments has not occurred. In the presence of loss of fluid from interstitial and cellular compartments, which would be more likely to take place in chronic volume loss or loss of vascular volume over a period of days, crystalloidal solutions tend to be preferred. Crystalloids are valuable primarily because of the potential of these solutions to diffuse outside the vascular compartments and into the interstitial space and intercellular compartments (Figure 14.3).[9–10]

Crystalloidal solutions, because of their enhanced ability to diffuse outside the vascular space, offer an increased value in expanding extravascular volumes as well as vascular volumes. This advantage, however, is considered by some clinicians to be a drawback. The volume of crystalloids required to replace vascular volume is roughly five times that of colloidal solutions.[11] For example, if 500 cc of normal saline or Lactated Ringers is administered, only about 100 cc will stay in the vascular space. The rest of the volume will diffuse outside the blood vessel into the interstitial and intercellular space. On the other hand, giving 500 cc of a colloidal

solution will generally result in the retention of the entire 500 cc in the vascular space (at least for the first 24 hours before renal and hepatic filtering mechanisms come into action).[12] The rapid volume expansion capability of colloidal solutions is a primary value that is seen in the settings of trauma and immediately postoperatively.

Both crystalloidal and colloidal solutions will improve vascular volume. Which agent is ideal is somewhat dependent on the clinical situation, but one must take into account some side effects that can occur with both types. The primary disadvantage of administering a crystalloidal solution is the need to administer large volumes to raise the vascular space to a level that may improve the cardiac output. Since extravascular accumulation of fluid occurs with crystalloidal solutions, the large increases in extravascular volume may be accompanied by marked weight gain.

The primary problem associated with colloidal solutions is the potential to leak large molecular structures into the extravascular space. In a patient who may have a pulmonary-capillary leak problem, such as ARDS, the colloidal solution will cause larger

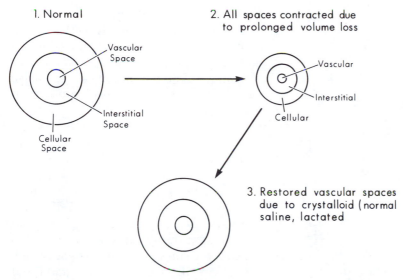

1. Normal

Vascular Space

Interstitial Space

Cellular Space

2. All spaces contracted due to prolonged volume loss

Vascular

Interstitial

Cellular

3. Restored vascular spaces due to crystalloid (normal saline, lactated)

FIGURE 14.3. Loss of volume in all fluid compartments may be best treated with crystalloidal agents.

amounts of fluid to exit the blood vessels than will the crystalloidal agents, causing a worsening of intrapulmonary shunting (Figure 14.4). In the adult respiratory distress syndrome, this might lead to a worsening pulmonary status. Crystalloidal agents have been demonstrated to cause less disruption to gas exchange in the patient with ARDS.[13-14] The extent of the potential problems associated with colloidal solutions versus crystallized solutions is somewhat controversial, with a wide degree of variation in opinions among clinicians concerning their preferences for different types of solutions. The key point to be made, regardless of the type of solution administered, is that one should note an improvement in the clinical condition. The primary clinical parameters to monitor are those that involve oxygenation: cardiac output, stroke volume, $Sa_{O_2}/S\bar{v}_{O_2}$, and lactate levels. Secondary signs such as improved renal function (increased urine output) usually are a reflection of the improved stroke volume and cardiac output.

Another factor to remember regarding crystalloidal and colloidal solutions is the difference in expense. Crystalloidal solutions tend to be relatively inexpensive, with

the actual cost (not charge) of administering a liter of normal saline or Lactated Ringers to be less than $10.00. Colloidal solutions, on the other hand, can be much more expensive. Albumin, for example, may cost in excess of $100.00 (for 25 grams). Hetastarch is also expensive, although it usually costs about one third the amount of albumin. Because colloidal solutions tend to be more expensive, the use of crystalloidals may be a logical first attempt to expand vascular space. This point, however, is controversial and depends on how important the clinician believes the colloidal solution is to expanding the vascular space and thereby improving oxygenation.

Treatment of a High Preload

An increased preload is clinically evident by a decreased stroke volume and an increased pulmonary-capillary wedge pressure. Increased preload is most commonly the result of reduced left-ventricular contractility. Treatment of alterations in left-ventricular strength is usually attempted by one of three methods: (1) reduction in the preload through the administration of diuretics or vasodilators, (2) improvement in

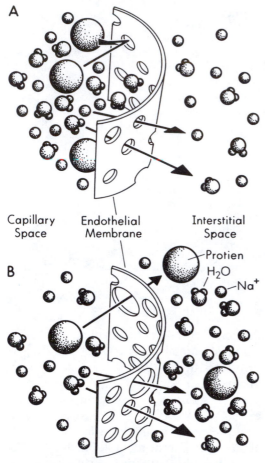

A

B

Capillary Space   Endothelial Membrane   Interstitial Space

Protien
H₂O
Na⁺

FIGURE 14.4. Changes in capillary permeability determines extravascular fluid levels. Note, under normal conditions (A), large molecules such as proteins are held in the capillary. When permeability of the capillary changes, such as in sepsis and ARDS, capillary permeability increases. This allows proteins and other substances that normally control fluid movement to move into the interstitial space. The result is an increase in fluid outside the blood vessel.

contractility, and (3) reduction of the systemic vascular resistance (SVR).

Reduction of Preload

As preload is increased to levels beyond what is normally accepted for adequate stroke volume, levels generally in excess of 18 mm Hg, reduction of the preload is attempted in an effort to increase stroke volume. Subsequently, all interventions that reduce preload are assessed for their impacts by their effects on stroke volume. Two

major categories of drugs are given to reduce preload: diuretics and vasodilators. Examples of these agents are contained in Table 14.2.

Removal of fluid from the vascular space is most commonly done with diuretic therapy. Intravenous (IV) diuretics primarily used include furosemide (Lasix) and other loop diuretics.[15] The theory behind the administration of diuretics is that the removal of fluid reduces the amount of fluid returning to the heart and causes the Starling's curve to shift to the left (Figure 14.5). This shift in the Starling's curve should cause an improvement in left-ventricular function and stroke volume. Vasodilators are administered with the same theory in mind, but work by a different mechanism. The mechanism for vasodilators such as nitroglycerin is a reduction in preload, which occurs through blood-vessel relaxation. The relaxation of venous vessel tone results in the subsequent pooling of blood in the venous system. Since venous blood accounts for approximately 80% of total blood volume, agents that alter venous tone have the marked potential to reduce the amount of blood volume returned to the heart.[16] This

TABLE 14.2.   Preload Reducing Agents

	Doses	Route
Vasodilators		
Diltaizem (Cardizem)	180–360 mg/day q 6–8 hr	Oral
Nifedipine (Procardia)	40–240 mg/day q 6–8 hr	Oral
Nitroglycerine (Nitrostat)	10–400 mcg/min	IV
Diuretics		
Furosemide (Lasix)	10–600 mg/day divided doses	IV/oral
Ethacrynic acid (Edecrin)	50–150 mg/day 2–3 times daily	IV/oral
Bumetanide (Bumex)	.5–10 mg/day	IV/oral
Chlorothiazide (Diuril)	1000–2000 mg/day	Oral
Zaroxolyn (Matolazone)	5–20 mg/day	Oral

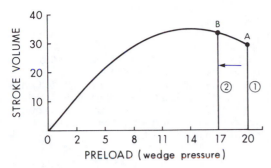

FIGURE 14.5. Shifting Starling's curve to improve contractility. (1) Initial clinical starting point, with a wedge pressure of 20 mm Hg. Treatment with preload reducers started at this time. (2) If preload reduction takes place (wedge of 17 mm Hg), the stroke volume improves. (A) Depressed contractility caused by overstretching of the ventricular muscle. (B) Improved contractility location on Starling's curve.

TABLE 14.3. Inotropic (Contractility) Agents

Drug	Dose
Dobutamine	1–20 mcg/kg/min
Dopamine	1–5 mcg/kg/min, renal dose
	5–10 mcg/kg/min, inotropic
	> 10 mcg/kg/min, vasopressor (Dopamine has overlapping responses at each dose.)
Amrinone	.75 mg/kg, loading dose
	5–10 mcg/kg/min

temporary reduction allows the heart to improve performance.

Preload reduction is attempted primarily through diuretics and vasodilators. One may assess the effect of preload reduction by comparing the changing preload (pulmonary-capillary wedge pressure) and its effect on the cardiac output and stroke volume. Reduction in preload is only successful if cardiac parameters such as stroke volume also improve. Without improvement in the cardiac parameters, systemic oxygenation is unlikely to improve.

Inotropic Therapy

Inotropic therapy, from a theoretical point of view, should be one of the primary treatments instituted to try and improve cardiac output. Inotropic therapy centers on sympathetic stimulation, although new categories of agents such as phosphodiesterase inhibitors have potential advantages in improving contractility status.[17–19] Examples of inotropic agents are included in Table 14.3.

While theoretically inotropes offer the best approach to improving cardiac output (except with hypovolemic patients), inotrope value has not been validated in research.[20] The lack of marked improvement with inotropic therapy, particularly long-

term improvements in cardiac outputs, may be the result of many factors, including loss of sympathetic stimulation responses in the heart over prolonged periods of time or changes in sympathetic response to stimulation.[21–22] For whatever reason, inotropic therapy is not always as successful as desired. The clinician must always note the stroke volume on the administration of an inotrope. An improvement will occur if the treatment is effective.

It is important for the clinician to note the changes in stroke volume rather than noting only the cardiac output and the PCWP. Inotropic therapy primarily affects stroke volume, but changes in heart rate can also occur, which may increase cardiac output and mask a change in stroke volume (see Example 1). The parameter that must be measured whenever assessing changes in the contractility strength is the stroke volume. Another potential measure, ejection fraction, is becoming clinically available and can also help assess contractility (see Example 2).

Inotropic therapy is commonly based on a person's overall hemodynamics, including blood pressure. For example, in the person whose blood pressure is close to normal, the most common treatment is with drugs such as dobutamine. Dobutamine, primarily a beta stimulator, has the best chance of improving stroke volume in the patient with simple contractility problems. Simple contractility problems are manifested by low stroke volume but are compensated by an increase in end diastolic volume and in-

Example 1

A 48-year-old man is admitted to the ICU with an R/O anterior MI. A pulmonary-artery catheter is placed to monitor hemodynamics. At 1700, dobutamine (5 mcg/kg) is started to increase cardiac output and decrease the PCWP. At 1800, the following values are obtained. Based on the 1700 and 1800 readings, has the dobutamine been successful?

	Time	
	1700	1800
BP	102/78	104/74
P	98	115
CO	3.90	4.58
CI	2.05	2.4
SV	40	40
SI	21	21
PCWP	21	18
CVP	12	10

ANSWER

The increase in cardiac output is due to an increase in heart rate, not contractility. Note that the stroke volume and stroke index are unchanged. The decrease in PCWP is not clinically significant since no improvement in stroke volume has occurred. While the increased cardiac output has increased oxygen transport, another inotrope would be a likely alternative treatment.

Example 2

A 77-year-old 60-kg woman is in the ICU with a diagnosis of congestive heart failure. She complains of orthopnea and has inspiratory crackles. She is given 20 mg of Lasix and is started on amrinone (2 mcg/kg/min after loading dose of 45 mg) at 1200. At 1300 she has no change in physical symptoms. Based on the following readings, have the interventions been effective?

	Time	
	1200	1300
BP	114/68	108/70
P	108	100
CO	3.4	3.9
CI	2.1	2.4
SV	31	39
SI	19	24
PCWP	22	17
CVP	11	7
EDV	175	175
Ejection Fraction	18%	22%

ANSWER

Based on the reduced heart rate and PCWP, and increased stroke volume/index and cardiac output/index, the therapy is likely improving the clinical status. The lack of improvement in clinical signs may be due to the lagging behind of the hemodynamic improvements, or it may indicate that further improvements in cardiac output and stroke volume are necessary. Notice how an improvement in ejection fraction also indicates an improvement in contractility.

creased SVR. These compensation mechanisms act to keep the blood pressure within normal limits. When compensation mechanisms have acted to keep the blood pressure near normal, agents such as dobutamine (and phosphodiesterase inhibitors such as amrinone) have their maximal impact.

When the systemic vascular resistance and increasing ventricular-muscle stretching cannot compensate for loss of cardiac output and the blood pressure falls, an agent such as dopamine, which has both beta and alpha stimulation properties, may be more effective. Improvements in both sympathetic stimulation and contractility will cause improvement in both stroke volume and systemic vascular resistance. Improvements in both contractility (stroke volume) and systemic vascular resistance act together to improve the blood pressure.

Agents such as dobutamine and dopamine can be employed together when a combination of low blood pressure and poor contractility exists. Any number of interactions between drug treatments can be employed in an attempt to increase cardiac performance. For example, in the normotensive patient administration of a preload reducing agent (such as Lasix) in combination with a contractility agent (such as dobutamine) is not uncommon (see Example 3). Whichever therapy is employed, the clinician must assess the impact on oxygenation. Measures of oxygenation serve as an end point in assessing the effectiveness of treatment.

Example 3

A 65-year-old man is in the ICU following gastric reaction. He as a history of CHF and is in the unit for postoperative management. At 2300, he complains of increasing shortness of breath. Based on the 2300 reading, 20 mg of Lasix is given, but no relief is afforded. Dobutamine at 4 mcg/kg/min is added at 2400. While he states he feels "somewhat better," nitroprusside is added at 0100. Based on the readings, has the addition of nitroprusside made a clinical improvement?

	Time		
	2300	2400	0100
BP	136/82	138/80	120/70
P	106	108	94
CO	4.1	4.3	4.8
CI	1.9	2.0	2.2
SV	39	40	51
SI	18	18.5	23
PCWP	24	24	20
CVP	13	12	4
		Dobutamine started	Nipride added

ANSWER

The addition of nitroprusside has resulted in a substantial improvement in cardiac output, stroke volume, and oxygen transport. The combination of dobutamine and nitroprusside appears to be very effective in this situation.

REDUCING SYSTEMIC VASCULAR RESISTANCE

When the cardiac output decreases, the normal response by the vasculature is to increase the tone or rigidity, causing an elevation in the systemic vascular resistance. Unfortunately, as the systemic vascular resistance increases, the potential exists to decrease the cardiac output through increased cardiac work. One therapy that may be employed in an attempt to improve cardiac output and stroke volume is to administer agents that may reduce the systemic vascular resistance and reduce myocardial work.[23] Agents used to reduce systemic vascular resistance are listed in Table 14.4. As the systemic vascular resistance is decreased, the clinician must again note if the treatment is effective by assessing if an improvement in

cardiac output or stroke volume has occurred. When pulmonary catheters are employed, rapid assessment of effectiveness can be made by measuring stroke volume. When utilizing SVR-reducing agents (such as nitroprusside) or angiotensin converting enzyme (ACE) inhibitors (such as captopril or enalapril), the cardiac output and stroke should be measured along with the SVR.[24] When administering agents that reduce the systemic vascular resistance, it is most important to note the effect on oxygenation through improvement in cardiac output and stroke volume. If the cardiac output or stroke volume does not change substantially, then a decrease in the systemic vascular resistance may not be effective. In addition, reduction of systemic vascular resistance without an increase in cardiac output may decrease the blood pressure. In a person with excessively high blood pressure, this is not a problem. However, in the patient with a border-line blood pressure, a further reduction could seriously impair the perfusion of major organ systems.

TREATMENT OF ABNORMAL HEART RATE (DYSRHYTHMIAS)

The treatment of abnormal heart rates centers on the attempt to return heart rates to within a normal range, which allows both adequate time for diastolic filling and a rate able to generate adequate cardiac output. To maintain heart rate within a normal range, one must accelerate the heart rate in the presence of a bradycardia or slow the heart rate in the presence of a tachycardia. Pharmacologic agents and physical methods that are used to treat abnormal heart rates are fairly extensive. The focus of this section will be to review the common mechanisms for treatment of abnormal heart rates. The emphasis will be on maintaining adequate cardiac output and oxygen transport. In-depth reviews of dysrhythmia treatment are available elsewhere.[25-26]

The treatment of dysrhythmias is better

TABLE 14.4. Treatment with Afterload Reducing Agents

Drugs of Choice	Dose	Route
Vascular Smooth Muscle Relaxants		
Sodium Nitroprusside (Nipride)	.5–10 mcg/kg/min	IV
Hydralazine (Apresoline)	40–200 mg/day	Oral
	10–40 mg	IV
Diazoxide (Hyperstat)	50–100 mg bolus	IV
Nitroglycerine	10–400 mc/min	IV
Alpha Inhibitors		
Clonidine (Catapres)	.2–.6 mg/day (divided doses)	Oral
Phentolamine (Regitine)	.1–2 mg/min	IV
Methyldopa (Aldomet)	500–2000 mg/day (divided doses)	Oral
	250–1000 mg/dose (q 6 hr)	IV
Trimethapan (Arfonad)	starts at 3–4 mg/min, up to 6 mg/min	IV
Prazosin (Minipress)	1–20 mg/day (divided doses)	Oral
Angiotenstion Converting Enzyme (ACE) Inhibitors		
Captopril (Capoten)	25–150 mg/day bid or tid	Oral
Enalopril (Vasotec)	5–40 mg/day bid	IV & Oral
Beta-Blocking Agents		
Metoprolol (Lopressor)	15 mg loading (in 3 doses, 2 min apart)	IV
	100–400 mg daily 50–100 mg q day–qid	Oral
Propanolol (Inderal)	1–3 mg	IV
	120–240 mg/daily (divided doses)	Oral
Labetalol (Trandate)	.25 mg/kg initial 50–200 mg total	IV
	400–2400 mg (divided doses)	Oral
Calcium-Channel Blocking Agents		
Diltiazem (Cardizem)	180–360 mg/day q 6–8 hr	Oral
Nifedipine (Procardia)	40–240 mg/day q 6–8 hr	Oral

(All dosages should be individualized per patient. Dosages listed are common clinical guides but may vary between patient.)

understood with the review of primary methods of how the common therapies act. There are three primary methods for treating dysrhythmias. These methods are (1) alteration of the sympathetic nervous system, (2) alteration of the parasympathetic nervous system, or (3) ion-flow regulating agents. While the exact mechanism of some of the pharmacologic agents used to treat dysrhythmias are not completely understood, if the concepts of how the agents work are understood, appropriate times for utilizing the agents will also be understood.

A review of each of these three treatments will be the focus of this next section.

Autonomic Nervous System (Sympathetic and Parasympathetic Nervous Systems)

The sympathetic and parasympathetic nervous systems make up the autonomic nervous system. The sympathetic nervous system has two primary receptor sites responsible for its action: alpha and beta cells. Alpha and beta cells can also be categorized further into α-1 and α-2 and β-1 and β-2 cells. For the purpose of dysrhythmia interpretation, the primary site of interest is the β-1 cell.

Alpha-1 and α-2 cells primarily affect the blood vessels. The effect of the α-1 and α-2 cells, is in regulation of the blood pressure. Stimulation of α-2 cells causes vasoconstriction, with a subsequent increase in a systemic vascular existence. Obstruction of α-2 cells causes vasodilation and a lowering of systemic vascular existence.

Beta cells are divided into β-1 and β-2 types. Beta-1 cells have three primary actions. The three effects of β-1 cells are (1) to increase the strength of the heart's contraction (inotropic response), (2) to change the rate of impulse formation (chronotropic), and (3) to alter impulse transmission (dromotropic). Stimulation of β-1 cells causes positive (increased) inotropic, chronotropic, and dromotropic responses. In other words, the strength of contractions increases, the heart rate increases, and the impulse transmission improves. Blockage or inhibition of β-1 cells causes the opposite effect, that is, negative inotropic, chronotropic, and dromotropic responses. The most important factor for regulating the heart rate is the chronotropic response. Beta-2 cells primarily act on blood vessels and smooth muscles (stimulation of β-2 cells is likely to produce vasodilation and bronchodilation). Inhibition of β-2 cells will increase blood vessels and bronchial muscle tone. While this is a brief and simplistic overview of the sympathetic nervous system, the understanding of the action of β-1 stimulation or inhibition is important when understanding treatment of dysrhythmias.

The parasympathetic nervous system acts on the heart primarily through the vagus nerve. The parasympathetic nervous system has the strongest effect on the heart rate and has the major action of slowing the heart rate through parasympathetic stimulation. The primary effect of inhibiting the parasympathetic nervous system is to increase the heart rate.

Cellular-ion-flow altering agents are pharmacologic agents that alter the flow of key ions into or out of the cells. Examples of ion-altering agents are drugs that change sodium inflow, potassium outflow, or calcium inflow to the cells during key times of depolarization of the heart muscle. A large number of agents are available that fit the cellular-ion-flow altering category.

These three categories of sympathetic and parasympathetic and ion-altering agents can form the basis for understanding dysrhythmia treatment. Other classifications exist, such as the Vaughn-Williams classification of categorizing drug types.[27] However, a presentation of the categories of sympathetic and parasympathetic and cellular-ion altering agents is presented as a practical guideline for treatment of dysrhythmias and maintenance of adequate oxygen transport.

Treatment of Slow Heart Rates (Bradycardias)

The treatment of slow heart rates centers on stimulation of the sympathetic nervous system or inhibition of the parasympathetic nervous system. Since the inhibition of the parasympathetic nervous system has the strongest effect on heart rates, parasympathetic inhibitors are most common in the treatment of slow heart rates. Atropine is the most common parasympathetic inhibitor recommended to initially attempt to raise the heart rate.[28] Sympathetic stimulators also can be effective in the treatment of bradycardias. Sympathetic agents are thought to act primarily in heart rates that are slowed because of conduction defects below the AV node. There is some evidence that parasympathetic nervous system fibers are not present below the AV node and in the ventricles.[29] Due to this lack of parasympathetic innervation of the ventricles, the sympathetic stimulants will work primarily on heart rates that originate from the ventricles, for example, ventricular escape rhythms and third-degree heart blocks. Bradycardias of these conditions are best treated with agents such as isoproterenol and epinephrine.[30] Any beta stimulant, such as isoproterenol and epinephrine, and to a lesser extent, norepinephrine, can be used to increase the heart rate. Isoproterenol is usually the preferred drug because of its major effect of beta stimulation with little or no alpha action. Avoidance of alpha stimulation is important in order to avoid vasoconstriction. Vasoconstriction will increase myocardial work through increasing systemic vascular resistance. Epinephrine and norepinephrine both have alpha-stimulating properties, which relegate these drugs to secondary choices in treatment of slow heart rates.

Treatment of Fast Heart Rate (Tachycardias)

Rapid heart rates can be divided into atrial and ventricular dysrhythmias. Atrial dysrhythmias are usually not as life threatening as ventricular dysrhythmias and are more likely to receive emphasis on pharmacologic treatment rather than electrical treatment, that is, unsynchronized or synchronized defibrillation. The emphasis in this section will be on the pharmacologic treatment of atrial dysrhythmias.

Atrial Dysrhythmias (Tachycardias)

Currently, atrial tachycardias can be divided into three different categories of fast responses. These responses include atrial tachycardia, also referred to as paroxysmal atrial tachycardia or supraventricular tachycardia (PSVT), atrial flutter, and atrial fibrillation. The agents utilized for these three differ slightly and will be identified during the discussion of each of the pharmacologic agents.

Atrial dysrhythmias can be treated through sympathetic inhibition or parasympathetic stimulation. Agents commonly used to treat atrial tachycardias are listed in Table 14.5. Parasympathetic stimulation can be accomplished with drugs such as edrophonium chloride or with physical stimulation. Physical stimulation includes carotid massage, Valsalvas maneuver, ocular pressure, and the application of cold water to the face. These physical measures all act to cause parasympathetic stimulation and can slow an atrial tachycardia.

Other agents used to slow a tachycardia are the beta inhibitors or beta blockers. Propranolol (Inderal) and esmolol (Brevibloc) are common beta blockers. The beta-blocking agents are relatively effective but are considered as a second-line treatment for atrial dysrhythmias.[31] Esmolol has an advantage over propranolol in that it has a much shorter half life; esmolol will wear off approximately 9 minutes after administration.[32] Propranolol has a span of action closer to 24 hours. The treatment of acute atrial tachycardia with shorter-acting agents is preferable when other pharmacologic agents might need to be administered. The short half life avoids some of the accumulative or additive effects of administering a second antidysrhythmic.

Most of the agents used to alter atrial tachycardias are centered in the ion-flow-control areas. Ion-flow-altering agents include sodium-potassium altering agents and calcium-channel agents. The treatment of paroxysmal supraventricular tachycardia (PSVT) initially is centered on calcium-channel agents such as verapamil (Isoptin, Calan). If the initial agent is a calcium-blocking agent, such as verapamil, the effect is generally short lived. Usually the effect of the drug will wear off within 20 minutes.[33] If no response is achieved by the calcium-channel agents, other agents, such as the sodium-potassium flow agents, can be employed. A digitalis preparation such as digoxin (Lanoxin) is a primary example of a sodium-potassium flow agent.[34]

Current guidelines for treatment of atrial tachycardia generally involve the administration of pharmacologic agents following physical attempts to slow the heart rate. For example, parasympathetic stimulation may include carotid massage as the first attempt to try and slow an atrial tachycardia. The physical maneuver is followed by a calcium-channel blocking agent, such verapamil,

TABLE 14.5. Agents to Treat Changes in Heart Rate

	Dose	Route
Bradycardias		
Atropine	.5–1 mg	IV push
Isoproterenol	2–10 mcg/min	IV drip
Secondary drugs		
Epinephrine	.5–1 mg	IV push
Norepinephrine	1–20 mcg/min	IV drip
Atrial Tachycardias		
Verapamil (Isoptin, Calan)	2.5–5 mg	IV push
	240–480 mg/day q 6–8 hr	Oral
Propanolol (Inderal)	1–5 mg, 1 mg/min	IV push
	120–240 mg/day highly variable	Oral
Esmolol (Brevibloc)	500 mcg/kg/min loading dose	IV drip
	50–200 mcg/kg/min maintenance	
Digoxin (Lanoxin)	up to 1.5 mg total	IV push
	.25–.5 mg q 8 hr	
	.125–.25 mg daily	Oral
Adenosine	0.5–.2 mg/kg	IV push
Ventricular Tachycardias		
Lidocaine	1 mg/kg	IV push
	3 mg/kg total	
	20–55 mcg/kg/min	IV drip
	or 1–5 mg/min	
Mexiletine (Mexitil)	300–400 mg, 10 mg/min	IV push
	.4–.8 mg/min	IV drip
	3–4 mg/kg	Oral
	200–400 mg q 8 hr	
Tocainide (Tonocard)	.5–1 mg/kg/min over 15–30 min	IV push
	200–800 mg q 8–12 hr	Oral
Flecainide (Tambocor)	200–400 mg/24 hr in 2 divided doses	Oral
Aprinidine	200–1000 mg/day	Oral
Bretylium (Bretylol)	5 mg/kg	IV push
	1–2 mg/min	IV drip
Procainamide	25–50 mg/min up to 1000 mg total	IV push
	12–25 mg/kg	
	2–4 mg/min	IV drip
Amiodarone	5 mg/ kg	IV push
	10–15 mg/kg/day for 3–5 days	
	1000–2000 mg daily for 1 week	Oral
	600–800 mg daily for next 1–3 weeks	
	400–600 mg daily thereafter	
Encainide (Enkaid)	200 mg max daily dose	Oral
	25–50 mg q 4–6 hr	
	1–2 mg/kg over 15 min	IV push
Disopyramide (Norpace)	100 mg q 8 hr	Oral
	200–300 mg q 12 hr	
Quinidine	15 mg/kg over 24 hr	Oral
	200–600 mg q 6 hr	

then by a sodium-flow-altering agent, such as digitalis. If these three therapies fail, the administration of a beta-blocking agent may be tried.

A recently introduced agent for treatment of atrial tachycardias is adenosine (Adenocard). Adenosine has the advantage of being extremely short acting, acting within

10 seconds.[35] The role of adenosine in atrial tachycardia is still developing, although it may eventually be the first pharmacologic agent administered.

Treatments for atrial flutter and atrial tachycardia have increased emphases on the sodium-altering agents such as digitalis preparations. Beta-blocking agents can also be employed to try and reduce the rapid response rates of atrial tachycardia and atrial fibrillation. Synchronized defibrillation, or cardioversion, is another category of treatment of atrial dysrhythmias. Cardioversion is employed either when a dysrhythmia fails to respond to pharmacologic intervention or in an attempt to avoid pharmacologic intervention.[36] The American Heart Association has developed guidelines for the use of cardioversion.[37] These guidelines basically address the need for explanation and sedation before cardioversion and the use of energy levels to accomplish cardioversion.

The key point to remember in the treatment of any atrial dysrhythmia is that the emphasis must be on reducing the heart rate to levels that will maintain adequate cardiac output. The primary danger of a fast atrial rate is the decreased filling time present in the ventricles as the rate increases. The decreased filling time will produce a low stroke volume. The rate where this decrease in stroke volume occurs varies according to several factors, including the contractility status of the heart. Generally heart rates in excess of 150 bpm have the potential to markedly reduce diastolic filling time. Treatments of abnormal heart rates should be encouraged if any evidence of a decrease in cardiac output occurs, that is, measurement of cardiac output reveals a decrease or the patient has some degree of hypotension.

Ventricular Dysrhythmias

The ventricular dysrhythmias of primary interest are ventricular tachycardia and fibrillation. Premature ventricular contractions (PVCs) can lead to either of the two situations but are treated with some of the same agents used to treat ventricular tachycardia. From an oxygenation perspective, PVCs are potentially dangerous but generally are not likely to alter cardiac output to the point that oxygenation is markedly disrupted. In this section, only ventricular tachycardia and fibrillation will be addressed.

Ventricular tachycardia can present in one of four ways:

1. asymptomatic
2. mild symptoms such as palpitations, chest pain
3. major symptoms, such as hypotension
4. absence of a pulse

In the first situation, the treatment focuses on using pharmacologic interventions (Table 14.5). The major agents utilized in this situation are Lidocaine, Bretylium or Pronestyl. In this situation, oxygenation has not markedly been altered since perfusion is still adequate to maintain cerebral oxygenation.

If the second situation develops, synchronized defibrillation (cardioversion) is applied, beginning at outputs of about 50 joules and increasing to a maximum of 360. Oxygenation is beginning to be impaired at this stage, to the point of producing noticeable symptoms. The urgency in treatment has increased, so the change in pharmacologic intervention to electrical has developed.

If the third situation develops, the defibrillation is administered in an unsynchronized manner, usually again starting at 50 joules. The oxygenation disturbance in this scenario is severe, producing a change in blood flow to the point of hypotension. The situation is deteriorated to the point that the risks of unsynchronized defibrillation are less than the disturbance produced by the problems in oxygenation.

In the fourth situation, unsynchronized defibrillation is administered, starting at 200 joules. Essentially, no blood flow is occuring with the net result of imminent widespread cell death. Ventricular fibrillation is essentially treated the same way as ventricular tachycardia without a pulse.

The treatment of any abnormal heart rate is centered on restoring a normal cardiac output and stroke volume. The assessment of the effectiveness of any of these treatments must include a hemodynamic assessment, which will include measurements of the cardiac output and stroke volume or estimations of their effects. While this session has only superficially covered key concepts with regard to dysrhythmia intervention, the ground work is laid to understand how dysrhythmia control is important in regulating and maintaining oxygen transport through the cardiac output.

SUMMARY

Four primary methods are employed to increase cardiac output: (1) preload manipulation (preload reduction in left-ventricular failure patients or preload stimulation in the hypovolemia patient), (2) improvement of contractility, (3) reduction of systemic vascular resistance (afterload), and (4) maintenance of the heart rate. Agents for improving cardiac output can be used independently or in combination with each other. The most likely reason to increase cardiac output is to improve overall oxygenation. Therefore, an increase in cardiac output cannot be viewed as successful unless overall improvement of oxygenation occurs. Overall oxygenation improvement can be monitored by assessing both oxygen transport and consumption and by assessing other oxygenation parameters such as serum-lactate levels. One common mistake made in hemodynamic monitoring is to look at cardiac output independently of oxygenation assessment. This overlooks the primary reason for improving the cardiac output—to improve oxygenation. The clinician must be aware that hemodynamics and oxygenation are intricately related and cannot be separated.

REFERENCES

1. Sprung CV. *The Pulmonary Artery Catheter: Methodology and Clinical Application.* Baltimore: University Park Press, 1983, 117.
2. Daily EK, Schroeder JS. *Techniques in Bedside Monitoring.* St. Louis: CV Mosby, 1989, 96.
3. Altschule MD. "Invalidity of using so-called Starling curves in clinical medicine." *Persp Biol Med* 1983;26:171.
4. Charette AL. "Bridging the gap between hemodynamics and monitoring." *Crit Care Nurs Clin N Am* 1989;1:539.
5. Urban N. "Integrating hemodynamic parameters with clinical decision making." *Crit Care Nurse* 1986;6:48.
6. Daily EK. "Use of hemodynamics to differentiate pathophysiologic causes of cardiogenic shock." *Crit Care Nurs Clin N Am* 1989;1:589.
7. Ley SJ, Miller K, Skow P, Pessig P. "Crystalloid versus colloid fluid therapy after cardiac surgery." *Heart & Lung* 1990;19:31.
8. Rackow EC, Falk J, Fein IA, et al. "Fluid resuscitation in circulatory shock: A comparison of the cardiorespiratory effects of albumin, hetastarch, and saline solutions in patients with hypovolemic and septic shock." *Crit Care Med* 1983;9:839.
9. Meyers KA, Hickey MK. "Nursing management of hypovolemic shock." *Crit Care Nurs Q* 1988;11:57.
10. Ross AD, Angaran DM. "Colloids versus crystalloids—a continuing controversy." *Drug Intell Clin Phar* 1984;18:202.
11. Falk JL, Rackow EC, Weil MH. "Colloid and crystalloid resuscitation." *In* Shoemaker WC, Ayres S, Brenvik A, Holbrook PR, Thompson WL (eds). *Textbook of Critical Care.* Philadelphia: WB Saunders, 1989, 1060–61.
12. Falk JL, Rackow EC, Weil MH. "Colloid and crystalloid resuscitation." *In* Shoemaker WC, Ayres S, Brenvik A, Holbrook PR, Thompson WL (eds). *Textbook of Critical Care.* Philadelphia: WB Saunders, 1989, 1055.
13. Gallagher TS, Banner MJ, Barnes PA. "Large volume crystalloid resuscitation does not increase extravascular lung water." *Anesth Analg* 1985;64:324.
14. Petty TL. "Acute respiratory distress syndrome (ARDS)." *DM* 1990;36:1.
15. Levine SD. "Diuretics." *Med Clin N Am* 1989; 73:271.
16. Abrams J. "Nitrates." *Med Clin N Am* 1988;72:1.
17. Kelleher RM. "Cardiac drugs: New inotropes." *Crit Care Nurs Clin N AM* 1989;1:391.
18. Colucci WS, Wright RF, Braunwald E. "New positive inotropic agents in the treatment of congestive heart failure: Mechanism of action and recent clinical developments." *N Engl J Med* 1986; 314:290.
19. Lollgen H, Drexler H. "Use of inotropes in the critical care setting." *Crit Care Med* 1990;18:556.
20. LeJentel TH, Sonnenblock EH. "Should the failing heart be stimulated?" *N Engl J Med* 1984;310:1384.
21. Colucci WS, Leatherman GF, Ludmer PL, et al. "B-adrenergic inotrope responsiveness of patients

with heart failure: Studies with intracoronary dobutamine infusion." *Circ Res* 1987;61 (suppl 1): 182.

22. Saunders MR, Kostis JB, Frishman WH. "Inotropic agents in congestive heart failure." *Med Clin N Am* 1989;73:283.
23. Perret C. "Acute heart failure in myocardial infarction: Principles of treatment." *Crit Care Med* 1990;18:326.
24. Rotmensch HH, Vlasses PH, Ferguson RK. "Angiotension converting enzyme inhibitors." *Med Clin N Am* 1988;72:399.
25. Michelson EL, Dreifus LS. "Newer antiarrhythmic drugs." *Med Clin N Am* 1988;72:275.
26. Roberts WC (ed). *Cardiology 1989.* Boston: Butterworth, 1989, 235.
27. Vaughan Williams EM. "Classification of antiarrhythmic drugs." *In* Sandoe E, Flensted-Jensen E, Olesen E (eds). *Symposium on Cardiac Arrhythmias.* Sodertalje, Sweden: AB Astra, 1970, 449.
28. Gunnar RM, Bourdillon PD, Dixon DW, et al. "Guidelines for the early management of patients with acute myocardial infarction." *JACC* 1990;16:249.
29. Nelson WP. "Supraventricular dysrhythmias." *In*

Henning RJ, Grenvik A (eds). *Critical Care Cardiology.* New York: Churchill Livingstone, 1989, 58.
30. Schweitzer P, Mark H. "The effect of atropine on cardiac arrhythmias and conduction. Part 1." *Am Heart J* 1980;100:119.
31. Podrid PJ. "Antiarrhythmic drug therapy (part 1): Benefits and hazards." *Chest* 1985;88:452.
32. Anderson JL. "Esmolol for supraventricular tachyarrhythmias and other applications." *Practical Card.* 1987;13:5.
33. Sayers M, Humphries JO. "Tachyarrhythmias." *In* Shoemaker WC, Ayres S, Brenvik A, Holbrook PR, Thompson WL (eds). *Textbook of Critical Care.* Philadelphia: WB Saunders, 1989, 376.
34. Rinkenberger RL, Naccarelli GV. "Evaluation and treatment of narrow complex tachycardias." *Crit Care Clin* 1989;5:569.
35. Barratt C, Liker N, Griffith M, et al. "Comparison of adenosine and verapamil for termination of paroxysmal junctional tachycardia." *Am J Card* 1989;64:1310.
36. Vlay SC. "Acute and semiacute management of cardiac arrest." *Crit Care Clin* 1989;5:643.
37. American Heart Assn. "Electrical therapy in the malignant arrhythmias." *In Textbook of Advanced Cardiac Life Support,* 1987, 89.

15
Treatment of Oxygen Consumption and Cellular Oxygenation Disturbances

TREATMENT OF OXYGEN CONSUMPTION (V_{O_2})

The concept of treating oxygen consumption ranges from being relatively simplistic to complex. This range for treating disturbances in V_{O_2} is due to the still developing understanding of V_{O_2} treatment. Current oxygen-consumption treatment can be classified in two categories: (1) efforts to reduce oxygen consumption, and (2) efforts to increase oxygen consumption.

Reduction of Oxygen Consumption

Oxygen consumption may be treated in clinical situations in which an increased oxygen consumption is providing a threat to overall oxygenation. This is present primarily when an increased oxygen consumption cannot be met by an increase in oxygen transport. The primary assumption in this situation is that the cellular utilization and local blood flow of oxygen is intact, eliminating clinical conditions such as sepsis. Oxygen consumption increases cannot be offset and will be a problem when oxygen transport is limited, such as in patients who have limited cardiac outputs or low hemoglobin levels. Table 15.1 summarizes specific conditions under which oxygen transport is limited. When oxygen transport may be limited, avoiding increases in oxygen consumption may be beneficial.

Limitations of oxygen consumption have been demonstrated to improve arterial oxy-

TABLE 15.1. Conditions Limiting Oxygen Transport

Problem	Sample Conditions
Failure to increase cardiac output	Cardiomyopathy
	Myocardial infarction
	Congestive heart failure
Loss of hemoglobin	Anemia
	Hemorrhage
	GI bleed
	Trauma
	Postoperative bleeding
Loss of Pa_{O_2}/Sa_{O_2}	Increased intrapulmonary shunt
	ARDS

gen saturation.[1-2] The potential for reductions in V_{O_2} to improve cellular oxygenation has been demonstrated through $S\bar{v}_{O_2}$ monitoring in several studies.[3-5] The limitation of oxygen consumption is generally accomplished by determining whether the oxygen consumption is disproportionately elevated, such as with a fever, or needs to be reduced because of limited oxygen transport, such as in a person with acute respiratory failure. The methods to reduce oxygen consumption are summarized in Table 15.2.

The mechanisms for reducing oxygen consumption generally are focused on either reducing the causative agent, such as a temperature elevation, or reducing skeletal-muscle oxygen consumption. If the causative agent is an infection or inflammation, antipyretic or anti-inflammatory agents may be

TABLE 15.2.   Mechanisms to Reduce Oxygen Consumption

Category	Example
Skeletal muscle relaxants	Paralyzing agents
Antipyretics	Aspirin
Anti-inflammatory agents	Ibuprofen (Medipren)
Sedatives	Midazolam (Versed)
Removal of skeletal muscle work	Mechanical ventilation

TABLE 15.3.   Agents that Reduce Skeletal-Muscle Oxygen Demands (Paralyzing Agents)

Agent	Dose
Succinylcholine chloride (Anectine)	.3–1.1 mg/kg
Vecuronium bromide (Norcuron)	.08–.1 mg/kg initial dose
Pancuronium bromide (Pavulon)	.7–1 mcg/kg/min as a continuous drip

All agents are in the intravenous form.

used to reduce oxygen-consumption levels. Reduction in skeletal-muscle oxygen consumption is usually accomplished through sedation and paralysis or by mechanical methods (mechanical ventilation) of achieving muscle action. Any attempt to paralyze the patient must be accompanied by careful explanation to both the patient and family of what paralyzing agents will do. Simultaneous sedation is recommended. The clinician should always check to ensure that paralysis is accompanied by adequate sedation.

Reduction in Skeletal-Muscle Activity

The oxygen consumption of skeletal muscles can be a major factor in the amount of total oxygen utilized in the body. Reduction in the oxygen used by skeletal muscle can be focused in two directions: (1) remove all or most of skeletal-muscle activity or (2) support those muscles that are working excessively.

When attempting to remove most muscle activity, agents that act as a general muscle suppressant are administered. Examples of these agents are listed in Table 15.3. When muscle-relaxing agents are employed, the clinician is attempting to reduce overall oxygen consumption in order to improve the balance between oxygen transport and consumption. Success in achieving the improved balance should be measured both by decreases in V_{O_2} and improvement in oxygen balance measures such as $S\bar{v}_{O_2}$, lactate levels, and O_2 extraction rates.

One benefit of reducing skeletal muscle activity, particularly of the chest wall, is the potential to improve Sa_{O_2} and Pa_{O_2} values. When skeletal muscle activity of the chest wall is reduced, the potential exists for the lungs to expand more completely owing to the reduction in dynamic compliance.[6–7] Improved ventilation may rapidly occur to raise the Pa_{O_2} and Sa_{O_2}. In addition, the reduced skeletal-muscle oxygen consumption may allow for improving total oxygenation. The improvement in total oxygenation may be reflected in improved $S\bar{v}_{O_2}$ values. The improved $S\bar{v}_{O_2}$ levels can contribute to an increasing Pa_{O_2} and Sa_{O_2} level if a large intrapulmonary shunt is present (Chapter 3).

Another method to reduce skeletal activity of the chest wall involves the type of support mode utilized during mechanical ventilation. Of the three common types of modes used, AMV (assisted mandatory ventilation or assist/control), IMV (intermittent mandatory ventilation) or PSV (pressure support ventilation), AMV has the most support as a mode of reducing oxygen consumption during acute respiratory failure.[8–10]

AMV reduces V_{O_2} of the skeletal muscles through the removal of most of the inspiratory work associated with breathing. AMV does not, however, remove all of the inspiratory work. Some patient effort is required to open the demand valve in the ventilator in order to initiate the ventilator breath (Figure 15.1). PSV also reduces V_{O_2} of breathing by supporting the patient's inspiratory effort. PSV has not been employed as often,

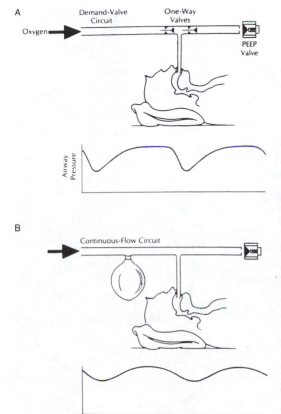

FIGURE 15.1. In assist/control mode of ventilation, work must be expended to overcome the resistance of the ventilator demand valve. Adapted from Tobin MJ. *Essentials of Critical Care Medicine.* New York: Churchill Livingstone, 1989.

though, as AMV in the setting of acute respiratory failure.

PSV has the potential to reduce V_{O_2} through an improved support of the initial inspiratory effort.[11] Once the inspiratory effort is initiated, PSV generates a supporting pressure throughout the inspiratory cycle. This support reduces the V_{O_2} of the skeletal muscle in the chest. At this point, however, PSV is not utilized in acute respiratory failure to the same extent as AMV. This may change if further studies indicate that PSV can maintain arterial oxygenation while reducing skeletal V_{O_2}. The key limitation to pressure-support ventilation is that it operates through pressure-limited ventilation. The high peak pressures seen in acute respiratory failure may cause variable tidal volume (V_T) with each PSV breath. The variability in V_T limits the use of PSV in acute respiratory distress.

When using mechanical ventilation as a support mode, the clinician should attempt to maintain alveolar ventilation at the lowest respiratory rate possible. The lower the respiratory rate, the lower the V_{O_2} of chest skeletal muscles. For example, if the patient has a respiratory rate of 40 bpm on an IMV of 10, and a V_T of 800 cc, the ventilator is not providing enough support for the skeletal muscles. Changing to AMV alone will usually help this patient by replacing the 30 spontaneous breaths (total patient rate of 40 minus the IMV of 10 equals 30) with 800 cc ventilator-delivered breaths. The ventilator breaths, due to their volume usually being greater than spontaneous tidal volumes, will reduce the number of breaths necessary to maintain alveolar ventilation.

The change to AMV in this tachypneic patient may be all that is necessary to improve oxygenation. If oxygenation does not improve with the ventilator change, the use of sedation and paralyzing agents may be necessary.

When assessing the tachypneic patient receiving mechanical ventilation, the clinician must be aware of the potential for pressure trapping in the lungs, a concept referred to as auto-PEEP.[12] Air trapping occurs due to incomplete expiration at the time of the next inspiration. If pressure trapping in the lungs occurs, cardiac output may decrease. If the cardiac output is reduced, a decrease in oxygen transport is likely. Auto-PEEP can be detected by obstructing the expiratory port immediately after an inspiration is given (Figure 15.2). If auto-PEEP is present, the airway pressure will not return to baseline (either 0 or the PEEP level). In cases where auto-PEEP is present, the inspiratory time should be reduced or peak flow rate increased. Auto-PEEP may also benefit from sedation or paralysis in an attempt to overcome the voluntary work of the patient's respiratory muscles.

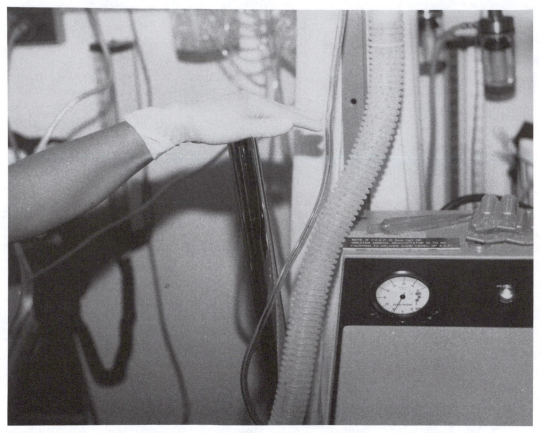

FIGURE 15.2.   Measurement of auto-PEEP by obstructing the expiratory circuit past the demand valve immediately before a mechanical ventilator breath is delivered.

Example 1

A 32-year-old woman is admitted to the ICU with the diagnosis of sepsis secondary to treatment of leukemia. She presently has the following clinical information available. She is restless and agitated. She has attempted to extubate herself several times and is now in soft restraints. She is frequently setting off the high pressure alarm on the ventilator due to her agitation. Her family requests your help in making her more comfortable.

Blood pressure	86/56	Pa_{O_2}	68
Pulse	126	Pa_{CO_2}	36
CO	9.8	pH	7.26
CI	5.8	HCO_3	18
PA	48/28	Lactate	3.0
PCWP	12	F_{IO_2}	.80
CVP	14	PEEP	+10

Mode of ventilation	AMV
Rate of AMV	12
Total rate	28
V_T	800

Based on the above information, what methods can be used to attempt to improve oxygen utilization and patient comfort?

ANSWER

This is a difficult situation to manage, although reducing V_{O_2} and improving patient comfort may be achieved through the same therapy. Sedation and, possibly, paralysis may be useful therapies. The sedation may make her more comfortable and also address a potential cause of agitation, that is, an oxygenation imbalance as reflected by the increased lactate level. In addition, therapies that may increase the cardiac output and oxygen transport may be employed. Agents such as fluid challenges or inotropes may be helpful. Assess the effectiveness of these therapies through systemic assessments, such as lactate levels.

Ideally, a more curative approach could be taken to correct the cause of the patient's sepsis. Unitl the cause of the sepsis is better understood, however, treatment will be more supportive than curative.

Example 2

A 68-year-old man is admitted to the ICU with the diagnosis of cardiogenic shock. He is restless and confused. He has the following set of data available. Based on this information, what measures can be used to reduce his V_{O_2}?

Blood pressure	80/50	Pa_{O_2}	66
Pulse	122	Pa_{CO_2}	36
Respiratory rate	38	pH	7.25
IMV	12	Lactate	2.8
V_T	800	CO	3.1
$F_{I_{O_2}}$	.80	CI	1.6
PA	42/28		
PCWP	26		
CVP	13		

ANSWER

One method of reducing oxygen consumption in this patient is to attempt to reduce the work of breathing. The respiratory rate of 38 bpm is likely too high given the limited cardiac output. The work of breathing can be reduced by changing from IMV to AMV (assist/control). The assist/control mode will remove some of the inspiratory work by replacing the patient's tidal volume with larger ventilator volumes. The increased tidal volumes should reduce the respiratory rate and V_{O_2}.

The low blood pressure makes sedation risky in this case. In addition, improving the oxygen flow to the brain by supporting the CO and CI is more likely to relieve the restlessness and confusion than is sedation.

Example 3

A 61-year-old woman returns from coronary-artery bypass grafting surgery. As she is warmed to normal body temperature, you note that she begins to shiver. As the shivering increases, her $S\bar{v}_{O_2}$ value begins to decrease.

	Time		
	1400 (Returning from Surgery)	1515 (Shivering Starting)	1530 (Shivering Worsening)
Sa_{O_2}	.99	.98	.97
$S\bar{v}_{O_2}$	.65	.60	.45
Blood pressure	108/78	118/82	116/80
Pulse	102	110	112
PA	28/13	26/14	28/14
PCWP	11	14	13
CVP	8	7	9
CO	3.8	4.1	4.1
CI	2.4	2.5	2.5

What treatment can be administered to improve the oxygenation?

ANSWER

Based on the $S\bar{v}_{O_2}$, the oxygenation is worsening, probably secondary to an increase in V_{O_2}. The increase in V_{O_2} can be treated with sedatives or paralyzatives. The $S\bar{v}_{O_2}$ can be trended to note the effect of the agents in reducing skeletal-muscle activity. Note the lack of compensation by cardiac output. The failure of the CO to increase in the face of an increasing V_{O_2} results in a worsening oxygenation.

Increase in Oxygen Consumption

Theoretically, the concept of increasing oxygen consumption is employed in situations where oxygen transport is dependent on oxygen consumption (see Chapter 9). Again theoretically, as oxygen consumption becomes dependent on oxygen transport, cellular hypoxia may be present. Some authors have suggested that one way to improve cellular oxygenation is to increase both oxygen transport and oxygen consumption.[13] Increasing both oxygen transport and consumption potentially reflects an improved cellular processing of oxygen. As cellular V_{O_2} increases, the metabolic capability of the cell returns to more normal levels.

While this approach to increasing V_{O_2} is somewhat controversial, the mechanisms for increasing oxygen consumption are also controversial. How to elevate the oxygen consumption is not clear. Currently, the only manner to increase V_{O_2} is to improve cellular blood flow, generally through fluid administration or inotrope therapy. Increased oxygen consumption as a treatment modality remains in the experimental field and as yet is not a practical clinical application.

IMPROVEMENT OF CELLULAR UTILIZATION OF OXYGEN

Support of the cardiac output or oxygen consumption is usually only a supportive rather than a primary therapy. Improvement in the cellular utilization of oxygen is perhaps one of the most important aspects of maintaining oxygenation. Unfortunately, at this point in time, the clinical capability to actually improve cellular utilization of oxygen is very limited. Due to the difficulty in improving cellular utilization of oxygen, treatment modalities are limited. Much of the proposed methods of improving cellular utilization of oxygen are still in the experimental phase. However, some of the potential mechanisms by which cellular oxygenation can be improved will be presented in this section. These mechanisms can be categorized in two areas: antibiotics and eicosanoids therapy.

Antibiotics

In the patient who has a septic pattern in which cellular dysoxia exists, the primary treatment is to find and address the cause of the sepsis. For example, if a person has an infection, antibiotics of the appropriate sensitivity are the goal. Common categories of antibiotics are presented in Table 15.4. Identifying the causative agent through blood or tissue cultures is a key step in initiating treatment of sepsis. Unfortunately, the use of antibiotics with cellular dysoxia, such as in sepsis, may not improve oxygenation. Unless the antibiotics are able to stop an infection from becoming a systemic response, simple killing of the originating antigen may not be adequate.[14]

If the antigen initiates a host reaction, potentially through substances such as endotoxin or antitumor-necrosing factor release, the imbalance at the cellular level now goes beyond the antigen reaction. A host-induced inflammatory response with potential injury to normal cells now exists. In order to treat host-induced inflammatory responses, the clinician must turn to more cell-oriented treatment. Treatment of inflammatory responses in response to antigenic stimulation is still in the experimental phase.

Cellular-Altering Agents

Since sepsis and conditions altering cellular oxygenation have been associated with increased release of arachidonic acid sub-

TABLE 15.4. Common Antibiotics Dosage and Classification

	Common Dosages (IV)
Penicillins	
Aqueous penicillin G	1–2 million U q 2–6 hr
Ampicillin	1–3 gm q 4–6 hr
Nafcillin	1–3 gm q 4–6 hr
Antipseudomonal Penicillins	
Carbenicillin	3–4 gm q 4 hr
Ticarcillin	3–6 gm q 4 hr
Mexlocillin	3–5 gm q 4–8 hr
Azlocillin	3 gm q 4 hr
Piperacillin	3 gm q 4 hr
Cephalosporins (Beta Lactams)	
First Generation	
Cefazolin—Ancef	.5–1 gm q 6–8 hr
Cephalothin—Keflin	.5–2 gm q 4–6 hr
Cephapirin—Cefadyl	.5–2 gm q 4–6 hr
Cephradine—Anspor, Velosef	.5–2 gm q 4–6 hr
Second Generation	
Cefamandole— Mandol	1–2 gm q 4–8 hr
Cefoxitin—Mefoxin	1–2 gm q 4–8 hr
Third Generation	
Cefotaxime—Claforan	1–2 gm q 6–12 hr
Ceftazidime—Fortaz	1–2 gm q 8–12 hr
Ceftriaxone— Rocephin	1–2 gm q 12 hr
Moxalactam—Moxam	1–2 gm q 6–12 hr
Aminoglycosides	
Streptomycin	.5–2 gm/day (IM)
Gentamicin	2 mg/kg
Tobramycin	2 mg/kg
Amikacin	7.5 mg/kg
Kanamycin	15 mg/kg/day
Other Categories	
Clindmycin	300–900 mg q 6–8 hr
Metronidazole	500–750 mg q 6–12 hr
Vancomycin	17.5 mg/kg, then 20– 30 mg/kg day
Erythromycin	.5–1 gm q 6–8 hr
Imipenem/Cilastatin	.25–1 gm q 6–8 hr

stances, such as thromboxane A_2 (TxA_2) and leukotrienes, therapies that inhibit cyclooxygenase (which generates TxA_2) have been suggested as possibly improving cellular oxygenation. Eicosanoid inhibitors, such as indomethacin or ibuprofen, have been suggested as potential treatment choices because of their abilities to block TxA_2 and leukotriene synthesis.[15] By blocking the TxA_2 and leukotriene synthesis (and their subsequent effects, such as alteration in capillary permeability, increased capillary clotting, and other inflammatory responses), eicosanoids may act to improve overall cellular oxygenation. Again, studies of eicosanoids have not demonstrated consistent clinical improvements.[16-19] The use of anti-inflammatory agents, such as steroids and aspirin, has been proposed, but we do not yet have consistent clinical research results to indicate that it is an improvement over current therapies.[20-22] The possibility of endogenous opiate release as a causative mechanism in the septic response has triggered investigation into opiate antagonists such as naloxone. This pathway, however, also has not been as promising as anticipated.[23-25]

One of the most exciting and controversial developments in the treatment of cellular oxygenation disturbances is monoclonal antibody application. While many monoclonal antibodies are being developed, only a few are likely to be released for clinical application in the near future. Two monoclonal antibodies likely to receive clinical approval are HA-1A and E5. Both are to be used in the treatment of gram negative sepsis. The advantage of the monoclonal antibody is the ability to specifically attack the cause of the septic process. Through this action, the septic cascade could more rapidly be halted.[26] The use of monoclonal antibodies offer one of the most promising therapies in the treatment of sepsis since the development of antibiotics.

A primary disadvantage of the monoclonal antibodies is the cost. The cost of these agents, approximately $4,000 per dose, has great potential to increase health care costs. Guidelines for using monoclonal antibodies are still being developed and will need to be sensitive to both the great potential for reducing the effects of sepsis and the cost of the drug.

Improving local blood flow has been suggested as possibly improving overall cellular disturbances in oxygenation. Much of the improvement in regional blood flow, however, is partially addressed in treatments that will increase cardiac output. Administering fluid boluses and inotropic agents, such as dobutamine, may help increase local blood flow. The administration of dobutamine and fluids may take place even in the presence of elevated cardiac outputs. While other agents may improve regional perfusion, none has reached the point of consistently demonstrating an improvement in overall oxygenation.

The concept of improving specific organ function, such as commonly used when treating a patient with an MI and attempting to improve myocardial oxygen supply, may eventually lie at the center of treatment in some forms of sepsis. If the organ that is primarily affected can be identified and treated specifically, the likelihood of improvement in oxygenation is enhanced. At this point in time, our clinical knowledge does not allow us to make such specific interventions.

One potentially useful model is the removal of endotoxins (and potentially other inflammatory substances) through the administration of agents that adsorb the inflammatory agent. Such a therapy would take place through plasmaphoresis. A chemical with known adsorptive properties for the inflammatory agent in question could be employed as a "filter." This filter could reduce the inflammatory response and mediate the response to conditions such as sepsis.

Unfortunately, no successful method to improve cellular-oxygen utilization currently exists, although a large amount of research in the area is occurring. The current therapy in patients with conditions such as sepsis remains supportive rather than curative.

REFERENCES

1. Field S, Kelly SM, Macklem PT. "The oxygen cost of breathing in patients with cardiorespiratory disease." *Am Rev Resp Dis* 1982;126:9.
2. Coggeshall JW, Marini JJ, Newman JH. "Improved oxygenation after muscle relaxation in adult respiratory distress syndrome." *Arch Intern Med* 1985; 145:1718.
3. Chiara O, Giomarelli PP, Biagioli B, et al. "Hyper-

metabolic response after hypothermic cardio-pulmonary bypass." *Crit Care Med* 1987;15:995.

4. Ralley FE, Wynands JE, Ramsay JG, et al. "The effects of shivering on oxygen consumption and carbon dioxide production in patients rewarming from hypothermic cardiopulmonary bypass." *Can J Anesth* 1988;35:332.

5. Zwischenberger JB, Kirsh MM, Dechert RE, et al. "Suppression of shivering decreases oxygen consumption and improves hemodynamic stability during postoperative rewarming." *Ann Thor Surg* 1987;43:428.

6. Westbrook PR, Stubbs JE, Sessler AD, et al. "Effects of anesthesia and muscle paralysis on respiratory mechanics in normal man." *J Appl Physiol* 1974;31:81.

7. Marini JJ. "Strategies to minimize breathing effort during mechanical ventilation." *Crit Care Clin* 1990;6:635.

8. Bolin RW, Pierson DJ. "Ventilatory management in acute lung injury." *Crit Care Clin* 1986;2:S85.

9. Scanlan CL. "Respiratory failure and the need for ventilatory support." *In* Scanlan CL, Spearman CB, Sheldon RL. *Egan Fundamentals of Respiratory Care.* 5th ed. 1990; 694.

10. Grum CM, Chauncey JB. "Conventional ventilation." *Clin Chest Med* 1988;9:37.

11. Saito S, Tokioka H, Kosaka F. "Efficacy of flow by during continuous positive airway pressure ventilation." *Crit Care Med* 1990;18:54.

12. Pepe PE, Marini JJ. "Occult positive end expiratory pressure in mechanically ventilated patients with airflow obstruction." *Am Rev Respir Dis* 1982; 126:166.

13. Kaufman BS, Rackow EC, Falk JL. "The relationship between oxygen delivery and consumption during fluid resuscitation of hypovolemic and septic shock." *Chest* 1984;85:336.

14. Neu HG. "General concepts on the chemotherapy of infectious diseases." *Med Clin N Am* 1987;71:1051.

15. Waxman K. "Pentoxifylline in septic shock." *Crit Care Med* 1990;18:243.

16. Petrak RA, Balk RA, Bone RC. "Prostaglandins, cyclooxygenase inhibitors, and thromboxane synthetase inhibitors in the pathogenesis of multiple systems organ failure." *Crit Care Clin* 1989;5:303.

17. Stroud M, Swindell B, Bernard GR. "Cellular and humoral mediators of sepsis syndrome." *Crit Care Nurs Clin N Am* 1990;2:151.

18. Lefer AM. "Eicosanoids as mediators of ischemia and shock." *Fed Proc* 1985;44:275.

19. Higgins TL, Chernow B. "Pharmacotherapy of circulatory shock." *DM* 1987;33:319.

20. Nicholson DP. "Review of corticosteroid treatment in sepsis and septic shock: Pro or con." *Crit Care Clin* 1989;51:23.

21. Sprung CL, Caralis PV, Marcial EH, et al. "The effects of high dose corticosteroids in patients with septic shock: A prospective controlled study." *N Engl J Med* 1984;311:1137.

22. Bone RC, Fisher CJ Jr, Clemmer TP, et al. "A controlled clinical trial of high-dose methylprednisolone in the treatment of severe sepsis and septic shock." *N Engl J Med* 1987;317:653.

23. Zimmerman JJ. "Therapy for overwhelming sepsis—clues for treating disease and not just the symptoms." *Crit Care Med* 1990;18:118.

24. Hackshaw KV, Panker GA, Robers JW. "Naloxone in septic shock." *Crit Care Med* 1990;18:47.

25. Gurll NJ. "Naloxine in endotoxic shock: Experimental models and clinical perspective." *In* Reichard S, Wolfe R (eds). *Advances in Shock Research.* New York: Alan R Liss, 1982, 63.

26. Bone RC. "A critical evaluation of new agents for the treatment of sepsis." *JAMA* 1991;266:1686.

16
Clinical Reviews

In this chapter, clinical review situations summarizing some of the key features of the text are provided for your interpretation. The clinical scenarios presented are taken from each chapter, with the scenario referenced to the chapter in case you wish to review the answer. This chapter is designed to help you synthesize the important clinical material presented in the text. Good luck in interpreting the following scenarios. The answers to all examples may be found at the end of the chapter.

	51	72
PaO_2	51	72
SpO_2	.85	.94
F_{IO_2}	.70	.70

0900 is the initial set of information. 1000 is after the addition of 8 cm of PEEP. Based on the information given, has the PEEP accomplished its primary purpose (namely, to improve oxygen transport)?

(Chapters 11 and 12)

Example 1

A patient of yours has just been changed from a high-flow face mask at a F_{IO_2} of 40% to nasal cannula at 5 liters per minute. The patient is breathing shallowly. What would you estimate his F_{IO_2} to be on the 5 l/min flow rate?

(Chapter 12)

Example 3

A 64-year-old woman is in the ICU with the diagnosis of exacerbation of COPD, primarily chronic bronchitis. She has been in the unit for one day and has been placed on postural drainage and triple antibiotics. Physically, she has peripheral and circumoral cyanosis, with a BP of 134/88, P 106, RR 28, temperature 38°C. You place a finger oximeter on her and note that she has a SpO_2 value of .91. Based on the above information, what is her oxygenation status?

(Chapter 11)

Example 2

A 62-year-old woman with the diagnosis of acute respiratory failure has the following information available.

	Time	
	0900	1000
BP	110/72	100/66
P	90	103
Hgb	11 gm/dl	11 gm/dl

Example 4

Assume you are the charge nurse in the ICU for the shift. A new nurse assigned with you asks why the oxygenation status of the patient in bed 2 is so bad and bed 1 is so good. What would you explain to this nurse based on the information she has given you?

	Bed 1	Bed 2
PaO_2	130	67
Hgb	12	15

175

	Bed 1	Bed 2
Sa_{O_2}	99%	90%
$F_{I_{O_2}}$	60%	30%
Ca_{O_2}	15.91	18.09
$Pa_{O_2}/F_{I_{O_2}}$ ratio	217	223

(Chapters 3 & 4)

Example 5

Three new admissions have taken place in the last eight hours. Based on the information below, which of the three has the worst oxygen transport?

	Post Code	Angina	Emphysema
Pa_{O_2}	76	112	56
Hgb	13	12	13
Sa_{O_2}	93%	98%	88%
CO	4	3	5
Ca_{O_2}	16.2	15.76	15.32

(Chapters 6 & 7)

Example 6

A 42-year-old, 70-kg man was admitted to the ICU yesterday following a fall from his two-story house while painting. He suffered blunt trauma to his left chest with fractures of ribs 4–6. He also sustained a head injury, resulting in loss of consciousness and disorientation. The disorientation continues to this point. He has had unstable vital signs, resulting in the placement of a pulmonary-artery catheter. Below are his most recent sets of clinical data and current treatments. At what point is his oxygenation status optimal?

	Time		
	1800	2000	2200
Pa_{O_2}	58	190	79
Hgb	12	11	14
Sa_{O_2}	88%	100%	94%
$F_{I_{O_2}}$	30%	100%	50%
CO	5	4	4
V_{O_2}	220	250	275
$S\bar{v}_{O_2}$	68%	56%	59%
$Pa_{O_2}/F_{I_{O_2}}$	193	190	158
Ca_{O_2}	14.15	14.74	17.63
D_{O_2}	708	590	705
O_2 extraction	31%	42%	39%
Consumable O_2	566	472	564

(Chapters 3 & 7)

Example 7

A 73-year-old man was admitted to the ICU two days earlier with the diagnosis of acute inferior myocardial infarction. At 0130, he begins to complain of shortness of breath. Breath sounds reveal an increase in posterior crackles. The house officer recommends that the $F_{I_{O_2}}$ be increased from 30% to 60%.

Upon noting the improved Pa_{O_2} at 1430, the physician elects not to recommend any further treatments. The patient is now dozing in a semi-sitting position, supported by pillows. Crackles in the lungs are unchanged. Do you agree with the position of no further treatments?

	Time	
	0130	0230
Pa_{O_2}	76	112
Sp_{O_2}	.95	.99
Hgb	13	13
Sa_{O_2}	93%	98%
$F_{I_{O_2}}$	.30	.60
$S\bar{v}_{O_2}$	64%	51%
$Pa_{O_2}/F_{I_{O_2}}$ ratio	253	187

(Chapters 2, 3, & 10)

Example 8

A 49-year-old woman is admitted to the ICU from the emergency room with chest pain unrelieved by rest or nitroglycerine. She states she was at her office when the chest pain started, unrelated to activity. An oximetry pulmonary-artery catheter is inserted to help direct therapy. At 1100, the chest pain markedly diminished, following the administration of 6 mg of morphine sulfate. In an attempt to increase the cardiac index, nitroprusside is added at 1200. Based on the following information, has the addition of the nitroprusside improved the oxygenation status?

	Time	
	1100	1230 (After Nipride Added)
BP	112/76	108/76
P	110	100
CI	2.4	2.3
PA	38/23	39/22
PCWP	19	21
CVP	12	13
Sp_{O_2}	.95	.95
$S\bar{v}_{O_2}$	.59	.64

(Chapters 10 & 14)

Example 9

A 56-year-old, 82-kg man is in the ICU following abdominal aortic aneurysm repair. You note that his respiratory rate is rapid (32 bpm) and tidal volume appears normal. The increased minute ventilation from the respiratory rate can be due to either an increased oxygen consumption or an increased dead space. Based on the information presented below, what is the most likely cause of the increased minute ventilation and respiratory rate?

Ve	15 l/min
CO	7 l/min
$S\bar{v}_{O_2}$	.66
Sa_{O_2}	.94
Hgb	12

(Chapters 8 & 11)

Example 10

A 34-year-old woman is in the ICU following a motor-vehicle accident. She sustained a fractured left humerus and blunt abdominal trauma, and required a splenectomy and three units of whole blood. She returns from the OR at 0200. At 0300, her finger oximeter decreases to 92% from 98%. The following data exist to compare the situation at 0100 and 0200. Based on the given data, the physician elects to increase the F_{IO_2}. How effective will the increase in F_{IO_2} be for this patient?

	Time	
	0100	0200
Pa_{O_2}	90	69
Pa_{CO_2}	37	39
pH	7.40	7.35
$S\bar{v}_{O_2}$	.64	.46
Pv_{O_2}	37	25
Sa_{O_2}	.96	.92
F_{IO_2}	.50	.50
Hgb	10.7	11.1
CO	5.1 l/min	4.4 l/min

(Chapter 3)

Example 11

An 81-year-old man was admitted to the ICU with the diagnosis of congestive heart failure. He has a pulse oximeter on his index finger to assess hemoglobin-saturation levels. The nurse on the shift noted that the Pa_{O_2} was 68 while the pulse oximeter value read 96%. Since the Sp_{O_2} value

appeared elevated for this Pa_{O_2}, he sent a blood sample to the lab for comparison. The following information was returned:

Sp_{O_2} at the time of the sample	96%
Sa_{O_2} from the lab	91%
Carboxyhemoglobin	2%
Methemoglobin	2%

Based on this difference between the Sp_{O_2} and the Sa_{O_2}, the nurse requests that the pulse oximeter not be used on this patient. Is this a valid request?

(Chapters 5–10)

Example 12

A 61-year-old woman is admitted to the ICU with the diagnosis of pneumonia. She is placed on mechanical ventilation with the following settings:

Mode	CMV
Vt	750 cc
RR	12
F_{IO_2}	50%

On the above settings, the following physical signs and blood gases are present:

Time 2000	
BP	110/72
P	90
Pa_{O_2}	51
F_{IO_2}	.70

Based on the 2000 set of information, 8 cm H_2O of PEEP is added. The following information is available two hours after the addition of 8 cm of PEEP.

BP	92/58
P	112
Pa_{O_2}	72
F_{IO_2}	.70

Based on the information given, has the PEEP improved oxygen transport?

(Chapters 7 & 12)

Example 13

A 67-year-old, 75-kg man is in the ICU with surgery for a colon resection. He developed respiratory distress postoperatively and required continued intubation and mechanical ventilation. On the second post-op day, a tentative diagnosis of adult respiratory distress syndrome is made. Currently his ventilator settings are

Vt	750 cc
Mode	IMV
RR	12
Total RR	30
F_{IO_2}	.80
PEEP	12 cm H_2O

A physical examination reveals slight cyanosis of the eyelids, diffuse crackles in both lungs, and 20-lb weight gain over the past two days. Blood gases and hemodynamic data reveal the following:

Pa_{O_2}	51 mm Hg
Pa_{CO_2}	34 mm Hg
pH	7.33
Sp_{O_2}	90%
$S\bar{v}_{O_2}$	64%
Hgb	10.4
Lactate	1.9 mmol
BP	86/56
P	112
CO	4.0
CI	2.0
PA	48/26
PCWP	11
CVP	4

Based on the above information, is this person's oxygenation status at a clinically dangerous level?

(Chapters 7 & 11)

Blood gases are

Pa_{O_2}	64 mm Hg
Pa_{CO_2}	35 mm Hg
pH	7.34
Sp_{O_2}	95%
$S\bar{v}_{O_2}$	71%

Hemodynamic values are

CO	8 l/min
CI	5.2 l/min
PA	28/14 mm Hg
PCWP	12 mm Hg
CVP	4 mm Hg
Hgb	11.2 gm/dl

Lactate levels are 5.4 mmol/l.

Based on this information, the intrapulmonary shunt is markedly elevated. Is the large intrapulmonary shunt more dangerous than the oxygenation status?

(Chapters 3, 9 & 10)

Example 14

A 71-year-old woman is admitted to the unit with the diagnosis of sepsis following pancreatic surgery. She presently is unresponsive except to painful stimuli. She is on mechanical ventilation with the following settings:

Vt	800 cc
RR	12
Mode	assist/control
F_{IO_2}	80%

Vital signs are

BP	88/62
P	118
RR	28
Temp	39

Example 15

A 73-year-old man was admitted to the ICU in cardiogenic shock. He was placed on mechanical ventilation with the following settings:

Time	1900
Mode	IMV
RR	10 bpm
Vt	800 cc
F_{IO_2}	.80
Total RR	36 bpm

He had the following set of clinical and laboratory data available at that time:

BP	78/50
P	128
CO	3.0
CI	1.6
PA	38/24
PCWP	22
CVP	18
$S\bar{v}_{O_2}$	.46
Hgb	13.4
Pa_{O_2}	58
Sa_{O_2}	.89
Pa_{CO_2}	28
pH	7.27

In order to try to improve overall oxygenation and reduce oxygen consumption, he is switched to assist/control ventilation with the same settings.

Following the change, the following information is available:

Time	2000
Mode	CMV
RR	10 bpm
Vt	800 cc
F_{IO_2}	.80
Total RR	24 bpm

BP	86/52
P	124
CO	3.2
CI	1.7
PA	40/25
PCWP	24
CVP	16
$S\bar{v}_{O_2}$	.52
Hgb	13.4
Pa_{O_2}	59
Sa_{O_2}	.90
Pa_{CO_2}	26
pH	7.29

Based on this information, has the oxygen consumption fallen since the change to assist/control ventilation?

(Chapters 8 & 15)

Example 16

A 56-year-old woman is in the ICU with the diagnosis of GI bleeding. Her husband found her at home lying on the floor in a pool of blood. She was unresponsive upon arrival to the hospital. She was intubated in the emergency room and is presently on a ventilator with the following settings:

Mode	IMV
RR	12 bpm
Vt	850 cc
F_{IO_2}	.50
Total RR	18

Upon arrival to the ICU, she was hypotensive. No active bleeding was noted at that time. Vital signs and intial laboratory data revealed:

BP	88/54
P	115
Pa_{O_2}	168
Sa_{O_2}	.99
Sp_{CO_2}	1.00
Hgb	8.4 gm/dl

An oximetry pulmonary-artery catheter was placed, revealing the following information:

CO	4.3
CI	2.6
PA	23/10
PCWP	6
CVP	2
$S\bar{v}_{O_2}$	.58

During your shift, you note the presence of blood developing in the nasogastric tube. You repeat a set of vital signs and hemodynamic data and Find the following:

BP	90/60
P	117
Pa_{O_2}	160
Sa_{O_2}	.99
Sp_{CO_2}	1.00
CO	4.7
CI	2.8
PA	24/12
PCWP	8
CVP	2
$S\bar{v}_{O_2}$	.54

In your discussion of the situation with the house officer, it is thought that no problem exists at this time due to the unchanged Sp_{O_2} and Sa_{O_2} with an increase in cardiac output. What is your assesment of the oxygenation status of this patient?

(Chapters 4 & 10)

Example 17

A 62-year-old man is admitted to the ICU with the diagnosis of rule-out myocardial infarction. He presently has mild shortness of breath upon lying flat. He has a oximetric pulmonary-artery catheter in place and at 1600 he has the following information:

Pa_{O_2}	81
Sa_{O_2}	.94
Hgb	13
$S\bar{v}_{O_2}$	.55

BP	94/56 mm Hg
P	110 bpm
CO	4.23 l/min
CI	2.22 $l/min/m^2$
PA	32/21 mm Hg
PCWP	19 mm Hg
CVP	12 mm Hg

Dobutamine is started at 3 mcg/kg/min, based on the above information. Repeat readings at 1800 reveal

BP	100/62 mm Hg
P	106 bpm

CO	4.61 l/min
CI	2.40 l/min/m²
PA	34/22 mm Hg
PCWP	21 mm Hg
CVP	14 mm Hg
$S\bar{v}_{O_2}$	.64
Pa_{O_2}	.79 mm Hg
Sa_{O_2}	.94
Hgb	13 gm/dl
V_{O_2} (measured with exhaled gases)	205 cc/min

Based on the above information, answer the following questions:

1. Is the dobutamine therapy working?
2. When performing thermodilution measurements, you note that the cardiac-output values are fluctuating between 3.2 and 6 l/min. How can you determine the cardiac output with the above data?

(Chapters 8 & 14)

ANSWER (Example 1)

A rule of thumb for estimating F_{IO_2} on nasal cannula is that for every liter the flow rate increases, the F_{IO_2} increases 3–4%. In this case, a 5-l/min flow rate would increase the F_{IO_2} by:

$$3 \times 5 = 15\%$$

or

$$4 \times 5 = 20\%$$

Considering room air is 21% oxygen, the new F_{IO_2} can be estimated. The new F_{IO_2} is between 36% and 41% (15% + 21% = 36%, or 20% + 21% = 41%).

In this patient, however, the respiratory pattern is shallow. One disadvantage of low-flow systems is the influence of the breathing pattern on the F_{IO_2}. Since the patient is breathing shallowly, the F_{IO_2} will be higher than anticipated. The exact F_{IO_2} will not be known, although the F_{IO_2} is likely higher than the 41% expected.

ANSWER (Example 2)

The PEEP has accomplished one purpose, the elevation of the Pa_{O_2} and Sp_{O_2}. However, it is unclear whether overall oxygen transport has increased. Without a measurement of cardiac output, the oxygen transport is unknown. However, the physical assessment reveals a lower systolic blood pressure and an increased heart rate, both possible signs of a decreased stroke volume. A lower stroke volume may be an indication of a decreased cardiac output. If the cardiac output is reduced, oxygen transport may be reduced rather than enhanced by the im-proved Pa_{O_2}/Sp_{O_2} levels. The clinician is wise to re-assess oxygen transport parameters at a lower level of PEEP.

ANSWER (Example 3)

The presence of cyanosis and the Sp_{O_2} value of .91 indicate probable hypoxemia. The normal blood pressure and slight tachycardia may reflect a normal cardiac output. Not enough information is available to make a complete oxygenation assessment; however, a normal cardiac output would protect against most forms of decreased oxygen content. The patient is unlikely to be at risk for decreased oxygen transport and she is probably safe. The tachycardia may reflect a response to the temperature. A guideline for heart-rate changes secondary to temperature elevations is for each one degree increase in temperature, the heart rate increases by 15 bpm. Reducing the temperature to normal may decrease this patient's heart rate to near 90 bpm.

ANSWER (Example 4)

The explanation can be provided in many ways, with one of the first being that not enough information is present to assess oxygenation. A second response is to make sure that oxygenation is understood. Oxygenation refers to the cellular supply of oxygen. In this case, from the information provided and calculating the arterial oxygen content (Ca_{O_2}), the person in bed 2 has more oxygen in his/her blood than does the person in bed 1. In addition, based on the Pa_{O_2}/F_{IO_2} ratio, they have similar degrees of intrapulmonary shunting. While they both have below normal Pa_{O_2}/F_{IO_2} ratios, indicating larger-than-normal intrapulmonary shunts, they are not markedly different in the degree of lung dysfunction.

From the available data, the person in bed 2 does not have worse "oxygenation." A review with the new nurse of the importance of hemoglobin in oxygen transport would be helpful. Another point which may be helpful is to review the limited role of the Pa_{O_2} in oxygen transport and its value in estimating the intrapulmonary shunt with estimates such as the Pa_{O_2}/F_{IO_2} ratio.

ANSWER (Example 5)

From the information presented, the patient with the worst oxygen transport is the patient with angina. When assessing oxygen transport, the most important factors to consider are the cardiac output and hemoglobin values. While Sa_{O_2} and Pa_{O_2} values have roles in oxygen transport, their roles are relatively small in comparison to hemoglobin and cardiac output. Both the post code (648 cc) and emphysematous patients (766 cc) have relatively normal oxygen-transport levels. On the other hand, the patient with angina requires aggressive oxygenation support in the form of increasing the cardiac output (473 cc O_{O_2}).

ANSWER (Example 6)

The oxygen extraction and $S\bar{v}_{O_2}$ values indicate that the most stable period for overall oxygenation was at 1800. This is most likely because of the better cardiac output and lower oxygen consumption exhibited at 1800. The clinician needs to continue investigating the reasons for the loss of hemoglobin and cardiac output at 2000 and 2200. There may be bleeding in the lung, although the $Pa_{O_2}/F_{I_{O_2}}$ ratio did not change substantially until 2200.

$S\bar{v}_{O_2}$ and O_2 extraction are likely reliable indicators of overall oxygenation, since no oxygen-consumption dependency on oxygen transport appears to exist (V_{O_2} and D_{O_2} appear to change independently of each other). At no time does a major threat to cellular oxygenation appear to exist. Based on the consumable oxygen levels, adequate stores of oxygen still exist on hemoglobin. However, whenever the oxygen-extraction levels increase, the clinician must investigate the potential reason.

ANSWER (Example 7)

Based on the worsening of the $S\bar{v}_{O_2}$ from 1330 to 1430, aggressive investigation of all aspects of oxygenation is warranted. For example, measuring the cardiac output is the most obvious assessment. Identifying the oxygen consumption would suggest whether work of breathing was partially responsible for the deterioration in oxygenation. The improvement in the Pa_{O_2} can be misleading. The Pa_{O_2} change was due simply to an increase in $F_{I_{O_2}}$. The intrapulmonary shunt may have worsened, based on the $Pa_{O_2}/F_{I_{O_2}}$ ratio, between 1330 and 1430. This patient should be actively assessed for further interventions that may improve oxygenation.

ANSWER (Example 8)

The improvement in the $S\bar{v}_{O_2}$ appears to indicate an improvement in oxygenation. Keep in mind, the adequacy of the cardiac output is measured by how much it affects oxygenation. The same evaluation of other cardiac parameters, such as the PCWP, holds true. In this case the cardiac index is less than normal both times. However, the nitroprusside may have improved local blood flow or altered oxygen consumption, allowing a borderline cardiac index to now be adequate. Further measures to improve the cardiac output are warranted, but the patient is likely safer from an oxygenation perspective at 1230 than at 1100.

ANSWER (Example 9)

Based on the above information, the oxygen consumption can be measured from the following formula:

$$(Ca_{O_2} - Cv_{O_2}) \times CO \times 10$$

From this formula, the oxygen consumption is measured as

$$4.5 \times 7 \times 10 = 315 \text{ cc/min}$$

This is a near-normal value for a large man. Based on the near-normal oxygen consumption, as well as the normal Pa_{CO_2} level, the increased minute ventilation and respiratory rate are secondary to an increased dead space. The clinician should aim to improve pulmonary function, not to directly treat oxygen consumption.

ANSWER (Example 10)

Based on the above information, treating this patient with oxygen therapy will not provide substantial improvement in her oxygenation. The reason for the lack of improvement with oxygen therapy is the same as the reason for the drop in the Pa_{O_2} and Sp_{O_2}. They were not due to an intrapulmonary shunt increase (a lung problem), but rather to a decrease in the $S\bar{v}_{O_2}$ value. Computing the intrapulmonary shunt (Qs/Qt) indicates that no major change in the Qs/Qt occurred between the two times.

$$Qs/Qt = \frac{Cc_{O_2} - Ca_{O_2}}{Cc_{O_2} - Cv_{O_2}}$$

0100 data:

$$Pa_{O_2} = .50 (760 - 47) - 37/.8 \qquad\qquad = 309$$
$$Cc_{O_2} = 10.7 \times 1.34 \times 1.00 + (.003 \times 309) = 15.2$$
$$Ca_{O_2} = 10.7 \times 1.34 \times .96 + (.003 \times 90) = 14.0$$
$$Cv_{O_2} = 10.7 \times 1.34 \times .64 + (.003 \times 37) = 8.6$$

$$Qs/Qt = \frac{15.2 - 14}{15.2 - 9.3} = .20$$

0200 data:

$$Pa_{O_2} = .50 (760 - 47) - 39/.8 \qquad\qquad = 307$$
$$Cc_{O_2} = 11.1 \times 1.34 \times 1.00 + (.003 \times 307) = 15.8$$
$$Ca_{O_2} = 11.1 \times 1.34 \times .92 + (.003 \times 69) = 13.9$$
$$Cv_{O_2} = 11.1 \times 1.34 \times .46 + (.003 \times 25) = 6.9$$

$$Qs/Qt = \frac{15.8 - 13.9}{15.8 - 6.9} = .21$$

Based on this information, the problem centers more on an oxygenation point. The decrease in the Pa_{O_2} is not caused by the worsening Qs/Qt, but rather to a decrease in $S\bar{v}_{O_2}$. Increasing the $F_{I_{O_2}}$ will not produce the expected change in the Pa_{O_2}, since the $S\bar{v}_{O_2}$ must be elevated first. The decrease in the $S\bar{v}_{O_2}$ indicates a problem with either oxygen transport or consumption. The exact answer is not known, although the clinician should determine whether problems exist in maintaining the cardiac output (it decreased from 5.1 l/min to 4.4 l/min).

ANSWER (Example 11)

The Sp_{O_2} and the Sa_{O_2} should not be the same, owing to a number of different types of hemoglobin detectable between the pulse and laboratory oximeters. The formula for comparing the measurements is

$$Sp_{O_2} = \frac{Sa_{O_2}}{1 - (COHgb + MetHgb)}$$

Inserting the data for the formula gives a comparison of Sp_{O_2} and Sa_{O_2}:

$$\frac{.91}{1 - (.02 + .02)} = .95$$

From this information, the Sp_{O_2} value of 96% is almost equal to the adjusted value of 95%. In this case, the oximeter is reading accurately and should be used for this patient. The clinician must remember that the Sp_{O_2} will routinely overestimate the Sa_{O_2} value because of the inability of the Sp_{O_2} measurement to account for all types of hemoglobin.

ANSWER (Example 12)

Based on the above information, the PEEP does not appear to have achieved the primary objective of increasing oxygen transport. Although the Pa_{O_2} increased, mild hypotension and tachycardia have developed, indicating a potential loss of cardiac output. While the exact cardiac output cannot be determined, the presence of a tachycardia and a decrease in systolic blood pressure represents a potential loss of stroke volume and cardiac output.

ANSWER (Example 13)

Not at this point. While hypoxemia and low cardiac indices are present, a low-normal $S\bar{v}_{O_2}$ and normal lactate levels provide an indication of adequate oxygenation. The low-normal $S\bar{v}_{O_2}$ tends to suggest an independence of V_{O_2} and D_{O_2}, and the normal lactate level indicates no major problem in the cellular processing of oxygen. The low Pa_{O_2} may be an inhibitor to driving pressure for oxygen diffusion into the cells, but at this point it does not appear to be a major problem (based on the $S\bar{v}_{O_2}$ and lactate values). Further computations of oxygenation, such as O_2 extraction, oxygen transport, and oxygen consumption, could be performed. These data are either borderline (D_{O_2}), normal (O_2e), or inconclusive (V_{O_2}). The physical signs reveal little that the laboratory data do not provide. Cyanosis, for example, indicates a low Sa_{O_2} The Sp_{O_2} of 90% usually overestimates the Sa_{O_2} by 2–3% and indicates a low Sa_{O_2}.

ANSWER (Example 14)

The intrapulmonary shunt by itself does not represent the danger to this patient. The intrapulmonary is a threat to oxygenation only if the Pa_{O_2} and Sa_{O_2} levels are decreased to dangerous levels. Both the Pa_{O_2} and Sa_{O_2} have been compensated by the increased $F_{I_{O_2}}$. The increased lactate level shows a major threat to overall oxygenation, likely caused by cellular inability to utilize oxygen, as illustrated by the above-normal oxygen transport (1117 cc/min), normal oxygen consumption (264 cc/min), and high $S\bar{v}_{O_2}$ and lactate levels. Treatments aimed at improving cellular use of oxygen are the priority in this patient.

ANSWER (Example 15)

Based on the above data, the oxygen consumption has decreased, from 231 to 221 cc/min. This decrease represents about a 5% reduction in V_{O_2}. While the change is not a major improvement in oxygenation, the therapy change to assist/control has allowed a partially successful treatment in oxygenation based on reducing respiratory-muscle requirements for oxygen.

The decrease can be obtained by computing V_{O_2} via the Fick equation. See below:

$$V_{O_2} = cardiac\ output \times \{arterial\text{–}venous\ oxygen\ content\} \times 10$$

1900 data:

$$Ca_{O_2} = 1.34 \times 13.4 \times .89 = 16\ cc/dl$$
$$Cv_{O_2} = 1.34 \times 13.4 \times .46 = 8.3$$
$$Ca_{O_2} - Cv_{O_2} = 7.7$$
$$V_{O_2} = 3.0 \times 7.7 \times 10 = 231\ cc/min$$

2000 data:

$$Ca_{O_2} = 1.34 \times 13.4 \times .90 = 16.2\ cc/dl$$
$$Cv_{O_2} = 1.34 \times 13.4 \times .52 = 9.3$$
$$Ca_{O_2} - Cv_{O_2} = 6.9$$
$$V_{O_2} = 3.2 \times 6.9 \times 10 = 221\ cc/min$$

ANSWER (Example 16)

Due to a decrease in the $S\bar{v}_{O_2}$ level, a potential deterioration of the oxygenation status is present. The Sp_{O_2} and Sa_{O_2} will not change unless the intrapulmonary shunt worsens. The primary problem in this patient is not lung function, but rather loss of hemoglobin. The loss of hemoglobin is probably caused by a redeveloping GI bleed. Finger oximetry will not pick up the loss of hemoglobin. Since hemoglobin is the most important aspect of arterial-oxygen content (Ca_{O_2}), blood gases and finger oximetry will not be useful in the assessment of Ca_{O_2}. The cardiac output is likely increasing to offset the loss of hemoglobin.

ANSWER (Example 17)

1. Based on the improvement in cardiac output, cardiac index, stroke volume (from 39 to 45 cc), stroke index (from 20 to 23 cc/m²), and $S\bar{v}_{O_2}$,

the dobutamine appears to be successful. The PCWP has not changed markedly and is not to be used as an indicator of failure of the dobutamine since the stroke volume/index has improved.

2. The cardiac output can be measured by using the Fick equation. From the oxygen consumption given and by computing the $Ca_{O_2} - Cv_{O_2}$ difference, the cardiac output is

$$CO = \frac{205/5.22}{10} = 3.93$$

The measured output differs from the Fick equation output. Reasons for the difference between the Fick equation and thermodilution methods include problems with tricuspid valvular competence, dysrhythmias, and technical issues. The Fick equation is considered the most accurate technique. Before assuming no change has occurred with the dobutamine therapy, one must obtain a Fick equation value on the 1600 readings as well.

Appendix
Nursing Diagnoses Appropriate for Patients with Oxygenation Disturbances

Pamela Becker Weilitz MSN (R), RN

NURSING DIAGNOSIS

A nursing diagnosis is "a clinical judgement about an individual, family, or community which is derived through a deliberate, systematic process of data collection and analysis. It provides the basis for prescriptions for definitive therapy for which the nurse is accountable. It is expressed concisely and it includes the etiology of the condition when known."

The role of the clinician treating patients with oxygenation disturbances is to assess, diagnosis, plan, implement, and evaluate the care given. The nursing diagnosis is selected based on the assessment. The clinician selects the appropriate nursing diagnosis using the definition of the diagnosis and the defining characteristics. Expected outcomes are developed with supporting interventions designed to assist the patient in reaching the outcomes. The expected outcomes are the points for evaluating the success of the therapy.

The following nursing diagnoses are appropriate for use with patients experiencing oxygenation disturbances. The definition of the diagnosis, defining characteristics, etiologies, expected outcomes and selected interventions are listed. A separate table lists possible related medical diagnoses by nursing diagnosis.

Activity Intolerance[2]

The state in which an individual has insufficient physiological or psychological energy to endure or complete required or desired daily activities.

Defining Characteristics
  Fatigue
  Dyspnea
  Inability to perform self-care activities
  Abnormal response to exercise
    tachycardia/bradycardia
    tachypnea
    changes in blood pressure
    decreased $S\bar{v}_{O_2}$
    oxygen desaturation
Etiologies
  Imbalance between oxygen supply and demand
  Hypoxemia

Expected Outcomes

The patient will be able to perform activities of daily living without breathlessness.

The patient will be able to verbalize energy conserving measures.

The patient will be able to identify physical signs and symptoms related to a decreased activity tolerance.

Interventions

Schedule activities and test to avoid breathlessness and fatigue.

Teach the patient pursed lip breathing and energy conservation techniques.

Monitor oxygen levels for desaturation with activity.

Monitor blood pressure, pulse and respiration during exercise.

Assess for placement in a pulmonary rehabilitation program.

Impaired Gas Exchange[2]

A state in which the individual experiences an imbalance between oxygen uptake and carbon dioxide elimination at alveolar-capillary membrane gas exchange area.

Defining Characteristics
  Confusion
  Somnolence
  Restlessness
  Irritability
  Inability to move secretions
  Hypercapnia
  Hypoxia
Etiologies
  Altered oxygen supply
  Alveolar-capillary membrane changes
  Altered blood flow
  Altered oxygen-carrying capacity of the blood

Expected Outcomes

The patient will maintain a Pa_{O_2} of > 60 mm Hg and a Sa_{O_2} of $> 90\%$, a pH of 7.35–7.45 with a Pa_{CO_2} between 35–45 mm Hg or at the patient's baseline.

Interventions

Monitor the patient for mental status changes, irritability and restlessness.
Monitor for signs of hypoxemia.
Provide assistance with removal of airway secretions.
Provide supplemental oxygen therapy to achieve the desired outcomes.
Monitor respiratory pattern and rate.
Monitor the patient with a history of carbon dioxide retention for increasing CO_2 related to oxygen administration.
Monitor heart rate and rhythm for irregularities.
Position patient to improve or optimize ventilation perfusion abnormalities.
Monitor pulmonary artery pressure and pulmonary vascular resistance for increases resulting from hypoxemia.

The AACN and Section on Nursing, American Thoracic Society have recommended that impaired gas exchange be further delineated as follows.

Impaired Gas Exchange: Hypercapnia[3]

The state in which an individual has a carbon dioxide pressure (Pa_{CO_2}) in arterial blood that is greater than normal with or without acidemia.

Defining Characteristics
  Headache
  Visual Disturbances
  $Pa_{CO_2} > 45$
  Decreased Pa_{O_2}
  Central Nervous System Changes
    somnolence
    stupor
    coma
  Cardiovascular changes
    bounding pulse
    flushed skin
    vasodilatation
Etiologies
  Alveolar hypoventilation
  Decreased V/Q ratio
  Increased VD/VT
  Severe intrapulmonary shunt
  Primary metabolic alkalosis

Expected Outcomes

The patient will have an arterial pH of 7.35–7.45 with a Pa_{CO_2} of 35–45 mm Hg or at the patient's baseline.

Interventions

Monitor the patient for mental status changes, irritability and restlessness.
Monitor respiratory pattern and rate.
Monitor heart rate and rhythm for irregularities.
Position patient to improve and/or optimize ventilation perfusion abnormalities

Impaired Gas Exchange: Hypoxemia[3]

The state in which an individual has an oxygen pressure (Pa_{O_2}) and/or saturation (Sa_{O_2}) in the arterial blood that is lower than the age-adjusted normal range at a given altitude.

Defining Characteristics
  Dyspnea
  Confusion
  Fatigue
  Oxygenation change

acute: $Pa_{O_2} < 60$ mm Hg or $Sa_{O_2} < 90\%$

chronic: $Pa_{O_2} < 55$ mm Hg or $Sa_{O_2} < 85\%$

Heart-rate change

Changes in respiratory pattern/rate

Neurobehavioral changes
  restlessness
  irritability
  somnolence
  coma

Increased PA pressure

Increased PVR

Activity intolerance

Cyanosis

Etiologies
  Alveolar hypoventilation
  Intrapulmonary shunting
  Low ventilation/perfusion ratios
  Diffusion impairment
  Decreased ambient oxygen concentration
  Decreased barometric pressure
  Carbon-monoxide poisoning

Expected Outcomes

The patient will achieve and maintain a Pa_{O_2} of > 60 mm Hg or a $Sa_{O_2} > 90\%$. For the patient with chronic hypoxemia, the Pa_{O_2} will be > 55 mm Hg and the Sa_{O_2} will be $> 85\%$.

Interventions

Provide supplemental oxygen therapy to achieve the desired outcomes.

Monitor for signs of hypoxemia.

Monitor the patient for mental status changes, irritability and restlessness.

Plan activities to reduce fatigue.

Monitor pulmonary artery pressure and pulmonary vascular resistance for increases resulting from hypoxemia.

Monitor respiratory pattern and rate.

Monitor the patient with a history of carbon dioxide retention for increasing CO_2 related to oxygen administration.

Provide assistance with removal of airway secretions.

Nursing Diagnosis	Possible Related Medical Diagnoses
Activity Intolerance	COPD
	Asthma
	Congestive heart failure
	Acute MI
Impaired Gas Exchange Hypercapnia	Severe COPD
	Metabolic alkalemia
	Pneumothorax
	Pulmonary edema
	ARDS
	Flail chest
	Neuromuscular dysfunction
Hypoxemia	ARDS
	Asthma
	Atelectasis
	Cardiogenic pulmonary edema
	COPD
	Pneumonia
	Pneumothorax
	Pulmonary embolus

REFERENCES

1. Shoemaker JK. "Essential features of nursing diagnosis." *In* Kim MJ, McFarland GK, McLane AM. *Classification of Nursing Diagnoses: Proceedings of the Fifth National Conference.* St. Louis: CV Mosby, 1984, 109.
2. Kim MJ, McFarland GK, McLane AM. *Pocket Guide to Nursing Diagnosis.* 4th ed. St. Louis: CV Mosby Yearbook, Inc., 1991.
3. Kurham R. (ed. in chief). *Outcome Standards for Nursing Care of the Critically Ill.* Laguna Nigel: American Association of Critical-Care Nurses, 1990.

Index